Soames' and Southam's
Oral Pathology

Soames' and Southam's Oral Pathology

FIFTH EDITION

Max Robinson

Senior Lecturer in Oral Pathology
School of Dental Sciences
Newcastle University
UK

Keith Hunter

Professor of Head and Neck Pathology
Department of Oral Pathology
School of Clinical Dentistry
University of Sheffield
UK

Michael Pemberton

Professor in Oral Medicine
University Dental Hospital of Manchester
Manchester University Hospitals NHS Foundation Trust
UK

Philip Sloan

Professor of Oral Pathology
School of Dental Sciences
Newcastle University
UK

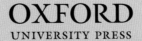

OXFORD
UNIVERSITY PRESS

OXFORD
UNIVERSITY PRESS

Great Clarendon Street, Oxford, OX2 6DP,
United Kingdom

Oxford University Press is a department of the University of Oxford.
It furthers the University's objective of excellence in research, scholarship,
and education by publishing worldwide. Oxford is a registered trade mark of
Oxford University Press in the UK and in certain other countries

Published in the United States of America by Oxford University Press
198 Madison Avenue, New York, NY 10016, United States of America

British Library Cataloguing in Publication Data

Data available

Library of Congress Control Number: 2017961371

ISBN 978-0-19-969778-6

Printed in Great Britain by
Bell & Bain Ltd., Glasgow

This book is dedicated to Professor Emeritus J. V. Soames and the late Professor Emeritus J. C. Southam who authored the first four editions.

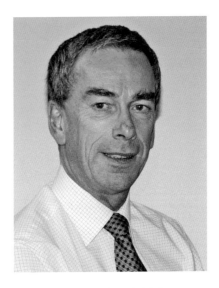

Professor Emeritus J. V. Soames
Newcastle University

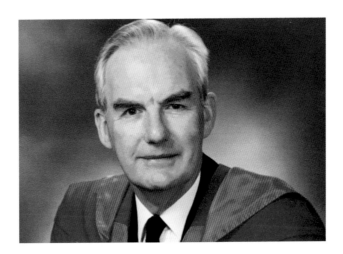

Professor Emeritus J. C. Southam
University of Edinburgh
1934–2015

Preface to the fifth edition

The fourth edition of *Soames' and Southam's Oral Pathology* was the culmination of a process of refinement of both content and production. Being tasked to produce a fifth edition was a major challenge for us. More than ten years has elapsed since the fourth edition was printed and as knowledge of the pathological mechanisms underlying oral diseases has advanced, new evidence-based management guidelines and therapies have become available. Accurate diagnosis is increasingly based on a multi-disciplinary approach involving the integration of rapidly evolving imaging techniques and molecular pathology tests. Sound diagnosis, however, is still based on an informed clinician taking an accurate history, making a thorough clinical examination, and selecting appropriate diagnostic tests. The modern dentalcare professional in training and in clinical practice has to contend with a vastly expanded knowledge base. Understanding of oral and maxillofacial pathology is essential if the clinician is to navigate successfully through clinical guidelines, make timely referrals to specialists, and provide good care for patients. The dental curriculum has changed to reflect this expansion of knowledge. High-quality specialist texts are now available that provide integrated clinico-pathological approaches to dental caries, periodontal diseases, temporomandibular joint disorders, and oral diseases in children. To reflect this we have chosen to reduce the content of chapters on these topics. Sections on certain diseases that have become less prevalent have been removed and new material on disorders that are more likely to be encountered nowadays has been added. This radically revised edition begins with an introductory chapter that outlines the importance of clinical assessment and how the synthesis of a differential diagnosis informs the selection of further investigations, including those provided by the cellular pathology laboratory. The subsequent chapters guide the reader through the various diseases that they may encounter in the oral cavity, starting with a comprehensive section on the oral mucosa, which leads on to an updated chapter on oral cancer and oral potentially malignant disorders. Diseases of the salivary glands are dealt with in the succeeding chapter. The text then follows the sequence of the pathology of teeth and supporting structures, including jaw cysts and odontogenic tumours, along with bone disorders. There are two new chapters: one that describes the important lesions that clinicians should recognize on the face and lips, and another that explores the differential diagnosis of neck lumps, which we consider to be an important part of the clinical examination. We conclude with a chapter on the oral manifestations of systemic disease, which highlights the importance of oral disease in the context of human disease. We hope that we have preserved much of the excellent content and character of the fourth edition. The radiology content has been updated by including examples of cross-sectional imaging. Virtually all the photomicrographs have been replaced with carefully selected images to illustrate key pathological features. We have continued the theme of tabulation and text boxes, which so enhanced the fourth edition, as we agree with our predecessors that these significantly aid learning.

We have pleasure in acknowledging the help we have received from our many colleagues. We particularly wish to express our gratitude to Dr Iain MacLeod, Dr Andrew Carr, and Tony Owens of the Department of Dental and Maxillofacial Radiology, Newcastle Dental School for providing many of the radiological images. Jan Howarth of the Department of Medical Illustration, Newcastle Dental School. Colleagues that have kindly provided photographs: Dr Nick Bown, Dr Ian Corbett, Professor Emeritus John Eveson, Dr Naika Gill, Dr Neil Heath Professor Clifford Lawrence, Dr Pia Nystrom, Professor Vinidh Paleri, Professor Paul Speight, and Dr Rachel Williams. Colleagues who have taken the time to critically review drafts of the manuscript: Dr Sonja Boy, Professor Justin Durham, Dr Giles McCracken, Professor Philip Preshaw, and Dr Marion Robinson.

MR, KH, MP, PS

Contents

Acknowledgements

Oxford University Press wishes to acknowledge the contribution of Professor J.V. Soames and Professor J.C. Southam to the popular textbook *Oral Pathology*, the fourth edition of which forms the basis of this work. This popular textbook has enlightened generations of dental students as we hope this new book does too.

Abbreviations

2WW	'2-week wait'
AB	Alcian blue
ACE	angiotensin-converting enzyme
ACTH	adrenocorticotrophic hormone
AIDS	acquired immune deficiency syndrome
ALL	acute lymphoblastic leukaemia
AML	acute myeloid leukaemia
AOT	adenomatoid odontogenic tumour
αMSH	α-melanocyte-stimulating hormone
BCNS	basal cell naevus syndrome
BPOP	bizarre parosteal osteochondromatous proliferation
BRONJ	bisphosphonate-related osteonecrosis of the jaw
CB–CT	cone beam–computed tomography
CEOT	calcifying epithelial odontogenic tumour
CLL	chronic lymphocytic leukaemia
CMC	chronic mucocutaneous candidosis
CML	chronic myeloid leukaemia
CMV	cytomegalovirus
CNS	central nervous system
CREST	syndrome calcinosis cutis, Raynaud's phenomenon, esophogeal dysfunction, sclerodactyly, and telangiectasia
CT	computerized tomography
CVS	cardiovascular system
CWT	'cancer waiting time'
DGCT	dentinogenic ghost cell tumour
DIGO	drug-induced gingival overgrowth
DLE	discoid lupus erythematosus
DMARDS	disease modifying anti-rheumatic drugs
DPAS	diastase periodic acid–Schiff stain
EBV	Epstein–Barr virus
EGFR	epidermal growth factor receptor
ESR	erythrocyte sedimentation rate
EVG	elastic van Gieson stain
FISH	fluorescence *in situ* hybridization
FNAB	fine-needle aspiration biopsy
FNAC	fine-needle aspiration cytology
GIT	gastrointestinal tract
GPA	granulomatosis with polyangitis
GUT	genitourinary tract
GVHD	graft versus host disease
HAART	highly active anti-retroviral therapy
HBA1C	glycosylated haemoglobin
HCV	hepatitis C virus
H&E	haematoxylin and eosin
HHV	humanherpes virus
HIV	human immunodeficiency virus
HL	hairy leukoplakia
HPV	human papillomavirus
HSP	heat shock proteins

HSV	herpes simplex virus
IMRT	intensity modulated radiotherapy
KS	Kaposi sarcoma
LCH	Langerhans cell histiocytosis
LP	lichen planus
MCH	mean cell haemoglobin
MCHC	mean cell haemoglobin concentration
MCV	mean cell volume
MMR	measles, mumps, rubella
MRI	magnetic resonance imaging
MRONJ	medication-related osteonecrosis of the jaw
MRSA	methicillin resistant *S. aureus*
NOS	not otherwise specified
NRBC	nucleated red blood cell
NSAIDS	non-steroidal anti-inflammatory drugs
NUG	necrotizing ulcerative gingivitis
NUP	necrotizing ulcerative periodontitis
OMIM	Online Mendelian Inheritance in Man
PAS	periodic acid Schiff stain
PET–CT	positron emission tomography–computed tomography
PTH	parathyroid hormone
PTLD	post-transplant lympho-proliferative disorder
PVL	proliferative verruous leukoplakia
PVNS	pigmented villo-nodular synovitis
RAS	recurrent aphthous stomatitis
RBC	red blood cell count
RCW	red cell distribution width
RS	respiratory system
SCC	squamous cell carcinoma
SCID	severe combined immunodeficiency
SLE	systemic lupus erythematosus
SLS	sodium lauryl sulphate
TMD	temporomandibular disorder
TMJ	temporomandibular joint
WBC	white blood cell count
WHO	World Health Organization
ZN	Ziehl–Neelsen stain

1

Diagnosis of oral disease

Chapter contents

Introduction

The most common oral diseases are dental caries and periodontal disease (Fig. 1.1). The diagnosis and treatment of these diseases are the focus of the majority of dentists, dental therapists, and dental hygienists. Nevertheless, it is the responsibility of the dental healthcare professional to provide a holistic approach to management that ensures both good oral and general health for their patients. A broad knowledge of the range of diseases that affect the oral cavity is essential and also an appreciation that oral disease may be the first sign of an underlying systemic disease. Before this knowledge can be applied, the clinician must obtain an accurate patient history and undertake a systematic clinical examination. These key clinical skills underpin both medicine and dentistry, and are an absolute requirement to formulate a differential diagnosis. The use of imaging modalities and laboratory tests are often required to reach a definitive diagnosis, and it is the justification and informed choice of these additional investigations that will facilitate a timely and accurate diagnosis. Following diagnosis, appropriate treatment can be instituted, the ideal outcome being a return to health or control of the patient's symptoms in recalcitrant chronic diseases.

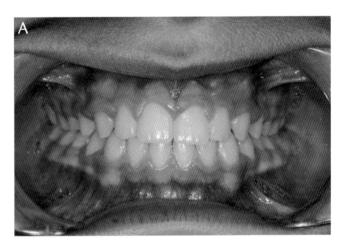
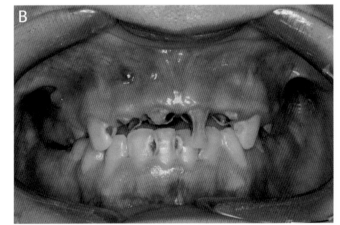

Fig. 1.1 The oral cavity in health and disease.

Obtaining an accurate history

History of the presenting problem

Obtaining a clear and precise clinical history is essential. The clinician must listen carefully to the information conveyed by the patient and then use direct questioning to collect additional data to construct an accurate picture of the patient's problem. This can be a significant challenge and requires excellent communication skills to build a good patient–clinician relationship.

The most common presenting problems relate to pain or the development of a lesion: swelling, lump, ulcer, or white/red patch. To establish a comprehensive pain history, the features listed in Table 1.1 should be addressed. Obtaining an accurate history for a lesion is dependent on the patient noticing the abnormality in the first instance and, as a consequence, the information may be rather vague; however, it is important to ascertain the key points listed in Table 1.2.

Medical history

A comprehensive medical history (Box 1.1) will identify any concurrent disease that may be relevant to the presenting oral condition

Table 1.1 Pain history

Features	Descriptors
Site	Anatomical location
Severity	Excruciating, severe, slight pain
Onset	Recent, longstanding, acute, chronic, days, weeks months, years
Nature	Sharp, lancating pain, dull ache, niggling pain, irritation
Duration	Transient, constant, seconds, minutes, hours, days, weeks
Radiation	Radiation of pain to other anatomical sites
Aggravating factors	Temperature (hot and cold), pressure, friction, specific food and drink
Relief	Avoidance of aggravating factors, topical medicaments, analgesics (type, dosage, route of administration)
Associated features	Malaise, fever, lymphadenopathy, dizziness, headaches

Table 1.2 Establishing the history of a lesion

Features	Descriptors
Site	Anatomical location, single, multiple
Size	Estimate of size, increasing in size (slowly, rapidly), decreasing in size, fluctuates in size
Onset	Recent, longstanding, days, weeks, months, years
Initiating factors	Trauma, dentoalveolar infection
Associated features	Pain, bleeding, malaise, fever, lymphadenopathy

Box 1.1 The medical history

System
- Cardiovascular system (CVS)
- Respiratory system (RS)
- Haematological diseases
- Bleeding disorders
- Central nervous system (CNS)
- Eyes
- Ear, nose, and throat
- Gastrointestinal tract (GIT)
- Liver
- Genitourinary tract (GUT)
- Kidneys
- Musculoskeletal system
- Endocrine disease
- Medications
- Allergies
- Pregnancy
- Hospitalization
- History of cancer
- Blood-borne infectious diseases

(Chapter 10) and highlight any issues relating to proposed medical or surgical interventions.

Family history

Some diseases are heritable and have a characteristic pedigree that can be mapped over multiple generations, e.g. haemophilia. Other diseases show a preponderance to affect individuals within family groups, but it is difficult to predict which individuals will be affected and relatives may suffer to a greater or lesser extent. These familial traits may be heritable with variable genetic penetrance and expressivity, or may reflect exposure to similar environmental and social factors.

Social history

The social history may be of direct relevance to oral disease and general health. For example, tobacco consumption and alcohol abuse are risk factors for the development of oral cancer, as well as other systemic diseases, e.g. cardiovascular disease and liver disease. Factors such as occupation and personal status provide additional information and may influence the care plan.

Dental history

The previous dental history will help to build a picture of the patient's current state of oral health and their previous engagement with dental health services. The dental history may inform the acceptability of any proposed treatment.

A systematic approach to patient examination

The physical assessment of a patient starts when the patient enters the surgery. The clinician can gauge a number of subtle signs from the patient's general appearance and disposition. The clinician can quickly establish general health and mobility. Once seated, examination of the complexion and hands may reveal signs of systemic diseases, e.g. finger clubbing, nail abnormalities, skin diseases, and eye signs.

Routine examination of the oro-facial complex should include inspection and palpation of the neck. The sequence should commence with the submandibular triangle, which contains the submandibular gland and level I lymph nodes (level IA submental lymph nodes and level IB submandibular lymph nodes). This is followed by level II lymph nodes, superior part of the deep cervical chain, including the jugulodigastric lymph node and level II lymph nodes (levels IIA and IIB lymph nodes located anterior and posterior to the accessory nerve, respectively), level III lymph nodes (middle part of the deep cervical chain), level IV lymph nodes (the inferior part of the deep cervical chain, which includes the jugulo-omohyoid lymph node), and level V lymph nodes in the posterior triangle of the neck (Fig. 1.2). Finally, the mid-line structures of

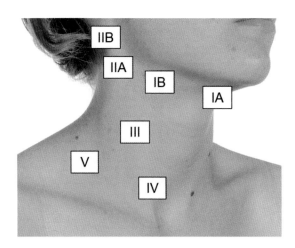

Fig. 1.2 The anatomical levels of the neck.

the neck, which include the larynx, trachea, and thyroid gland, should be examined. The presentation of lumps in the neck is covered in Chapter 9. Any lumps, e.g. enlarged lymph nodes, are described by anatomical site, size, consistency (cystic, soft, rubbery, or hard), relationship to underlying tissues (fixed or mobile), and whether palpation elicits pain. The parotid glands are also examined and palpated for any abnormalities.

The examination then focuses on assessment of the temporomandibular joints and the muscles of mastication to assess functional abnormalities and any muscle tenderness. The muscles of facial expression are also assessed, to establish facial nerve function. Any sensory neurological deficit over the distribution of the trigeminal nerve should be documented and mapped out.

The intra-oral, soft-tissue examination should include inspection of the vermillion border of the lips, labial and buccal mucosae, hard palate, soft palate, fauces and tonsils, the floor of the mouth, oral tongue, alveolar mucosa, gingivae, and teeth. The clinician should be aware of the regional variation of the mucosa within the oral cavity and recognize the normal anatomical structures that occasionally are mistaken for disease: Fordyce spots (intra-oral sebaceous glands), sublingual varices, lingual tonsil, and fissured tongue (Fig. 1.3). Documentation of lesions (lumps, ulcers, and patches) follows the schemes outlined in Tables 1.3 and 1.4.

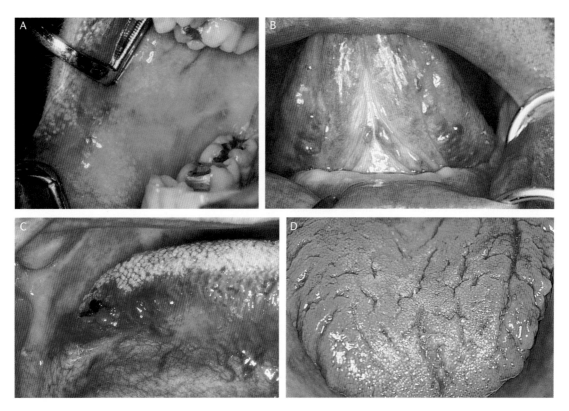

Fig. 1.3 Fordyce spots on the buccal and labial mucosa (A), sublingual varices (B), lingual tonsil (C), and fissured tongue (D).

Table 1.3 Description of a lump

Features	Descriptors
Site	Anatomical location, single, multiple
Size	Measurement
Shape	Polypoid, sessile
Surface	Smooth, papillomatous, rough, ulcerated
Consistency	Soft, firm, fluctuant, pulsatile, rubbery, indurated (hard)
Colour	Pink, red, white, yellow, brown, purple, black
Edge	Well defined, irregular, poorly defined
Attachment to adjacent structures	Mobile, tethered, fixed

Table 1.4 Description of an ulcer

Features	Descriptors
Site	Anatomical location, single, multiple
Size	Measurement
Shape	Round, stellate, irregular
Surface (base)	Smooth, granular
Consistency	Soft, firm, rubbery, indurated (hard)
Colour	Yellow, red, grey, black
Edge	Well defined, ragged, rolled margin
Attachment to adjacent structures	Mobile, tethered, fixed

Thinking about the differential diagnosis

Formulating a differential diagnosis requires the integration of information from the history and examination with a sound knowledge of oral and systemic diseases. There are several strategies that can facilitate this thought process. For example, the 'surgical sieve' can be used to generate a list of diseases according to aetiology and pathogenesis (Table 1.5). When considering a neoplasm, visualizing the anatomical structures in the vicinity of the lesion can also help to formulate the differential diagnosis (Table 1.6). With increasing experience and clinical acumen it is possible to focus a wide differential diagnosis, depending on subtle clinical findings and the likelihood of a particular disease at a specific anatomical site. For example, a swelling in the lower labial mucosa is most likely to be a mucocoele, whereas a similar swelling in the upper labial mucosa is more likely to be a benign salivary gland neoplasm. It is worth considering the maxim that common entities are more likely to be encountered than those that are rare. For instance,

Table 1.6 Basic classification of neoplasia by tissue type

Tissue type	Neoplasm	
	Benign	**Malignant**
Epithelium	Squamous cell papilloma	Squamous cell carcinoma
Melanocytes	Melanocytic naevus	Malignant melanoma
Fibrous tissue	Fibroma	Fibrosarcoma
Adipose tissue	Lipoma	Liposarcoma
Striated muscle	Rhabdomyoma	Rhabdomyosarcoma
Smooth muscle	Leiomyoma	Leiomyosarcoma
Blood vessels	Angioma	Angiosarcoma
Peripheral nerves	Neurofibroma Schwannoma	Malignant peripheral nerve sheath tumour
Bone	Osteoma	Osteosarcoma
Cartilage	Chondroma	Chondrosarcoma
Lymph nodes	None	Lymphoma
Salivary glands	Adenoma	Adenocarcinoma

Table 1.5 The surgical sieve

Trauma	Mechanical, thermal, chemical, radiation
Tumour (neoplastic)	Benign, malignant
Infection	Bacterial, viral, fungal, protozoal
Inflammatory	Autoimmune diseases
Inherited	Congenital disease
Iatrogenic	Dental or medical intervention
Idiopathic	Unknown cause
Systemic disease	Oral manifestation of systemic disease

an oro-facial swelling in a patient with a neglected dentition is most likely to be a dentoalveolar infection. If the clinical assessment indicates that the lesion is benign, then the differential diagnosis should focus on infective causes, hyperplastic lesions, and benign neoplasms. Conversely, clinical signs and symptoms of a destructive lesion suggest malignancy.

Choosing and ordering investigations

Once a differential diagnosis has been formulated, ancillary investigations are typically required to arrive at the definitive diagnosis. Additional information may be obtained by imaging techniques: ultrasound, radiographs, computerized tomography (CT), and magnetic resonance imaging (MRI). In the majority of cases an accurate diagnosis will require the analysis of a biological sample by one of the laboratory-based medical specialties: haematology, clinical chemistry, immunology, medical microbiology, virology, cellular pathology (cytopathology and histopathology), and molecular pathology (cytogenetics and genetics).

Imaging techniques

The main imaging techniques used in the oro-facial complex are listed in Table 1.7. The decision to use imaging as part of the clinical examination is governed by three core principles: justification of the imaging technique, optimization of the radiation dose, and limiting the amount of

radiation exposure. In the UK, these principles are outlined in the Ionizing Radiation Regulations 1999 (IRR99) and the Ionizing Radiation (Medical Exposure) Regulations 2000 (IR(ME)R2000). The reader is referred to specialist texts on dental and maxillofacial imaging for detailed information on imaging techniques, and their applicability and interpretation.

Haematology, clinical chemistry, and immunology

The analysis of biological fluids, mainly blood and urine, can yield important information about the general health of the patient. A full blood count gives information about the constituents of the blood: the erythrocytes, leukocytes, and platelets (Table 1.8). Analysis of the haemoglobin, red cell count (RBC), and erythrocyte size (mean cell volume, MCV) may demonstrate that the patient is anaemic. Too few platelets, termed thrombocytopenia, indicates a risk of excessive bleeding.

Table 1.7 Imaging of the oro-facial complex

Imaging modality	Anatomical structures	Diseases
Intra-oral radiographs	Dentoalveolar complex	Dental caries and its sequelae
		Periodontal disease
Extra-oral radiographs	Skull Sinonasal complex Jaws	Odontogenic cysts/neoplasms Bone diseases Sinusitis
Cone Beam–Computed Tomography (CB–CT)	Dentoalveolar complex Maxillary antrum	Odontogenic cysts/neoplasms Bone diseases Sinusitis
Ultrasound	Major salivary glands Cervical lymph nodes Thyroid gland Soft tissues of the neck	Sialolithiasis/sialadenitis Lymphadenopathy Thyroiditis, thyroid neoplasia
Sialography	Submandibular gland Parotid gland	Sialolithiasis/sialadenitis
Computerized Tomography (CT)	Head and neck tissues	Mainly used for neoplasia
Magnetic Resonance Imaging (MRI)	Head and neck tissues	Mainly used for neoplasia
Positron Emission Tomography–Computed Tomography (PET–CT)	Head and neck tissues	Mainly used for neoplasia

Table 1.8 A normal full blood count with reference range values

Haemoglobin	15.0	g/dl	(13.0 to 18.0)
Platelet count	223	$\times 10^9$/l	(150 to 450)
Haematocrit	0.460	l/l	(0.400 to 0.500)
Red blood cell count	4.85	$\times 10^{12}$/l	(4.50 to 5.50)
Mean cell volume	94.8	fl	(83.0 to 101.0)
Mean cell haemoglobin	31.0	pg	(27.0 to 34.0)
Mean cell haemoglobin concentration	32.7	g/l	(31 to 36)
Red blood cell distribution width	12.6	%	(10.0 to 14.0)
White blood cell count	6.5	$\times 10^9$/l	(4.0 to 11.0)
Neutrophil count	3.82 (58.77%)	$\times 10^9$/l	(2.0 to 7.0)
Lymphocyte count	2.16 (33.23%)	$\times 10^9$/l	(1.5 to 4.0)
Monocyte count	0.38 (5.85%)	$\times 10^9$/l	(0.2 to 0.8)
Eosinophil count	0.13 (2.00%)	$\times 10^9$/l	(0.04 to 0.4)
Basophil count	0.01 (0.15%)	$\times 10^9$/l	(0.00 to 0.1)
Nucleated red blood cell count	0.00 (0.00%)	$\times 10^9$/l	(0 to 0)

Increased numbers of leukocytes (WBC) may be caused by infection or leukaemia, whereas depleted leukocytes may identify a patient that is immunocompromised. Other blood tests include an assessment of the micronutrients required for haematopoiesis, the haematinics: iron, vitamin B_{12}, and folate, which are measured by the serum ferritin, serum vitamin B_{12}, and serum or red cell folate, respectively. These specific tests are important in understanding the cause of anaemia. Analyses of blood glucose and glycosylated haemoglobin (HbA1c) are required for the assessment of diabetes mellitus. Urinalysis is often used as a simple screen for diabetes, haematuria, and proteinuria. An autoimmune profile can be used to screen for autoimmune diseases, such as Sjögren's syndrome and systemic lupus erythematosus. Other immunological assays are important in the diagnosis of hypersensitivity reactions.

Medical microbiology and virology

Bacteria, viruses, and fungi can all cause infections of the oro-facial complex. Biological samples may include needle aspirates or swabs of pus, viral and fungal swabs, sterile saline oral rinses, and fresh tissue. Precise identification of the aetiological agent and determining the sensitivity of the microorganism to a variety of antimicrobial agents are core activities of the medical microbiology service.

Cellular pathology

Acquisition of material from a lesion, cells for cytopathology and tissue for histopathology, is the most common method of establishing a definitive diagnosis. A variety of methods can be used and are outlined in Table 1.9.

Cytology samples, collected by either an exfoliative method (e.g. brush biopsy) or fine-needle aspiration, can be used to prepare smears on glass slides, which are either air-dried or preserved in an alcohol-based fixative. Alternatively, brush biopsies and needle washings can be collected in proprietary liquid-based cytology fluid (e.g. SurePath, BD or ThinPrep, Hologic). Currently, brush biopsy of oral lesions is not widely used, as most clinicians proceed directly to tissue biopsy. However, the brush biopsy is a safe, simple, and

Table 1.9 Types of biopsy

Type of biopsy	Description	Sites	Examination
Exfoliative cytology	A sampling device is used to collect cells from a surface lesion.	Oral cavity	Cytology
Fine-needle aspiration biopsy (FNAB)	A 21-gauge (green) needle is used to sample a deep lesion. Ultrasound guidance can be used to ensure correct location of the needle.	Oral cavity Major salivary glands Lymph nodes Deep soft tissue of neck	Cytology
Incision biopsy	A scalpel is used to incise the tissue and sample a piece of the lesion.	Oral cavity Skin	Histology
Punch biopsy	An device, similar to a hole punch, is used to take a disc of tissue. Sizes: 2–6mm diameter.	Oral cavity Skin	Histology
Core biopsy	A large bore cutting needle is used to sample deep tissue producing a long thin core of tissue.	Major salivary glands Lymph nodes Deep soft tissue of neck	Histology
Open biopsy	In some circumstances it is necessary to visualize a deep lesion prior to biopsy and this is sometimes referred to as an 'open biopsy'.	Lymph node Salivary glands	Histology
Excision biopsy	Removal of all the diseased tissue with a small margin of healthy tissue.	Oral cavity Major salivary glands Lymph nodes	Histology
Resection	Typically a larger operation planned to remove all the diseased tissue with a margin of healthy tissue. The surgical site may require reconstruction with tissue from another part of the body.	Oral cavity Major salivary glands Lymph nodes	Histology

economic technique that is acceptable to patients. Multiple samples can be taken if there is multi-focal disease or it can be employed as an adjunct to visual surveillance during routine follow-up. The disadvantages of this technique mainly relate to adequacy of sample and whether the sample is representative of the lesion. Fine-needle aspiration biopsy (FNAB) is mainly used during investigation of a lump in the neck or one of the major salivary glands. It is a safe, simple, low-cost technique, which is usually tolerated by patients. Multiple needle passes can be employed to increase cellular yield, and some operators use ultrasound guidance to ensure adequate sampling. Diagnostic information can be provided rapidly, as there are only a few laboratory steps required to produce a slide for interpretation, and diagnostic accuracy is high. The disadvantages are similar to the brush biopsy and relate to the adequacy of the sample for diagnosis. A negative result does not exclude disease. It is important to appreciate that the information provided by the cytopathologist requires careful correlation with the clinical examination and any available imaging information.

A variety of techniques can be used to acquire tissue for diagnosis (Table 1.9). For oral mucosa, the majority of diagnostic biopsies are performed under local anaesthesia. Small, clinically benign lesions may be removed completely by excisional biopsy. For larger lesions, an incisional biopsy technique is used to sample a representative area or areas of the lesion, prior to planning further treatment. It is important to avoid injecting the local anaesthetic solution directly into the piece of tissue to be removed. The tissue sample should be handled with care to avoid distortion, causing stretch and crush artefacts. Routine biopsies are placed immediately in a fixative—typically neutral buffered formalin (10% formalin in phosphate buffered saline). Fixation prevents tissue desiccation and autolysis; it also hardens the tissue in preparation for laboratory processing. Occasionally fresh biopsy material is required for the laboratory investigation of oral blistering conditions (Chapter 2). Fresh material can be transported to the laboratory in damp gauze, a proprietary transport medium (provided by the pathology laboratory), or snap frozen in liquid nitrogen. Rapid diagnosis can also be attempted using fresh biopsy material. Surgeons sometimes employ this technique during an operation to ensure that the margins of the surgical defect are clear of cancer, which is referred to as intra-operative frozen sections.

When the specimen arrives in the laboratory, it is checked to ensure that it is correctly labelled and the accompanying request form is completed satisfactorily. The specimen is then assigned a unique specimen number and starts its journey through the laboratory. The specimen is retrieved from the container and described; this constitutes the macroscopic description. The pathologist may then slice the biopsy to ensure optimal sampling and places the tissue into cassettes ready for tissue processing and embedding (Fig. 1.4). The resultant formalin-fixed paraffin-embedded tissue block is then ready for sectioning on a rotary microtome (Fig. 1.5). Very thin (5 μm) sections are mounted on glass slides and stained with haematoxylin and eosin (H&E) (Fig. 1.6). Haematoxylin stains cell nuclei dark blue and connective tissue glycoproteins light blue; by contrast eosin stains the cytoplasm and connective tissue collagen fibres a reddish pink colour. The slides are then examined by the pathologist; in some instances a diagnosis can be rendered by examining the H&E stained sections alone. However, additional stains or immunohistochemistry may be required before a definitive diagnosis can be formulated (Table 1.10). The pathologist will describe the salient microscopic features and provide either a definitive diagnosis or a differential diagnosis in cases that require further clinico-pathological correlation. A typical histopathology report

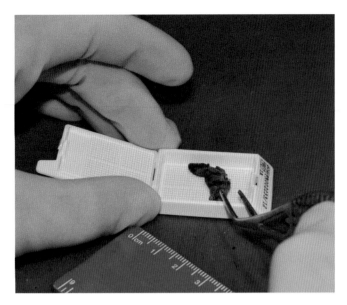

Fig. 1.4 A formalin-fixed biopsy placed in a cassette prior to processing.

is shown in Box. 1.2. The average time from biopsy to pathology report is around 7 days; however, it is possible to reduce the 'turn around time' to around 24 h for urgent biopsies. Large surgical resection specimens, particularly those containing bone that requires decalcification, can take up to a fortnight to report.

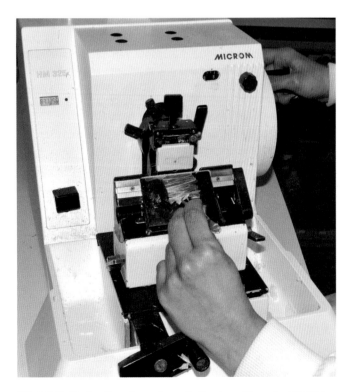

Fig. 1.5 Cutting sections from a formalin-fixed paraffin-embedded tissue block using a rotary microtome.

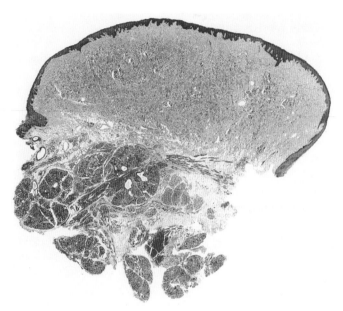

Fig. 1.6 Haematoxylin and eosin (H&E) stained section of a fibroepithelial polyp, with lobules of minor salivary gland on the deep aspect.

Molecular pathology

Increasingly, the identification of genetic abnormalities is being used to diagnose specific tumours and predict treatment response to targeted therapies. Chromosomal abnormalities, such as amplifications, translocations, and deletions, can be identified by cytogenetics (Chapter 4). Molecular biological techniques can be employed to identify genetic abnormalities such as loss of heterozygosity and specific gene mutations (Chapter 3). Molecular methods such as

Table 1.10 Histopathological investigations

Laboratory work	Description
Additional histological sections	The biomedical scientist will cut deeper into the tissue block, typically producing further histological sections, which are stained with H&E.
Histochemistry (Special stains)	Histochemistry is used to highlight a variety of biological materials in the tissue by using different staining techniques:
	Periodic Acid Schiff stain (PAS)—highlights carbohydrates
	Diastase PAS stain—highlights epithelial mucin and fungal hyphae
	Elastic van Gieson stain (EVG)—highlights elastin fibres and collagen
	Ziehl Neelsen stain (ZN)—used to identify acid-fast bacilli (tuberculosis)

Table 1.10 *Continued*

Laboratory work	Description
Immunohistochemistry	Immunohistochemistry employs antibodies to detect the location of antigens within the tissue sections. The location of the bound antibody is visualized using a chromogen, which typically produces a brown or red colour. In tumour pathology, the detection of specific antibodies helps the pathologist to refine the diagnosis by giving information about the differentiation of the malignant cells:
	Cytokeratins—epithelial cells
	Leukocyte common antigen (CD45)—lymphoid cells
	S100—melanocytes and neural elements
	Desmin—muscle cells
	Vimentin—mesenchymal cells
In situ hybridization	*In situ* hybridization is a method for detecting nucleic acids (DNA and RNA) in tissue sections. A labelled DNA probe hybridizes (sticks) to complementary nucleic acid sequences within the tissue section. The DNA probe is visualized using a similar chromogen-based signal amplification method as for immunohistochemistry:
	Immunoglobulin light chains (kappa and lambda)
	Epstein–Barr virus
	Human papillomavirus

Box 1.2 Pathology report

Clinical details

Polyp on left buccal mucosa for several years, 5mm diameter. Catches on teeth. Provisional diagnosis: fibroepithelial polyp.

Macroscopic report

Oral biopsy, left buccal mucosa: a cream piece of muscosa measuring $5 \times 3 \times 1$ mm. The mucosa bears a cream polypoid lesion measuring 3×3 mm to a height of 3 mm. The mucosa is bisected and both halves embedded in 1A for levels.

Microscopic report

Sections show a polypoid piece of mucosa. The squamous epithelium is hyperplastic and shows hyperkeratosis. The lamina propria is focally expanded by cellular fibrous tissue. The features are consistent with a fibroepithelial polyp. There is no evidence of neoplasia.

Interpretation

Left buccal mucosa; fibroepithelial polyp.

polymerase chain reaction and *in situ* hybridization can be used to detect virus infection in oral tissues, e.g. Epstein–Barr virus in hairy leukoplakia (Chapter 2) and high-risk human papillomavirus in oropharyngeal cancer (Chapter 3). Significantly, gene mutation screening is being used to 'personalize' targeted cancer drug treatment. Detection of BRAF gene mutations in malignant melanoma is used to select patients that may benefit from vemurafenib. Improving outcomes for patients with oral cancer requires a similar approach and will be built on an increased understanding of the molecular progression of the disease and the identification of 'drugable' molecular targets (Chapter 3).

Referring a patient to a specialist

The majority of dentists provide services in the primary care setting. It is important that the dental practitioner has the breadth of knowledge to identify oral lesions and conditions that require referral for specialist care. In the context of oral disease, patients are usually referred to secondary care for diseases that require further investigations in order to establish a definitive diagnosis and/or specialist medical or surgical interventions. When considering referring a patient, it is important to discuss the reasons with the patient and seek their consent. The referral letter should include patient details and a clear statement about the nature of the condition, including the clinical history, medical history, and clinical examination, along with a provisional or differential diagnosis. The information contained in the referral letter is used to allocate individual patients to appropriate appointment slots (urgent/routine). A patient that presents with a lesion that is considered to be clinically malignant should be clearly marked as urgent. It is recommended that urgent referral letters are accompanied by either a telephone call to the specialist unit or a secure FAX communication of the referral letter. This strategy will ensure that the patient is able to access the specialist care that they require quickly. In the UK, such patients follow a care pathway that is known as the '2-week wait' (2WW) or 'cancer waiting time' (CWT), which means that patients with suspected cancer will receive a hospital outpatient appointment within 2 weeks of their urgent referral. The UK National Cancer Plan indicates that no patient should wait longer than 1 month from an urgent referral for suspected cancer to the beginning of treatment, except for good clinical reasons.

Documenting clinical information

It is important that all stages of the diagnostic process are accurately documented in the clinical notes. The record must include dated clinical entries with any radiographs, laboratory reports, and copies of correspondence. Maintaining a proper record is not only good practice, it also is essential for clinical governance and is invaluable for the resolution of medico-legal claims.

Key points **Diagnosis of oral disease**

- Oral disease is common
- Oral disease may be the first sign of an underlying systemic disease
- Take time to establish an accurate clinical history
- Adopt a systematic approach to patient examination
- Radiological investigations should adhere to the principles of justification, optimization, and limitation of radiation exposure
- Analysis of patient samples by laboratory-based medical specialties are usually required to render a definitive diagnosis
- Maintain accurate, contemporaneous clinical records

2

Diseases of the oral mucosa

Chapter contents

Normal oral mucosa

The oral mucosa lines the oral cavity and comprises a surface squamous epithelium with underlying lamina propria. Below the mucosa is the submucosa, which is composed of fibrous tissue and adipose tissue, and contains lobules of minor salivary glands and neurovascular bundles. In places, there is no submucosa and the lamina propria is continuous with periosteum, forming the resilient mucoperiosteum that covers the maxilla and mandible.

The microanatomy of normal oral mucosa

The squamous epithelium is composed of keratinocytes arranged in layers: there is a basal cell layer that rests on the basement membrane, a prickle cell layer, and usually a keratinized layer (Fig. 2.1). The keratinocytes are attached to each other by desmosomes and the basal keratinocytes are attached to the basement membrane by hemi-desmosomes. The basement membrane is important in maintaining the integrity of the mucosa by sticking the squamous epithelium to the underlying lamina propria (Fig. 2.2). There are two patterns of keratinization: parakeratosis and orthokeratosis. In parakeratinized epithelium the surface keratinocytes become flattened and the nucleus becomes dark and shrunken (pyknotic). These terminally differentiated squamous cells are eventually lost at the surface by desquamation. In orthokeratinization, there is a granular cell layer (containing numerous keratohyaline granules) between the prickle cell layer and the keratinized layer. The surface squames become flattened and do not contain any discernible nuclear material. Whilst the majority of cells in squamous epithelium are keratinocytes, there are also accessory cells such as melanocytes, Langerhans cells, and neurosensory cells (Merkel cells and taste buds).

The lamina propria is the connective tissue that lies immediately below the epithelium (Fig. 2.1). It is divided into the superficial papillary layer (sometimes referred to as the corium) and the deeper reticular layer. The lamina propria is composed of fibrous tissue with a rich neurovascular supply and contains fibroblasts that elaborate collagen and elastin fibres along with other extracellular matrix proteins. The lamina propria also contains components of the mucosal immune defence system such as Langerhans cells, macrophages, mast cells, and lymphocytes.

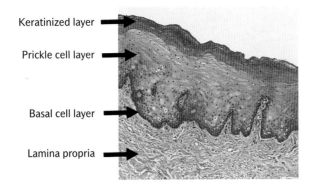

Fig. 2.1 Microanatomy of oral mucosa showing the stratification of the squamous epithelium.

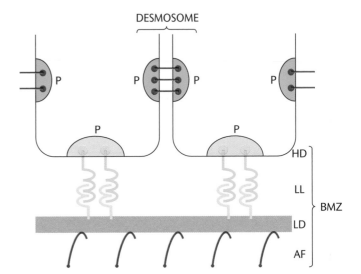

Fig. 2.2 Ultrastructural organization of desmosomes, hemi-desmosomes, and the basement membrane zone. The inter-cellular attachments of keratinocytes are mediated by desmosomes comprising opposing attachment plaques (P) and inter-cellular adhesion proteins. The attachment of the squamous epithelium to the lamina propria is mediated by hemi-desmosomes (HD) and proteins of basement membrane zone (BMZ). Adhesion proteins from the hemi-desmosome attachment plaque interact in the lamina lucida (LL) with adhesion proteins from the lamina densa (LD). Type IV collagen of the LD interacts with type VII collagen of the anchoring fibrils (AF), which in turn interact with collagen in the underlying lamina propria.

Regional variation of normal oral mucosa

The clinical appearance of the oral mucosa is dependent on the thickness of the epithelium, the amount of surface keratinization, melanin (and other) pigmentation, and the vascularity of the lamina propria. There are three main mucosal patterns: lining mucosa, masticatory mucosa, and specialized mucosa.

Lining mucosa

The vermillion border of the lip is the transition zone between the skin and the oral mucosa, and is covered by thin, orthokeratinized squamous epithelium. The labial mucosa, buccal mucosa, floor of the mouth, and the ventral surface of the tongue are covered by a non-keratinized squamous epithelium, which varies in thickness (Fig. 2.3A). In the floor of the mouth, the epithelium is thin and the epithelial–mesenchymal interface is rather flat with fewer, shallower rete processes than in buccal or labial mucosa. The lining mucosa is perforated by the ducts of the minor and major salivary glands.

Masticatory mucosa

The hard palate and gingiva are covered by keratinized masticatory mucosa (Fig. 2.3B). The mucosa is firmly bound down to the underlying bone surface to produce a mucoperiosteum (sometimes called the attached mucosa). The palate is mainly covered by orthokeratinized

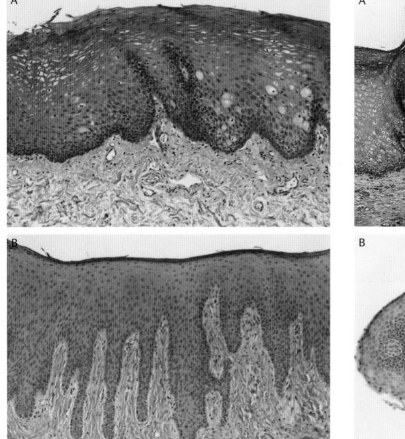

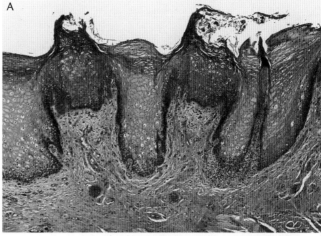

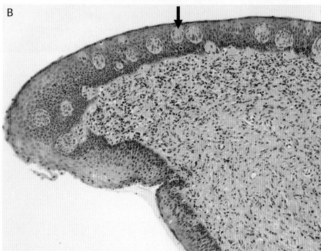

Fig. 2.3 Histology of non-keratinized lining mucosa (A) and keratinized masticatory mucosa that has a thin layer of parkeratin on the surface (B).

Fig. 2.4 Histology of specialized mucosa. Dorsum of tongue with filiform papillae on the surface (A). A foliate papilla with taste buds in the epithelium (arrow) and a subgemmal neurogenous plaque filling the lamina propria (B).

squamous epithelium. The attached gingiva and the external part of the free gingiva are variably covered by parakeratinized and orthokeratinized squamous epithelium. The gingiva that lies adjacent to the crown of the tooth is lined by sulcular epithelium, which is non-keratinized. Clinically, the attached gingiva forms a scalloped border with the alveolar mucosa (Fig. 1.1A), which is covered by a thin non-keratinized squamous epithelium.

Specialized mucosa

The mucosa of the dorsum of the tongue is organized into structures called papillae, most of which are filiform papillae (Fig. 2.4A). The filiform papillae give the dorsum of the tongue its characteristic 'velvety' surface. There are also numerous fungiform papillae, which have a dome-shaped appearance and are variably covered by non-keratinized and keratinized squamous epithelium. Circumvallate papillae are arranged in a V-shaped line just anterior to the sulcus terminalis at the junction of the posterior and middle-thirds of the tongue, with a deep sulcus around their circumference. They are usually covered by non-keratinized squamous epithelium with taste buds on the walls of the

papilla. At the base of the trough there are the serous glands of von Ebner. Foliate papillae are located on the postero-lateral aspect of the tongue and are folds of non-keratinized squamous epithelium that also contain numerous taste buds (Fig. 2.4B). The nerve fibres that supply the taste buds form a dense plexus in the lamina propria, termed subgemmal neurogenous plaques. In addition, the foliate papillae may have focal areas of mucosa associated lymphoid tissue called lingual tonsil.

Features variably present in normal oral mucosa

It is important, clinically, to be able to recognize normal variants in the appearance of the oral mucosa. Patients who are anxious may become concerned that such features are signs of disease and will require reassurance.

Leukoedema

The oral mucosa has a translucent, milky whiteness with a slightly folded appearance. The condition is more evident in persons with

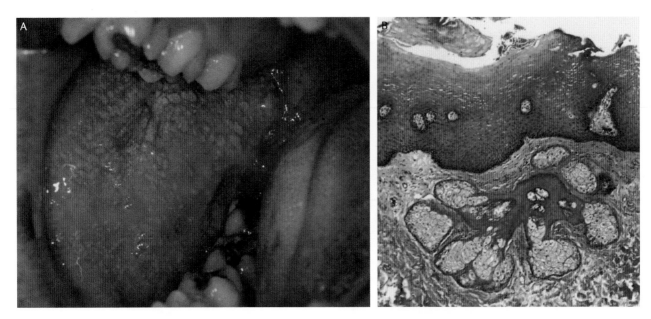

Fig. 2.5 Prominent Fordyce spots on the buccal mucosa. Histology shows a mucosal sebaceous gland (Fordyce spot).

racial pigmentation. Histologically, the epithelium is thicker than normal with broad rete processes, and the cells in the superficial part of the prickle cell layer appear vacuolated and contain considerable quantities of glycogen. Leukoedema is regarded as a variation of normal oral mucosa.

Fordyce spots

Sebaceous glands in the oral mucosa are called Fordyce spots or granules, and are usually seen as separate, small, yellowish bodies beneath the surface in the mucosa of the upper lip, cheeks, and anterior pillar of the fauces, usually with a symmetrical distribution (Fig. 2.5). The glands are present in most adults, but the number of glands varies greatly between individuals. The prevalence and number in the upper lip increase around puberty, and there may be greater prominence of these glands in the buccal mucosa in later life. The glands are situated superficially in the mucosa and consist of a number of lobules of sebaceous cells grouped around one or more ducts. Sebaceous glands do not appear to have any function in the oral cavity, and no significant pathological changes are associated with them.

Sublingual varices

The prevalence of varicosities of the branches of the sublingual veins increases with age (Fig. 1.3B). The varices have no clinical significance and may be related to smoking and cardiovascular disease. Similar lesions are occasionally seen elsewhere in the oral cavity and on the lips.

Lingual tonsil

Lingual tonsillar tissue, composed of mucosa-associated lymphoid tissue, is mainly located on the postero-lateral aspect of the tongue and may be associated with vertical folds of mucosa, sometimes referred to as foliate papillae (Fig. 2.6). Diseases of lingual tonsillar tissue are

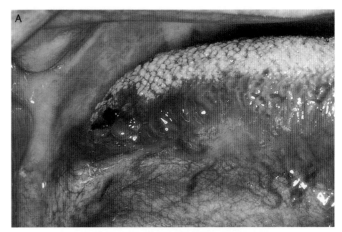

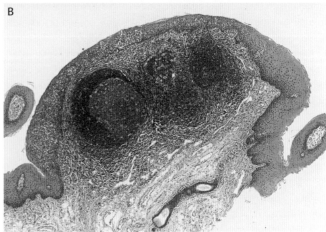

Fig. 2.6 Lingual tonsil located on the postero-lateral part of the tongue. Histology shows organized mucosa-associated lymphoid tissue just below the epithelium.

uncommon, but they may become enlarged as a result of trauma from teeth or dentures, or undergo reactive lymphoid hyperplasia secondary to local inflammation or infection. Occasionally, lingual tonsillar crypts may become obstructed and undergo cystic dilatation as a result of accumulation of squamous debris. Mucosa-associated lymphoid tissue may also be found in the floor of the mouth, where they appear as small pink papules.

Age changes in oral mucosa

Although a variety of changes may occur in the oral mucosa of the elderly, distinguishing those attributable only to ageing from those due to systemic disease, nutritional deficiencies, or the side-effects of medication is difficult. Atrophic changes have been reported in lingual mucosa related to a reduction in epithelial thickness with increasing age. However, this may not apply to other oral mucosal surfaces. The question of whether increased keratinization of the oral mucosa occurs in old age has not been resolved. Oral mucosal connective tissues become more fibrosed, less vascular, and less cellular with age. As a result, certain local oral mucosal lesions are reported to occur more frequently in the elderly, examples being sublingual varices, increased prominence of Fordyce spots, and relative enlargement of foliate papillae.

Diseases of the oral mucosa

For a description of the histopathological terms used in this chapter see Table 2.1.

Geographic tongue (benign migratory glossitis)

This condition has a reported prevalence of 1% of the population and there is often a family history. The disorder occurs over a wide age-range and presents both in children and adults. It is of unknown aetiology, but geographic tongue has been reported in patients with psoriasis and it is possible that these disorders share the same underlying genetic predisposing factors.

Clinically, geographic tongue presents as irregular, partially depapillated, red areas on the anterior two-thirds of the dorsal surface of the tongue and is associated with loss of the filiform papillae, the fungiform papillae remaining as shiny, dark-red eminences. The margins of the lesions are often outlined by a thin, white line or band (Fig. 2.7A). The affected areas may begin as small lesions only a few millimetres in diameter, which, after gradually enlarging, heal and then reappear in another location. The condition may regress for a period and then recur. It is usually symptomless but there may be some irritation associated with acidic and spicy foods.

Histological examination shows the epithelium at the edges of the lesions to be acanthotic with a dense, neutrophil infiltration throughout the epithelium and the lamina propria (Fig. 2.7B). In the centres of the lesions, the desquamating cells on the surface are lost and there is underlying chronic inflammatory cell infiltration composed of macrophages, lymphocytes, and plasma cells.

Table 2.1 Histopathogical terms

Term	Description
Hyperkeratosis	Increased thickness of the keratin layer.
Hyperplasia	Increase in cell numbers by mitosis and/or decrease in apoptosis. Epithelial hyperplasia refers to thickening of the epithelium.
Atrophy	Decrease in size of cell, tissue, or organ. Epithelial atrophy refers to thinning of the epithelium, usually associated with loss of rete processes.
Acanthosis	Epithelial hyperplasia in which the increased thickness is due to an increased number of cells in the prickle cell layer, producing broadening and lengthening of the rete processes.
Acantholysis	Loss of adhesion of keratinocytes in the prickle cell layer causing the epithelium to 'fall apart'.
Dysplasia	Increase in cell growth and altered differentiation, producing an overall change in architecture of tissue.
Neoplasia	Growth disorder characterized by genetic alterations that lead to loss of the normal control mechanisms that regulate cell growth and differentiation. Neoplasia can be benign or malignant.
Hamartoma	A hamartoma is a non-neoplastic overgrowth of tissue that is disordered in structure and is composed of tissues indigenous to the anatomical site. Hamartomas have a limited growth potential.

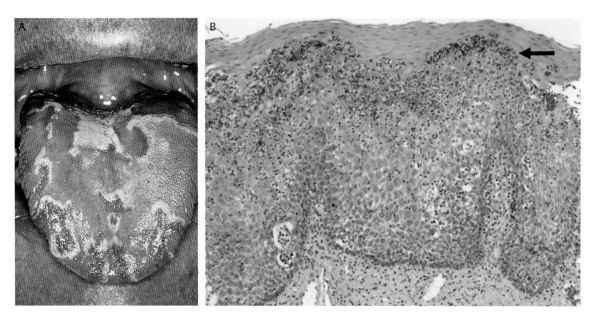

Fig. 2.7 Geographic tongue showing areas of white and red mucosa. The squamous epithelium shows hyperkeratosis and acanthosis, and contains numerous acute inflammatory cells (neutrophils). Most of the neutrophils are located just below the keratinized layer (arrow).

Reactive hyperplastic lesions

Localized hyperplastic lesions of the oral mucosa are common and usually represent exuberant production of repair tissue (granulation tissue and fibrous scar tissue) as a consequence of tissue damage and attendant chronic inflammation. Although several named lesions are distinguished either on clinical or histological grounds, it is important to appreciate that most are essentially variations of the same basic disease process.

Fibroepithelial polyp

The fibroepithelial polyp is a very common lesion occurring over a wide age-range. It arises mainly in the buccal mucosa (particularly along the occlusal plane), lips, and tongue, and presents as a firm, pink, painless, pedunculated or sessile polypoid swelling varying in size from a few millimetres to a centimetre or more in dimension (Fig. 2.8A). Minor trauma is thought to be an important initiating factor and occasionally the surface is white due to frictional keratosis. Ulceration is not a feature unless the patient has traumatized the polyp.

Histologically, the lesion comprises a core of dense, relatively avascular and paucicellular fibrous tissue, which has a scar-like quality (Figs 1.6 and 2.8B). Thick, interlacing bundles of collagen fibres are the dominant feature and they blend with those of the adjacent normal tissue through the base of the lesion. Fibroblasts are scanty, although plump, angular, and occasionally multinucleate forms are sometimes observed, particularly in the sub-epithelial zone. When such prominent fibroblasts are present, the polyp may be referred to as a 'giant cell fibroma'. The surface of a fibroepithelial polyp is covered by squamous epithelium, which may vary in thickness and show areas of hyperkeratosis in response to frictional irritation. Typically, there is little inflammatory cell infiltration and the lesion can be regarded as an exuberance of reparative scar tissue.

Denture-associated lesions

The term 'denture irritation hyperplasia' is applied to hyperplastic mucosa related to the periphery of an ill-fitting denture. The lesions may be single or multiple and most frequently present as one or several broad-based, leaf-like folds of tissue embracing the over-extended flange of the denture (Fig. 2.9). They usually arise in the depths of the sulci but can involve the inner surfaces of the lips and cheeks, and the palate along the posterior edge of an upper denture. When the lesion occurs in the palate under a denture, it becomes flattened and leaf-like, and is commonly referred to as a 'leaf fibroma' (Fig. 2.10A). Denture-associated lesions occur more frequently in relation to lower than upper dentures, and more often in females than males. Most of the patients have worn ill-fitting dentures for many years. Clinically, the hyperplastic tissue is usually firm in consistency and not grossly inflamed, but there may be ulceration at the base into which the flange of the denture fits.

Another reactive mucosal condition frequently associated with the wearing of ill-fitting dentures is papillary hyperplasia of the palate (Fig. 2.10B). These lesions are especially encountered in patients who wear their upper denture constantly. Although the pathogenesis is still uncertain chronic trauma, poor oral hygiene and *Candida* infection have been implicated.

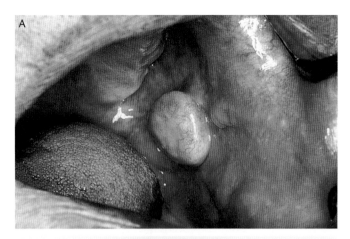

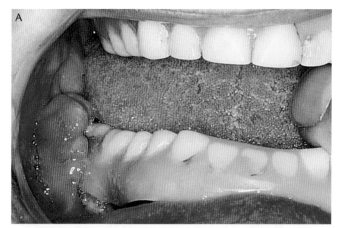

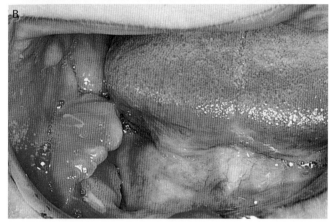

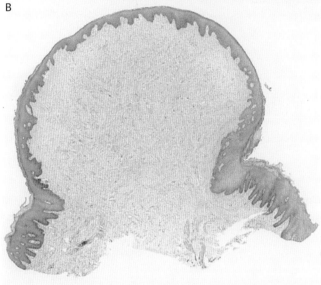

Fig. 2.9 Denture irritation hyperplasia.

Fig. 2.8 Fibroepithelial polyp. Histology shows a nodule of fibrous tissue covered by squamous epithelium.

Pyogenic granuloma

Pyogenic granuloma is a reactive vascular lesion. Although the majority of pyogenic granulomas in the oral cavity arise on the gingiva, the lesion can occur at other sites, e.g. the tongue, and buccal and labial mucosa (Fig. 2.11A), usually as a result of trauma.

Histologically, the pyogenic granuloma is characterized by vascular proliferation, which may take the form of rather solid sheets or lobules of endothelial cells with little evidence of canalization or of numerous small vessels and large, dilated, thin-walled vascular spaces (Fig. 2.11). The vascular element is supported by a delicate and often oedematous cellular fibrous stroma. Inflammatory cell infiltration is variable and usually prominent beneath areas of ulceration. An epithelial collarette around the base is typically present.

Epulides

Reactive hyperplastic lesions arising from the gingiva receive the designation 'epulis'. Although the term is not specific and literally means 'on

the gum', by common usage it implies a localized, chronic, inflammatory hyperplasia of the gingiva. Epulides are common; they present as localized, gingival enlargements but are hyperplastic and not neoplastic lesions. Most arise from the interdental tissues. Trauma and chronic irritation, particularly from sub-gingival plaque and calculus, are considered to be the main aetiological factors.

The lesions share several common clinical features: they are all more common in females than males, particularly so in the case of vascular lesions; most occur anterior to the molar teeth; and they are slightly more common in the maxilla than the mandible. They may recur if local precipitating factors are not identified and eliminated or, particularly in the case of the giant cell epulis, if the lesion has not been completely excised in the first instance. Reported recurrence rates differ considerably between series. Recurrence of the fibrous epulis is relatively uncommon, assuming that the cause has been removed. By contrast, the ossifying fibrous epulis and the giant cell epulis are more prone to recur.

Fibrous epulis

The fibrous epulis presents as a firm, pedunculated or sessile lesion, which is of similar colour to the adjacent gingiva (Fig. 2.12A), although this depends on the degree of vascularity and inflammation within the lesion. The surface may be ulcerated, in which case it will be covered by a yellowish fibrinous exudate. The epulis occurs over a wide age-range but most arise in children and young adults.

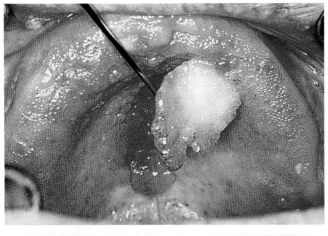

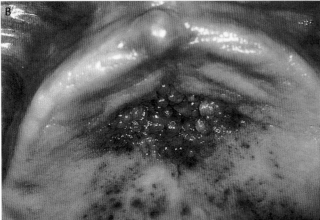

Fig. 2.10 'Leaf fibroma' and papillary hyperplasia of the palate.

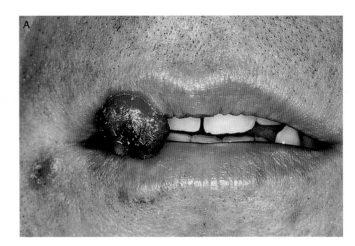

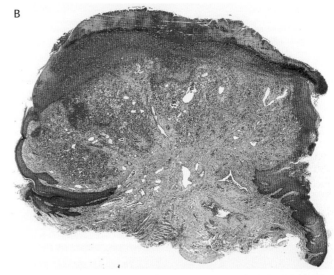

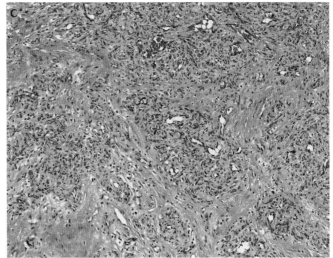

Fig. 2.11 Pyogenic granuloma. The surface is ulcerated and covered by a thick fibrinous crust. Below the crust is a highly vascular lesion.

Histologically, the lesion usually comprises varying amounts of richly cellular fibroblastic tissue with mature collagen fibres (Fig. 2.12B). There is a variable inflammatory cell infiltrate, predominantly of plasma cells and lymphocytes. Around one-third of cases contain amorphous deposits of calcification and/or trabeculae of metaplastic bone within the fibroblastic tissue (Fig. 2.12C). The term ossifying fibrous epulis may be used for this histological variant, which is most common on the maxillary labial gingivae and has a tendency to recur. Such lesions have previously been termed 'peripheral ossifying fibroma'; however, as the lesion is reactive rather than neoplastic, this terminology should not be used.

Vascular epulis

A vascular epulis is essentially a pyogenic granuloma on the gingiva and is commonly associated with pregnancy, when the term pregnancy epulis is often used. It presents as a soft, bright red swelling (Fig. 2.13), which is often ulcerated. Haemorrhage may occur either spontaneously or on minor trauma. The lesions occur over a wide age-range but there is a peak incidence in females of child-bearing age. Lesions occurring in pregnancy can arise at any time from the first to the ninth month, although onset is usually around the end of the first trimester. They gradually increase in size, but after delivery may regress spontaneously or decrease in size and assume the clinical and histological features of a fibrous epulis. Lesions excised during pregnancy also frequently recur and for these reasons it may be preferable to delay surgical treatment until after the birth of the child. The histological features are those of a pyogenic granuloma.

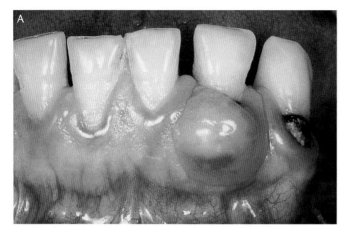

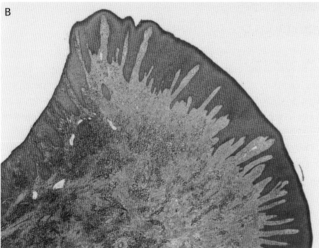

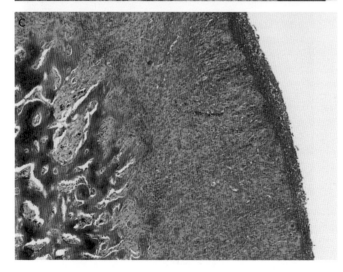

Fig. 2.12 Clinical appearance of a fibrous epulis (A). Histology shows a typical fibrous epulis (B) and an ossifying fibrous epulis with an ulcerated surface (C).

Giant cell epulis

The giant cell epulis is uncommon and accounts for only around 10% of epulides. It is also known as peripheral giant cell granuloma because it has identical histopathological features to central giant cell granuloma

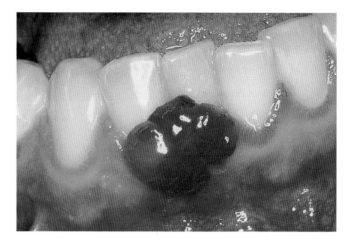

Fig. 2.13 Vascular epulis.

and also 'brown tumours' of hyperparathyroidism, both of which should be excluded in order to render a diagnosis of giant cell epulis. The name pertains to the preponderance of multinucleate giant cells within the lesion. It occurs over a wide age-range with a peak incidence in the second decade in males and the fifth decade for females. The lesion can arise anywhere on the gingiva or alveolar mucosa in dentate or edentulous patients but most occur anterior to the molar teeth. Females are affected about twice as frequently as males, and slightly more occur in the mandible than in the maxilla.

Giant cell epulis presents as a pedunculated or sessile swelling of varying size, which is typically dark red/purple in colour and commonly ulcerated. In dentate areas of the jaws, the lesion usually arises interdentally and may have an hour-glass shape with buccal and lingual swellings joined by a narrow waist between the teeth (Fig. 2.14A). Radiographs are required for a definitive diagnosis since it is possible for a central giant cell granuloma to perforate the cortex of the bone and present as a peripheral lesion (Chapter 7). By contrast, radiographs of a giant cell epulis will only demonstrate superficial erosion of the underlying alveolar process.

Histopathological examination shows focal collections of multinucleated osteoclast-like giant cells lying in a richly vascular and cellular stroma (Fig. 2.14). The collections of giant cells are separated by fibrous septa. A narrow zone of fibrous tissue, often containing dilated blood vessels, also separates the core of the lesion from the covering squamous epithelium. The giant cells are numerous and show variation in size, shape, and number of nuclei. Large numbers of vascular channels of varying diameter are found throughout, and extravasated red blood cells and deposits of haemosiderin are common. The mononuclear stromal cells are ovoid or spindle-shaped and comprise a mixture of fibroblasts, macrophages, and endothelial cells.

The pathogenesis of the giant cell epulis is unknown, but it is generally accepted that it is a reactive hyperplasia and, like other hyperplastic conditions of the oral mucosa, trauma may be an important aetiological factor. An origin from periosteum rather than gingiva has been suggested since the lesion can cause superficial erosion of the alveolar bone and occurs in edentate, as well as dentate, areas of the jaws. Very rarely the lesions may be multiple, associated with systemic disorders such as hyperparathyroidism (Table 2.2).

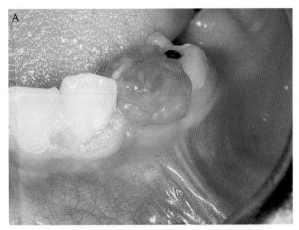

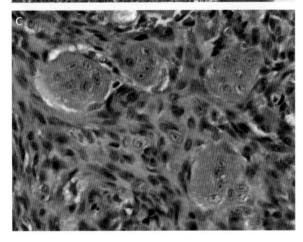

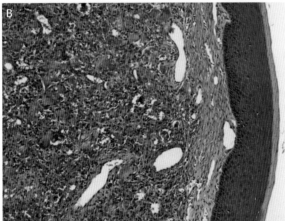

Fig. 2.14 Giant cell epulis. Histology shows a highly vascular lesion that contains characteristic multinucleated giant cells.

Key points Epulides

- Localized gingival hyperplasia
- Reactive to local irritation
- May recur unless predisposing factors removed
- Fibrous and vascular epulides represent exuberant repair tissue
- Vascular epulis may mature to fibrous epulis
- Giant cell epulis is clinically and histologically distinct

Table 2.2 Classification of hyperparathyroidism

Type	Features
Primary	Increased parathyroid hormone (PTH) secretion due to disease of the parathyroid gland, e.g. parathyroid adenoma.
Secondary	Increased PTH secretion due to chronic hypocalcaemia, seen in vitamin D deficiency or renal failure.
Tertiary	Long-term secondary hyperparathyroidism results in parathyroid hyperplasia and loss of calcium sensitivity, seen in renal failure.

Squamous cell papilloma

Squamous cell papilloma is a common benign tumour that can occur anywhere on the oral mucosa. Most occur in adults but they may also be seen in children. Papillomas vary in size and may be either pedunculated or sessile. They present as warty or cauliflower-like growths with a white or pink surface, depending on the amount of keratin present (Fig. 2.15A).

Histological examination shows finger-like processes of hyperplastic squamous epithelium supported by thin cores of vascular connective tissue (Fig. 2.15B). The epithelium may show hyperkeratosis.

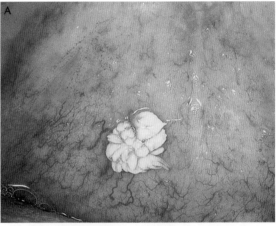

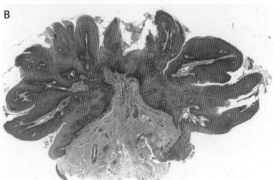

Fig. 2.15 Squamous cell papilloma. Histology shows hyperplastic squamous epithelium covering finger-like projections of fibro-vascular tissue.

Mitotic figures are often seen in the basal layer of the epithelium, but features of epithelial dysplasia are not present. Most, if not all, squamous cell papillomas are caused by human papillomavirus (HPV) infection. There are distinct variants of squamous cell papilloma, such as verruca vulgaris (common wart), condyloma acuminatum (venereal wart), and Heck's disease, which are associated with certain HPV genotypes; however, laboratory testing to identify HPV is not routinely conducted. Malignant transformation is not a feature of oral squamous cell papilloma.

Verruca vulgaris (common wart)

Verruca vulgaris may present as single or multiple lesions. They appear white because of hyperkeratosis and are seen most often in children when they may be associated with autoinoculation from warts on the skin of the fingers and lips. Lesions are most commonly seen on the vermillion border, labial mucosa, and anterior tongue. Histologically, they consist of verrucous processes of proliferating, acanthotic, hyperkeratotic squamous epithelium supported by thin cores of vascular connective tissue. The hyperplastic rete processes at the periphery of the wart usually slope inwards towards the centre of the lesion. On the surface there are spikey tiers of parakeratin and orthokeratin. Koilocyte-like cells are usually seen in the granular cell layer. Common warts are usually associated with infection by HPV-2, -4, -11, and -40.

Condyloma acuminatum (venereal wart)

These warts mainly occur in the ano-genital region of sexually active adults but may be seen on the oral mucosa, presenting as multiple pink nodules that grow and coalesce to form soft, pink, usually sessile papillary lesions similar in colour to the surrounding mucosa (Fig. 2.16). Condyloma acuminatum is associated with HPV-6, -11, and -16.

Focal epithelial hyperplasia (Heck's disease)

This condition was originally described in native North Americans and Inuits but occurs in other racial groups and in immunocompromised patients. It is characterized by multiple, small, elevated epithelial plaques or polypoid lesions, most frequently involving the lower lips and buccal mucosa. HPV-13 and -32 appear to be specific to oral focal epithelial hyperplasia.

Verruciform xanthoma

Verruciform xanthoma is an uncommon lesion that occurs most frequently on the masticatory mucosa of the gingiva and hard palate. Clinically, it presents as a flat or slightly raised, but otherwise symptomless, lesion with a papillary/warty surface and varies in size. Histopathology shows hyperplastic epithelium thrown into papillary projections, with the connective tissue papillae filled by lipid-containing xanthoma cells (Fig. 2.17). The xanthomatous infiltrate is sharply limited to the papillary lamina propria. The aetiology of the disorder is unknown and there are no known associations with other diseases.

Key points Intra-oral lumps

- Use a systematic approach when assessing a lump
- Lumps arising from the gingiva or alveolus require radiographic examination
- The majority of lumps are reactive hyperplastic lesions
- Neoplasms are less common
- Biopsy is required for a definitive diagnosis

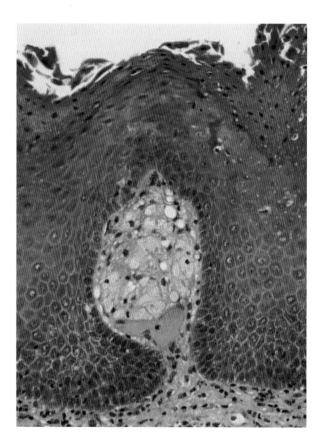

Fig. 2.17 Verruciform xanthoma showing lipid-containing foam cells filling the papillary lamina propria.

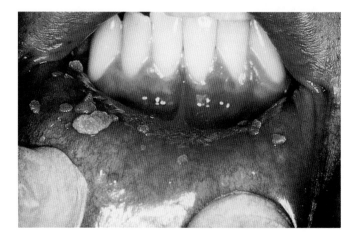

Fig. 2.16 Condyloma acuminatum.

Benign soft-tissue tumours

Soft-tissue tumours are derived from mesenchymal components of the connective tissues. A great variety of benign and malignant soft-tissue tumours and tumour-like lesions have been reported in the oral cavity but, with few exceptions, they are rare (Table 2.3). Clinically, most of the benign soft-tissue tumours present as swellings that may be indistinguishable from hyperplastic mucosal lesions. Histologically, oral soft-tissue tumours resemble their counterparts occurring at other sites in the body. The various lesions will be discussed under their tissues of origin. The malignant soft-tissue tumours are covered briefly in Chapter 3.

Fibrous tissue

Fibroma and myofibroma

The majority of fibrous lesions that occur in the oral cavity are reactive hyperplastic lesions. Nevertheless, occasionally, true fibromas may arise. Distinction from hyperplasia is problematic, but a circumscribed mass of fibrous tissue with an apparently inherent growth potential (i.e. larger size than usual for hyperplasia) and recurrence following excision are indicative of a benign fibrous neoplasm or fibroma. In the oral cavity, the fibroblasts often express smooth muscle actin and are termed myofibroblasts. If these specialized cells are predominant in a tumour, the term myofibroma is used. Another tumour-like growth that contains

myofibroblasts is nodular fasciitis, which often has a short history of worrisome, rapid growth. The aetiology is not known, but the myofibroblasts have a characteristic chromosomal translocation: t(17;22) (p13;q13). Nodular fasciitis is benign and tends to regress following surgical intervention.

Adipose tissue

Lipoma

In the oral cavity, lipomas present as soft, yellowish-coloured swellings, most commonly in the cheek and tongue (Fig. 2.18). A typical feature of a lipoma is that the tumour floats in the fixative solution when dropped into a pathology specimen pot. On histopathological examination the tumour consists of a circumscribed mass of mature adipose tissue supported by varying amounts of fibrous stroma.

Vascular tissue

Haemangioma and vascular malformations

Haemangiomas and vascular malformations are common lesions that are generally accepted to be hamartomas rather than neoplastic. They occur more commonly in the head and neck region than in any other part of the body, and most are present at birth or arise in early childhood, although some (malformations) may not be noticed until old age.

The majority of haemangiomas appear within the first few weeks of life. Precursor lesions include erythematous macules and localized telangiectasias. The clinical hallmark of haemangioma is its defined growth phases: namely, an initial highly proliferative phase followed by involution. Clinically, haemangiomas in children present as a bright red, non-compressible papule, nodule, plaque, or destructive mass. The lesion cannot be evacuated of blood, which distinguishes them from vascular malformations. When deeper seated, the lesions may, however, appear as flesh-coloured masses. Thirty percent of

Table 2.3 Basic classification of soft-tissue tumours affecting the oral cavity

Tissue type	Benign	Malignant
Fibrous tissue	Fibroma Myofibroma	Fibrosarcoma Low-grade myofibroblastic sarcoma
Adipose tissue	Lipoma	Atypical lipomatous tumour Liposarcoma
Vessels	Haemangioma Lymphangioma	Angiosarcoma Haemangioendothelioma Kaposi sarcoma
Perivascular	Solitary fibrous tumour	Malignant solitary fibrous tumour
Nerve	Neurofibroma Schwannoma	Malignant peripheral nerve sheath tumour
Smooth muscle	Leiomyoma	Leiomyosarcoma
Striated muscle	Rhabdomyoma	Rhabdomyosarcoma
Mesenchymal cells (not otherwise specified)	Ectomesenchymal chondromyxoid tumour	Alveolar soft part sarcoma Synovial sarcoma Hyalinizing clear cell sarcoma

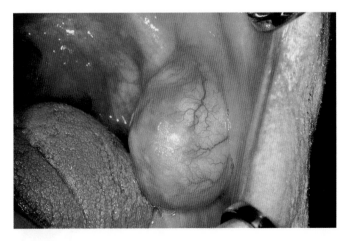

Fig. 2.18 Lipoma, note the yellowish appearance.

haemangiomas will completely resolve by age 3 years, 50% by age 5 years, 70–90% by age 7 years, and almost all haemangiomas will be completely involuted by 12 years of age.

Vascular malformations are developmental vascular anomalies that result from errors in vascular morphogenesis. All vascular malformations are present at birth but they become clinically evident at different times of life. On the basis of their clinical appearance, natural history, and histopathology, vascular malformations are divided into arterio-venous, capillary, lymphatic, venous, and combined lesions. The spaces are lined by endothelium and contain erythrocytes. Thrombosis and calcification may occur. Some lesions, particularly in infants, may be more solid, extremely cellular, and consist of sheets of endothelial cells with little evidence of canalization. Angiomatous malformations may also involve arteries and veins, and some lesions consist almost entirely of thick-walled vessels.

Vascular malformations, in contrast to haemangiomas, enlarge very slowly, proportionately with the growth of the child, and persist throughout life, never showing spontaneous regression. They are compressible and the vascular lesion can be emptied of its contents by pressing on it. Oral vascular malformations occur most commonly in the lips, tongue, cheeks, or palate, and vary considerably in size and shape. They are characteristically dark reddish-purple in colour (Fig. 2.19A), of soft consistency, and may present as a smooth, flat, or raised lesion of the mucosa that typically blanches on pressure. The lesions are usually symptomless. A history of recent increase in size may be due to haemorrhage, thrombosis, or inflammation. In addition to the mucosa, oral haemangiomas may also involve muscle, bone, and the major salivary glands.

Vascular malformations are usually solitary, although multiple lesions may occur and, rarely, these may be part of a generalized angiomatous syndrome, such as Sturge–Weber syndrome (OMIM 185300) (Fig. 8.5). This congenital disorder is characterized by the combination of lesions of the face over one or more branches of the trigeminal nerve, and may also affect the cerebral meninges over the cerebral cortex. Lesions may also occur in the oral mucosa or alveolar bone, and excessive bleeding may occur if teeth are extracted in the affected area.

Lymphangioma

Lymphangiomas are less common than haemangiomas but, like the latter, are considered to be hamartomas rather than neoplasms. They are usually present at birth or arise in early childhood and, although they can occur anywhere in the oral mucosa, they are seen most frequently in the tongue (Fig. 2.20A). Trauma to a lymphangioma may give rise to inflammation, calcification, or a sudden increase in size.

Histologically, the lesion consists of capillary or, more commonly, cavernous, endothelial-lined spaces containing lymph fluid. A rather typical feature of superficially located lesions is that the lymphatic spaces extend close up to the overlying epithelium, which they may cause to bulge (Fig. 2.20B). Clinically, the surface of such lesions manifests numerous papillary projections or small nodular masses.

Cystic hygroma (Fig. 9.10) is an extensive lymphangiomatous malformation that presents in infancy and commonly affects the neck (Chapter 9).

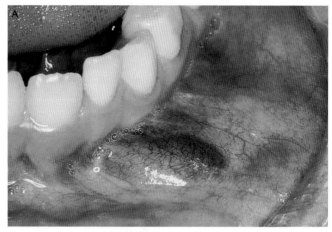

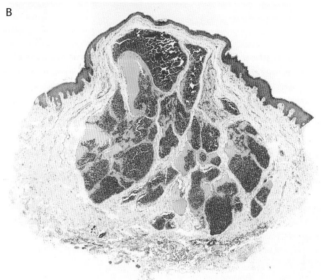

Fig. 2.19 Vascular malformation. Histology shows a complex network of interconnecting blood-filled cavities.

Neural tissue

The main tumours of peripheral nerves, which arise from the nerve sheath, are neurofibroma and Schwannoma (neurilemmoma). Traumatic neuromas are non-neoplastic, tumour-like masses of neural tissue.

Neurofibroma

Neurofibromas are benign tumours that may present as a solitary lesion or occur as multiple tumours associated with neurofibromatosis type 1 (OMIM 162200) (Fig. 2.21). Oral lesions occur in a small proportion of cases as mucosal swellings involving, most frequently, the tongue and gingiva or, more rarely, as intra-osseous growths, usually in the mandible. Malignant change in neurofibromas is a well-recognized complication in patients with neurofibromatosis. Malignant change in solitary lesions is very rare.

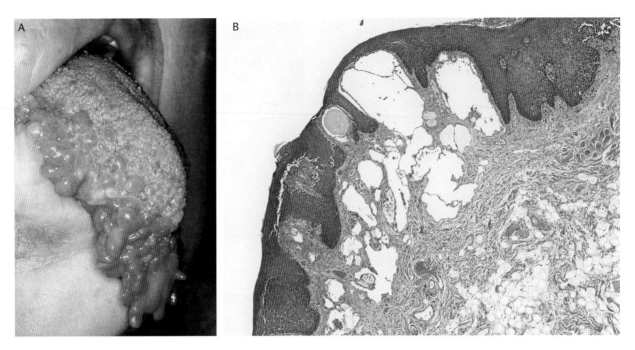

Fig. 2.20 Lymphangioma. Histology shows a complex network of lymphatic channels that are located just below the epithelium.

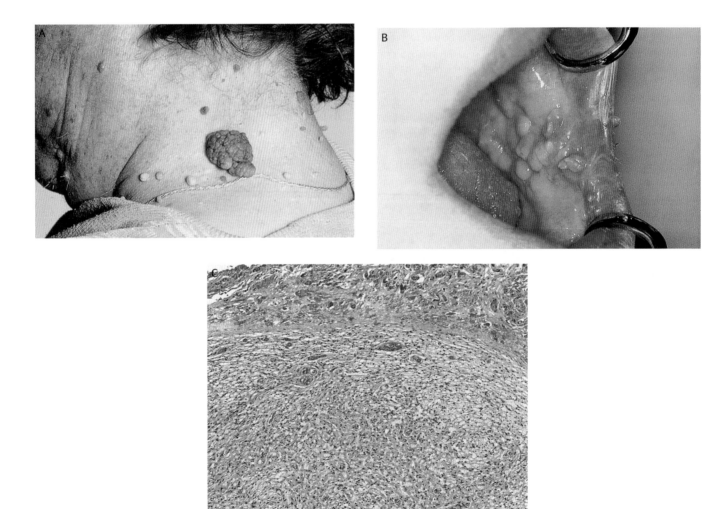

Fig. 2.21 Neurofibromatosis. Histology shows a circumscribed nodule of benign spindle cells.

Histologically, neurofibromas show considerable variation, but consist of a mixture of Schwann cells and fibroblasts with varying amounts of collagen and ground substance (Fig. 2.21). A few nerve fibres run through the lesion, which may be circumscribed or diffuse. Lesions arising within or around the nerve trunk consist of a mass of convoluted nerves surrounded by a proliferation of Schwann cells and fibroblasts. Clinically, this has been described as feeling like a 'bag of worms' on palpation of the lesion. This pattern is referred to as a plexiform neurofibroma and is characteristic of neurofibromatosis.

Schwannoma

Schwannoma (neurilemmoma) is a benign, encapsulated tumour. The neoplastic cells are arranged in two distinct patterns: Antoni A areas composed of haphazardly arranged spindle cells and Antoni B areas where the cells are arranged in parallel bundles with stacking up or palisading of the nuclei, called a Verocay body (Fig. 2.22). Unlike the neurofibroma, nerve fibres do not run through the lesion but may be associated with the capsule.

Traumatic neuroma

Traumatic neuroma is a non-neoplastic, disorganized overgrowth of nerve fibres, Schwann cells, and scar tissue occurring at the proximal end of a severed nerve (Fig. 2.23). It represents an exaggeration of the normal process of nerve regeneration and usually presents as a small nodule that can give rise to pain on pressure. It is uncommon in the oral cavity, which is surprising considering the frequency with which nerves are severed as a consequence of tooth extraction and other common minor surgical procedures, but is more often seen after damage to large-diameter nerves (e.g. lingual nerve during

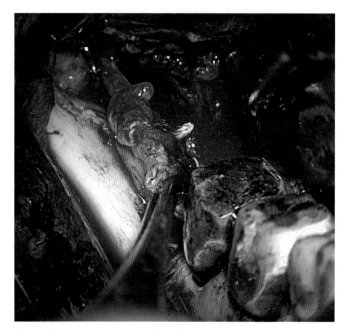

Fig. 2.23 Traumatic neuroma of the lingual nerve.

third molar extraction) and in skin after surgery for neck dissection or parotidectomy.

Solitary circumscribed neuroma

This lesion most often presents as a small, rubbery nodule on facial skin, but intra-oral lesions do occur, most commonly on the palate. These tumours arise from the perineurium of the nerve. They are benign and excision is curative.

Mucosal neuromas in multiple endocrine neoplasia syndrome type IIB

Patients with multiple endocrine neoplasia syndrome type IIB develop mucosal neuromas, which are tumour-like malformations of peripheral nerves (OMIM 162300) (Chapter 10).

Granular cell tumour

Clinically, the granular cell tumour presents as a painless, slow-growing swelling that arises most commonly on the dorsum of the tongue (Fig. 2.24). It occurs over a wide age-range and is slightly more common in females. Multiple tumours may occur. Current evidence supports a neural origin for the granular cell tumour.

Histologically, the lesion is non-encapsulated and consists of sheets and strands of large cells with granular, eosinophilic cytoplasm (Fig. 2.25). Striated muscle fibres lying between the granular cells may give the impression of invasion, but the lesion is benign. The covering squamous epithelium commonly shows pseudo-epitheliomatous hyperplasia (epithelial hyperplasia that may be mistaken for carcinoma; Fig. 2.25). Complete excision is required and incomplete removal is associated with recurrence.

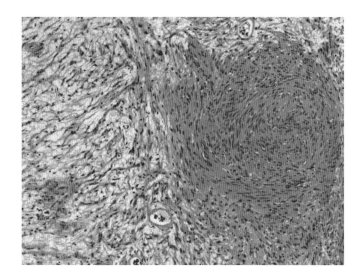

Fig. 2.22 Schwannoma showing loose Antoni A areas (left side) and Antoni B areas with Verocay body formation (right side).

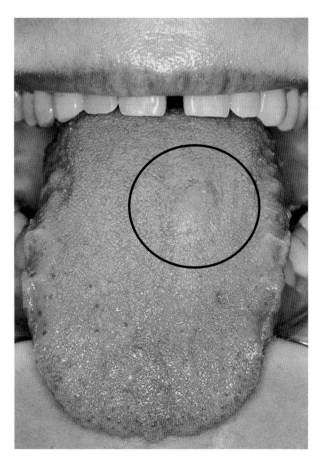

Fig. 2.24 Granular cell tumour on the dorsum of the tongue.

Muscle tissue

Benign tumours of either smooth or striated muscle are rare in the oral cavity. Leiomyomas are smooth-muscle tumours and in the oral cavity most arise from the walls of blood vessels (angiomyomas). Rhabdomyomas have also been reported but are very rare.

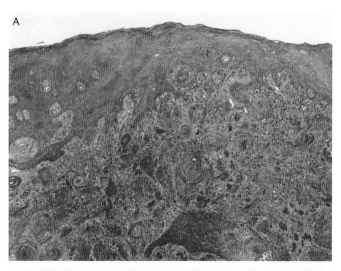

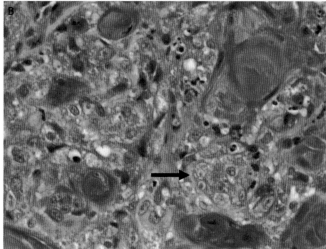

Fig. 2.25 Histology of a granular cell tumour showing pseudo-epitheliomatous hyperplasia (A) and granular cells (arrow) between the strands of pink epithelium (B).

Infections of the oral mucosa

Infections of the oral mucosa are very common and are caused by bacteria, viruses, and fungi, with other rarer causes outside the scope of this book.

Bacterial infections

The most common diseases of the oral cavity caused by bacterial are dental caries and periodontal disease (Chapter 5). Considering the enormous number of bacteria and bio-diversity (including pathogens), it is remarkable how few bacterial infections affect the oral mucosa. The paucity of oral mucosal bacterial infections reflects the natural defence mechanisms operating within the oral environment, maintaining homeostatic regulation of the oral microbiome.

Mycobacteria infection

Tuberculosis is caused by *Mycobacteria*, usually *M. tuberculosis*, but *M. bovis* and other atypical *Mycobacteria* may also cause disease in humans. Worldwide, the disease is once again increasing in incidence, mainly due to HIV infection and the development of multiple antibacterial-resistant strains.

Globally, about 9 million people develop pulmonary tuberculosis each year, but oral infection is uncommon. Primary lesions of the oral mucosa may occur, but secondary infections from infected sputum in a patient with pulmonary tuberculosis are more likely. The commonest presentation is a chronic, painless, undermined ulcer on the dorsum of the tongue (Fig. 2.26), covered with a greyish-yellow slough, but other types of ulcer and granulating gingival lesions have also been described.

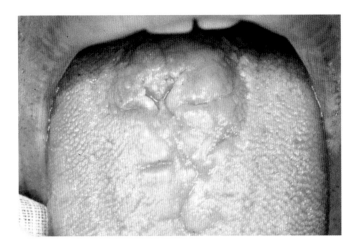

Fig. 2.26 Tuberculous ulcer on the dorsum of the tongue.

Patients may also present with tuberculous lymphadenitis, most frequently affecting the cervical nodes, but the intra- and para-parotid groups are occasionally involved (Fig. 9.4A).

Diagnosis usually follows identification of caseating epithelioid granulomas in a biopsy (Fig. 9.4B). *Mycobacteria* must be identified in Ziehl–Neelsen stained sections, by microbiological culture or by polymerase chain reaction, before a definitive diagnosis can be established.

Leprosy is another infection caused by *Mycobacteria: M. leprae*. It is rare in Northern Europe and America but endemic in certain tropical areas. Oral lesions occur almost exclusively in the lepromatous-type of the disease. They present as nodular inflammatory masses that tend to ulcerate and heal with fibrosis. The palate, anterior gingiva in the maxilla, and the tongue are most often affected. Oral lesions are usually secondary to nasal involvement. Lip involvement, clinically resembling oro-facial granulomatosis, has also been reported.

Syphilis

Syphilis is caused by the spirochaete *Treponema pallidum*. The incidence in Western countries declined markedly during the twentieth century, but incidence has risen since 2000, particularly in men who have sex with men. Syphilis presents in three distinct clinical stages, each of which may include oral lesions:

Primary: the oral primary lesion (chancre) may form on the lips, tongue, or other oral mucosal site (Fig. 2.27A). It is a shallow, painless ulcer with an indurated base. The regional lymph nodes are also enlarged. It heals spontaneously in 3–6 weeks. Histologically, the features are of non-specific ulceration, but the inflammatory infiltrate is often dominated by plasma cells, which may cluster around blood vessels.

Secondary: lesions appear about 2–3 months after initial infection. A generalized skin rash is the predominant feature and may be accompanied by oral lesions, including multiple, flat areas of ulceration termed 'mucous patches', which most commonly occur on the tongue. These may coalesce to produce lesions of irregular outline called 'snail-track ulcers'. This may then progress to the *latent phase* in which there is serological evidence of infection, but without symptoms.

Tertiary: this stage may develop many years after the initial exposure and is characterized by the development of areas of necrosis called

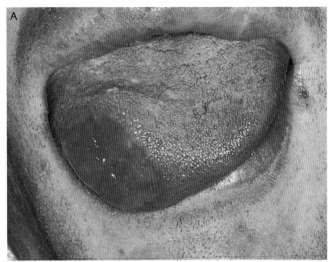
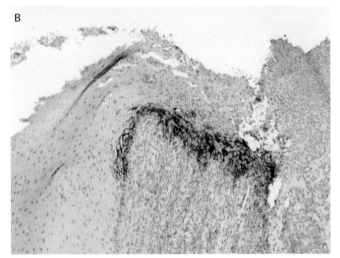
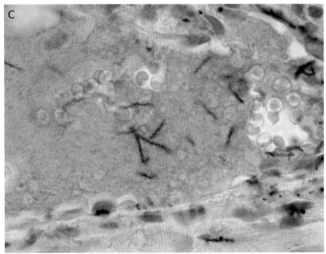

Fig. 2.27 Chancre in primary syphilis (A). Immunohistochemistry at the edge of a chancre highlighting *Treponema pallidum* infection (B); high magnification shows individual spirochaetes (C).

gummas. These are destructive lesions and, especially when developing on the hard palate, may lead to perforation into the nasal cavity. Oral mucosal white lesions may develop, which have an increased risk of developing into squamous cell carcinoma.

Congenital: exposure to syphilis *in utero* is termed congenital syphilis. This is now rare in Western countries, but in developing countries it is still an important cause of miscarriage, stillbirth, or neonatal infection. Congenital syphilitic infection is associated with destructive abnormalities of the facial skeleton and characteristic dental abnormalities, including Hutchinson's incisors and Moon's/mulberry molars (Fig. 5.5).

Viral infections

The main viral infections of the oral mucosa are listed in Table 2.4. Lesions associated with human immunodeficiency virus (HIV) are discussed in Chapter 10. The most common viral infections of the oral mucosa are caused by viruses of the herpes family (Table 2.5).

Herpes simplex virus infection

Primary infection with HSV is common and is transmitted by droplet spread or contact with the lesions. It occurs predominantly in young children and in the majority of cases is sub-clinical or causes a mild pharyngitis. However, in some patients it presents as primary herpetic gingivo-stomatitis. Infection is usually with HSV type 1 but infection with HSV type 2 (more common in genital lesions) may also occur.

Following an incubation period of about 5 days, the patient complains of prodromal symptoms of malaise and fever, and within a day or two the mouth becomes uncomfortable with the development of numerous small vesicles on any part of the oral mucosa and lips. There is also, usually, a widespread inflammation of the gingiva, which is erythematous and oedematous (Fig. 2.28). The vesicles soon ulcerate and become secondarily infected by bacteria; this is accompanied by cervical lymphadenitis. Fresh crops of vesicles may develop over the next

Table 2.4 Viral infections of the oral mucosa

Virus	Disease
Herpes simplex virus	Primary herpetic gingivostomatitis Herpes labialis
Varicella zoster virus	Chickenpox Shingles
Coxsackie virus	Herpangina Hand, foot, and mouth disease
Measles virus	Measles
Rubella virus	German measles
Epstein–Barr virus	Hairy leukoplakia
Human papillomavirus	Verruca vulgaris Condyloma acuminatum Focal epithelial hyperplasia HPV-related epithelial dysplasia HPV-related squamous cell carcinoma

Table 2.5 Herpes family viruses

HHV-1	Herpes simplex virus-1 (HSV-1)
HHV-2	Herpes simplex virus-2 (HSV-2)
HHV-3	Varicella zoster virus (VZV)
HHV-4	Epstein–Barr virus (EBV)
HHV-5	Cytomegalovirus (CMV)
HHV-6	Roseolovirus
HHV-7	Roseolovirus
HHV-8	Kaposi sarcoma-associated herpes virus

few days, but the systemic symptoms begin to subside about the sixth day with the oral lesions taking 10–14 days to resolve. Circumoral crusting lesions on the lips and other extra-oral lesions may also be present, particularly in children (Fig. 2.28).

Histologically, the vesicles are located within the epithelium (intra-epithelial vesicles) and are caused by destruction of infected keratinocytes (Fig. 2.29). Initially, the cells become swollen and have eosinophilic cytoplasm and large, pale vesicular nuclei—changes described as 'ballooning degeneration'. Giant cells containing many such nuclei also form as a result of fusion of the cytoplasm of infected cells. The balloon cells and multinucleate giant cells can sometimes be identified in smears taken from an intact vesicle or from one that has recently ruptured (Fig. 2.30). The lamina propria shows a variable inflammatory infiltrate.

Secondary (recurrent) infections occur in about 30% of those who have had a primary infection, either clinical or sub-clinical. This is due to reactivation of the virus, which, following the primary infection, has remained latent in the sensory ganglion of the trigeminal nerve (Box 2.1). Systemic symptoms are usually absent because of the immunity acquired during the primary infection.

Herpes labialis ('cold sore') is the most frequent type of recurrent infection (Fig. 2.31), and appears as clusters of vesicles on the mucocutaneous junction of the lips a few hours after prodromal symptoms of itching or tingling. The vesicles rupture within a short time and become crusted. They usually heal in 7–10 days. Recurrences may be triggered by a number of different stimuli, including mild, febrile infections such as the common cold, ultraviolet light, mechanical trauma, menstruation, stress, and immunosuppression. Recurrent intra-oral lesions occur occasionally, almost always on the hard palate or gingiva.

Diagnosis and treatment

When required, diagnosis can be achieved by detecting HSV by polymerase chain reaction from material taken on a swab from the lesion. A rising IgM antibody titre in the blood against HSV can also help to establish the diagnosis.

In the immunocompetent individual, the primary infection is usually treated supportively with paracetamol analgesia, as required, maintenance of fluid intake, and a soft diet. Intra-orally, chlorhexidine mouthwash minimizes secondary infection with bacteria and controls plaque

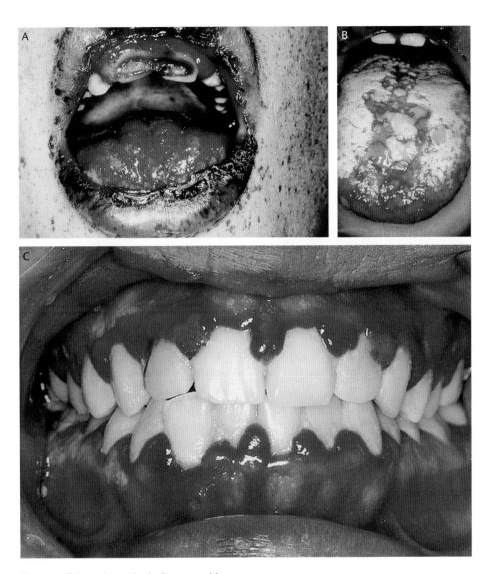

Fig. 2.28 Primary herpetic gingivo-stomatitis.

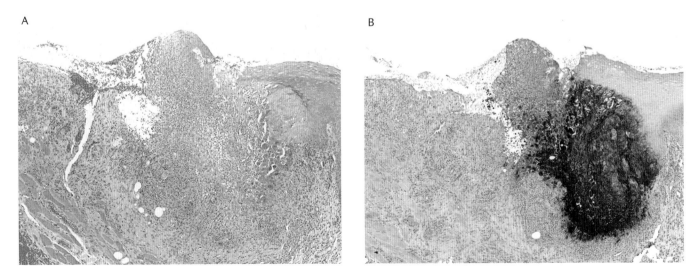

Fig. 2.29 Herpetic ulceration showing destruction of the surface epithelium and the production of an acute inflammatory exudate. Immunohistochemistry can be used to demonstrate herpes simplex virus infection (dark-brown stained area).

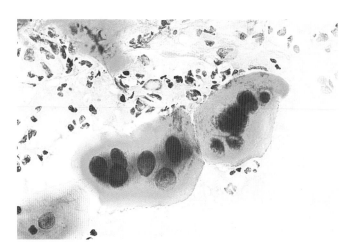

Fig. 2.30 Cytopathic changes and multinucleate cells in a smear from a herpetic vesicle.

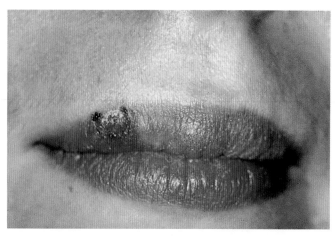

Fig. 2.31 Herpes labialis (cold sore).

accumulation if toothbrushing is painful. Benzydamine mouthwash can be used as a topical analgesic.

In the immunosuppressed or immunocompromised individual, or in severe herpetic gingivostomatitis, anti-viral drugs may be required. Systemic aciclovir five times daily is effective. Newer anti-virals such as valciclovir, with less frequent dosing regimes, are also effective.

Prevention of herpes labialis can be improved by the wearing of sunblock on the lips in individuals susceptible to ultraviolet light activation. Treatment of herpes labialis in immunocompetent patients is usually with frequent application of topical anti-viral agents applied as early as possible to the developing lesion, ideally when prodromal changes of sensation are felt in the lip and before vesicles appear. Penciclovir cream may be more effective than acyclovir cream. Systemic anti-viral treatment is required for frequent recurrences, recurrent intra-oral lesions, or in the immunocompromised.

Key points Herpes simplex virus

Primary herpetic gingivostomatitis

- Febrile illness precedes appearances of oral lesions
- Acute gingivitis
- Vesicles present on erythematous mucosa
- Vesicles quickly break down to form painful ulcers
- Lesions often seen on circumoral skin and lips
- Bilateral cervical lymphadenitis
- Self-limiting infection
- Supportive care: soft diet, hydration, paracetamol

Secondary herpetic infections

- Cold sores occur around the lips and occasionally intra-orally
- Precipitated by sunlight, local or generalized immunosuppression
- Topical anti-viral agents can be used to treat cold sores

Box 2.1 Herpes simplex virus latency

- Latency is a characteristic property of the herpes viruses.
- During primary infection HSV gains access to sensory neurons and viral DNA is transported to the trigeminal ganglion.
- In the ganglion transcription of HSV DNA changes to a latency associated transcript. This balance between the host and the virus is probably related to cell-mediated immunity.
- Factors that impair the host's immune response disturb the balance, allowing transcription of HSV DNA until the balance is restored.
- Viral particles travel down the axons to the nerve endings, where they may be shed asymptomatically into the mouth or re-infect epithelial cells, where there is transition to a lytic transcriptome.
- Damage to epithelial cells, e.g. trauma/UV radiation, may favour re-infection.
- Immunity to HSV does not protect against recurrent infection, but systemic symptoms are absent/minimal.

Varicella zoster virus infection

Primary infection by VZV (chickenpox) may produce lesions on the oral mucosa, especially the soft palate and fauces, which may precede the characteristic skin rash. The oral lesions usually present as small ulcers. Intact vesicles are seldom seen but when examined histologically show cytopathic effects indistinguishable from those of herpes simplex.

Zoster (shingles) is the manifestation of recurrent VZV infection and in this respect is similar to recurrent herpes simplex infection, except that repeated attacks of zoster are unusual. The virus remains latent in the sensory ganglia and may be reactivated spontaneously or when the host defences are depressed. Severe infection may be seen in immunocompromised patients. The lesions are localized to the distribution of one or more sensory nerves. The characteristic unilateral vesicular eruption is frequently preceded by prodromal symptoms of pain and paraesthesia for up to 2 weeks. When the trigeminal nerve is involved, the ophthalmic division is most frequently affected. Involvement of the

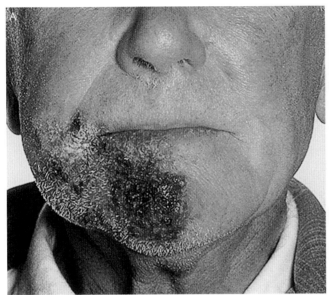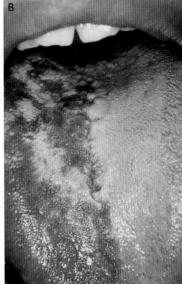

Fig. 2.32 Shingles (recurrent varicella zoster virus infection) affecting the right mandibular division of the trigeminal nerve; note the lesions are restricted to the dermatome of the nerve.

second or third division causes facial pain and the patient may complain of toothache-like pain, followed by the development of vesicles in the distribution of associated nerve branches (Fig. 2.32). The vesicles may be entirely intra-oral, where they rapidly ulcerate and become secondarily infected by bacteria. The disease usually runs a course of about 14 days. If zoster involves the geniculate ganglion of the facial nerve, the patient may develop Ramsay–Hunt syndrome, which is characterized by facial paralysis with a rash and other variable symptoms and signs such as tinnitus, hearing loss, nausea, vertigo, and nystagmus. The most distressing complication of zoster is post-herpetic neuralgia, probably caused by fibrosis in and around the sensory nerves and ganglia.

Treatment

Treatment of shingles with systemic anti-virals (such as acyclovir, famciclovir, or valciclovir) can reduce the severity and duration of pain, and reduce complications. Whenever possible, treatment with the anti-viral should be started within 72 h of the onset of the rash and continued for 7–10 days. Severely immunocompromised patients may require parenteral anti-viral medication, such as acyclovir by intravenous infusion. In addition, intra-oral lesions of shingles should also be managed with supportive therapy, chlorhexidine mouthwash twice daily and benzydamine mouthwash, as required. Treatment of post-herpetic neuralgia is usually with a tricyclic antidepressant (such as amitriptyline) or with certain anti-epileptic drugs (such as gabapentin or pregabalin).

Key points Varicella zoster virus

Chickenpox

- Common childhood infection
- Numerous small vesicles on the skin that burst and crust over
- Oral mucosal lesions also present

Shingles in the oro-facial region

- The pre-eruptive phase may simulate toothache
- Lesions are restricted to the dermatomes of the trigeminal nerve
- Post-herpetic neuralgia may persist for months or years

Epstein–Barr virus infection

EBV is associated with an array of diseases. Infectious mononucleosis (glandular fever) caused by the EBV occurs predominantly in teenagers and young adults, and is transmitted by contact with saliva, especially by kissing, either from an infected patient or a healthy carrier. The disease is characterized by fever, malaise, cervical lymphadenitis, and enlargement of the tonsils (Chapter 9). Petechial haemorrhages at the junction of the soft and hard palates, and inflammation and ulceration of the oral mucosa, may also be present. EBV is associated with oral hairy leukoplakia (Chapter 10). In the head and neck region, EBV infection is found in nasopharyngeal carcinoma and some haematological malignancies (Chapter 3).

Coxsackie virus infection

Herpangina is caused by various types of Coxsackie A virus. The infection is seen most commonly in children and is characterized by the sudden onset of a mild illness with fever, anorexia, sore throat, and dysphagia. Vesicles, which rapidly break down into ulcers 1–2 mm in diameter, are seen on the tonsils, soft palate, and uvula (Fig. 2.33). The symptoms persist for 2–3 days.

Hand, foot, and mouth disease is also caused by various types of Coxsackie A virus, especially type 16. It occurs predominantly in children and is transmitted in conditions of close association, such as within households or at school. The disease is characterized by

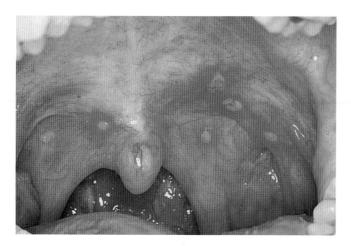

Fig. 2.33 Herpangina.

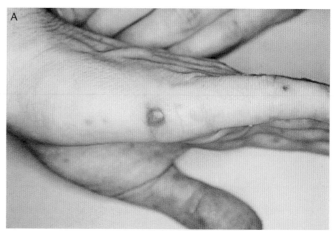

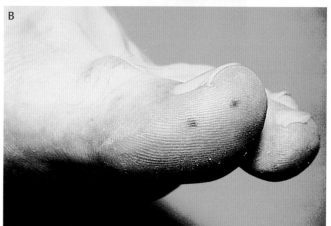

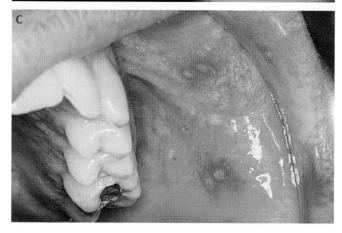

Fig. 2.34 Hand, foot, and mouth disease.

shallow oral ulcers together with vesicles and ulcers on the hands and feet (Fig. 2.34). It usually lasts about 7–10 days.

Measles

Measles is caused by a paramyxovirus infection and predominantly affects children. Incidence is rising due to recent reductions in immunization uptake. Prodromal symptoms may resemble a common cold and are accompanied by the appearance of Koplik spots on the oral mucosa, especially the buccal mucosa. They present as pin-point bluish-white spots against an erythematous background, and range from few in number to several hundred. They are likely to be overlooked, particularly as they start to disappear, as the characteristic skin rash develops some 3–4 days later (Chapter 8).

Fungal infection

The fungal infections of the oral mucosa most frequently encountered are those due to the dimorphic fungal species of the genus *Candida*. Of these, *C. albicans* is the principal species associated with infection, but other species such as *C. glabrata* and *C. tropicalis* are also pathogenic in humans. *Candida* species are commensal organisms in the mouth of about 40% of the population. Carriage rates are increased in the presence of systemic disease, in pregnancy, tobacco smokers, and denture wearers. The primary oral reservoir for the organism in carriers is the dorsum of the tongue.

Candida species are notorious opportunistic pathogens whenever the balance between the host and the organism is disturbed. Both local and systemic factors are important in the pathogenesis of *Candida* infections (Table 2.6). Such factors act by altering the host–organism balance and the defence mechanisms of the oral cavity in health.

Clinical presentation of oral candidosis

A variety of *Candida* infections involve the oral mucosa and perioral tissues, and the classification used in this chapter is summarized in Table 2.7. This distinguishes between acute and chronic oral/perioral infections and also includes forms where the oral infection is a manifestation of a generalized systemic candidosis. In addition, *Candida* may be found in association with other mucosal

lesions, e.g. median rhomboid glossitis. For any patient with *Candida* infection it is important to identify underlying predisposing factors (Table 2.6).

Pseudomembranous candidosis

Pseudomembranous candidosis is usually an acute infection that tends to occur at the extremes of age. It occurs in up to 5% of newborn infants, when it is associated with immature antimicrobial defences. In this situation, *Candida* transmission takes place from mother to baby in the

Table 2.6 Risk factors for *Candida* infection

Risk category	Risk factor	Example
Local factors	Mucosal trauma	Denture Orthodontic appliance
	Appliance wearing and poor hygiene	Denture Orthodontic appliance
	Diet	Carbohydrate-rich diet
	Tobacco	Smoking
Age	Neonates/infants	
	Old age	
Medications	Broad-spectrum antibiotics	Amoxicillin
	Steroids	Steroid inhalers Systemic steroids
	Cytotoxic agents	Cisplatin
Xerostomia	Medications	Antidepressants and others
	Sjögren's syndrome	
	Radiotherapy	Head and neck cancer
Genetic syndromes	Reduced immunity	Polyglandular autoimmune syndrome
Systemic disease	Endocrine	Diabetes mellitus Cushing's syndrome
	Infection	HIV
	Haematological	Anaemia Haematinic deficiency

birth canal. The infection is also seen in about 10% of elderly debilitated patients.

The disease presents clinically as a soft, white coating on the affected mucosa (Fig. 2.35A), which can be wiped away to leave a red, raw, and often bleeding base. Lesions may occur on any mucosal surface of the mouth and vary in size from small drop-like areas to confluent plaques covering a wide area. Examination of stained smears prepared from the white pseudomembrane reveals epithelial and inflammatory debris matted together by *Candida* hyphae and yeasts (Fig. 2.35B).

Persistent thrush may be seen in immunocompromised individuals, e.g. in patients with AIDS or on immunosuppressive drugs, in which case it is described as chronic pseudomembranous candidosis.

Erythematous candidosis

Acute erythematous candidosis is seen most commonly on the dorsum of the tongue in patients undergoing prolonged broad-spectrum antibiotic or corticosteroid therapy, but it may develop after only a few days of topical application of an antibiotic. Antibiotic therapy alters the oral bacterial flora, allowing resistant organisms, such as *Candida*, to flourish, and the condition is sometimes referred to as antibiotic sore mouth. It presents as a red and often painful area of oral mucosa, most commonly on the dorsum of the tongue, which may also appear depapillated (previously the condition was referred to as acute atrophic candidosis). The palate is also often involved.

Chronic erythematous candidosis is most commonly associated with denture wearing and is also known as denture stomatitis or denture sore mouth (Fig. 2.36). This is regarded as a secondary candidal infection of tissues modified by the continual wearing of dentures (or orthodontic appliances) and is associated with poor oral hygiene. The condition, which almost invariably affects the palate, is characterized clinically by clearly delineated chronic erythema and oedema of the mucosa directly covered by the denture. The fitting surface of the denture is the reservoir of infection and improved denture hygiene is key to the management of this condition, in order to avoid re-infection. Modification of other

Table 2.7 *Candida* infections of the oral mucosa

	Type	Form	Synonym
Primary	Acute	Pseudomembranous	Thrush
		Erythematous/atrophic	Antibiotic sore mouth
	Chronic	Pseudomembranous (protracted forms seen in immuno-compromised patients)	Thrush
		Erythematous/atrophic	Denture stomatitis
		Hyperplastic	Candidal leukoplakia
	Candida-associated lesions	Angular cheilitis	
		Median rhomboid glossitis	
Secondary	Muco-cutaneous candidoses	See Box 2.2	

predisposing factors in the medical history or of a high-carbohydrate diet may also be required.

Chronic hyperplastic candidosis

This form of candidosis presents clinically as a persistent white or mixed white-red patch on the oral mucosa that cannot be removed by scraping (Fig. 2.37). Lesions are seen most frequently on the buccal mucosa adjacent to the labial commissures and present as roughly triangular, often bilateral, white plaques. Less frequently, the palate or tongue may be involved. In many patients there is a strong association with tobacco smoking.

Histologically, the epithelium shows hyperparakeratosis and prominent, irregular acanthosis (Fig. 2.38). The parakeratinized surface of the epithelium often contains numerous neutrophils, which may collect as microabscesses. *Candida* hyphae invade the parakeratin, but never penetrate deeper into the prickle cell layers. There is a mixed chronic inflammatory cell infiltrate in the lamina propria, in which plasma cells are often prominent.

Chronic hyperplastic candidosis typically resolves following systemic anti-fungal treatment (fluconazole). Persistent lesions that show epithelial dysplasia are sometimes referred to as 'candidal leukoplakia' and are considered an 'oral potentially malignant disorder' (Chapter 3).

Chronic muco-cutaneous candidosis

The chronic muco-cutaneous candidoses are a rare group of disorders characterized by persistent superficial *Candida* infections of mucosae, skin, and nails, the oral mucosa being involved in almost all cases (Box 2.2). Oral lesions resemble those seen in chronic hyperplastic candidosis and may involve any part of the mucosa (Fig. 2.39).

Candida-associated lesions

Angular cheilitis occurs predominantly in denture wearers and is seen in about 30% of patients with denture stomatitis and less frequently with other types of oral candidosis. In patients with no evidence of *Candida* infection, *S. aureus* or other bacteria may be involved. In some cases, combinations of these organisms are implicated. Clinically, angular cheilitis is characterized by soreness, erythema, and fissuring at the

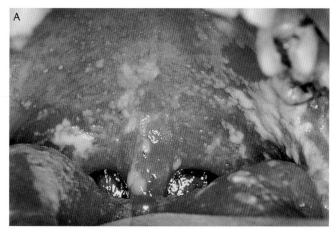

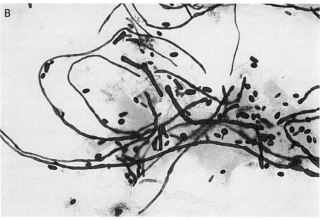

Fig. 2.35 Acute pseudomembranous candidosis (thrush) and a smear from the pseudomembrane showing tangled hyphae (Giemsa stain).

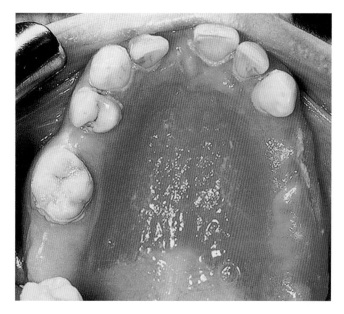

Fig. 2.36 Chronic erythematous candidosis (denture stomatitis).

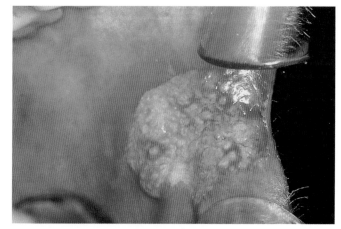

Fig. 2.37 Chronic hyperplastic candidosis.

A

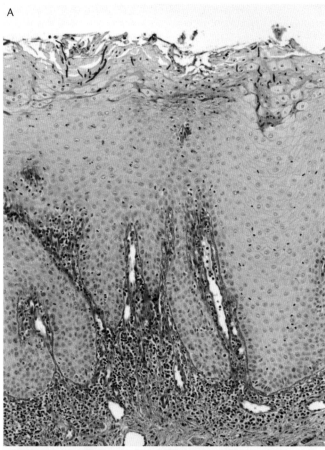

B

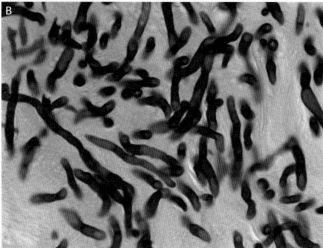

Fig. 2.38 Chronic hyperplastic candidosis showing fungal hyphae in the upper epithelial layers. High magnification of hyphae (Diastase PAS stain).

corners of the mouth (Fig. 2.40). Deep folds of skin at the angles of the mouth, which may be associated with loss of occlusal height in old age or result from incorrectly designed or old dentures, may be contributory factors. Nutritional deficiencies, in particular iron deficiency and deficiencies of riboflavin, folic acid, and of vitamin B$_{12}$, are predisposing factors in some cases.

Box 2.2 Sub-groups of chronic muco-cutaneous candidosis

- Familial CMC: early onset, autosomal recessive.
- Diffuse CMC: early onset, autosomal recessive/sporadic.
- Candidosis endocrinopathy syndrome: early onset, autosomal recessive/sporadic.
- Late-onset CMC: late onset, sporadic in patients with thymoma,
- CMC associated with primary immunodeficiency: early onset, sporadic/hereditary

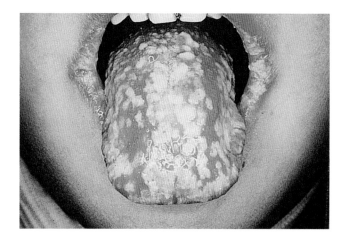

Fig. 2.39 Chronic muco-cutaneous candidosis.

Median rhomboid glossitis is a characteristic area of depapillation located in the mid-line of the dorsum of the tongue. The surface appears red in colour and may be smooth, nodular, or fissured (Fig. 2.41). It is usually asymptomatic. For many years it was regarded as a developmental anomaly, but most cases are associated with candidal infection. In some patients, usually smokers, an opposing ('kissing') lesion may be seen on the palate and the term 'multi-focal candidosis'

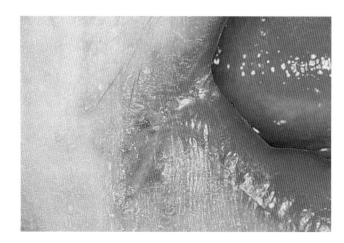

Fig. 2.40 Angular cheilitis.

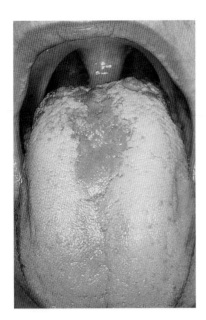

Fig. 2.41 Median rhomboid glossitis.

has been used to describe this. Histologically, the area is devoid of papillae and the surface is covered by parakeratotic acanthotic squamous epithelium. There is neutrophil infiltration of the parakeratin associated with candidal hyphae, and a chronic inflammatory cell infiltration of the lamina propria, often with some degree of fibrosis.

Diagnosis and treatment

Diagnosis of candidal lesions is based on clinical appearance and, where necessary, confirmation by special tests. Cytopathological examination of smears taken from affected mucosa to detect candidal hyphae, and levels of *Candida* colonization estimated from culturing microbiological swabs or oral rinses, can all be used.

Predisposing conditions favouring growth of *Candida* should be managed, where possible. Where candidosis is associated with a corticosteroid inhaler, rinsing the mouth out with water after using the inhaler may prevent recurrence. Where candidosis is associated with a denture, improving denture hygiene helps prevent re-infection. Chlorhexidine mouthwash has anti-candidal effects and can be used in the prevention and suppression of oral candidosis.

Oro-pharyngeal candidosis will frequently respond to topical therapy. Treatment with nystatin (in the form of a suspension) and miconazole (in the form of an oral gel) are effective in many cases. Miconazole is applied topically but it is absorbed to the extent that potential drug interactions, especially with warfarin, need to be considered. In unresponsive candidal infection, in immunocompromised patients, and in conditions where candidal hyphae penetrate the epithelium, systemic anti-fungal agents are needed. Fluconazole is effective. Itraconazole can also be used. Patients with recurrent infections, without known underlying causes, should be referred for investigation.

In angular cheilitis, predisposing factors require identification and management where possible. Where *Candida* is the causative organism, co-incident oro-pharyngeal candidosis frequently needs treatment as well to prevent re-infection via saliva. Miconazole cream has some antibacterial activity, as well as anti-fungal activity, and is usually effective. If *S. aureus* is the cause, sodium fusidate ointment can be used.

Key points *Candida* infection

- *C. albicans* is the principal species associated with infection
- Commensal organism in the oral cavity
- Carriage rates around 40%, reservoir dorsum of tongue
- Opportunistic pathogen
- 'Disease of the diseased', consider underlying systemic disease
- Topical anti-fungal agents: nystatin suspension and miconazole gel
- Systemic anti-fungal agent: fluconazole and itraconazole

Inflammatory ulceration and vesiculobullous diseases

An approach to the differential diagnosis of oral ulceration

Ulceration of the oral mucosa is common with a wide differential diagnosis (Table 2.8). As with all oral disease, it is important to take a careful history, including the duration of the lesion, initiating factors, periodicity, and symptomatology. This should be followed by a thorough clinical examination, focusing on the site distribution of the lesion(s), consistency and surface appearance, although in some cases lesions may not be available for examination at the time the patient presents. In many cases, the diagnosis can be made from the clinical history, but identification of a potential cause allows for its removal to see the effect on the lesion. Urgent biopsy, for an appointment within 2 weeks, is required for unexplained ulcers that do not heal after a period of 3 weeks (Box 3.18). A chronic traumatic ulcer that has been present for several weeks may mimic malignancy, particularly if it is crater-like with rolled edges and indurated because of fibrosis. In patients who have undergone therapeutic radiation for oral cancer, the development of a new ulcer at the site of the original malignancy may be difficult to differentiate from recurrent tumour. Radiation-associated ulcers tend to be painful, whereas this is not a common symptom of early recurrent malignant disease. In these circumstances biopsy is required to achieve a definitive diagnosis.

Table 2.8 Differential diagnosis of oral ulceration

Disease process	Cause	Examples
Developmental	Inherited genetic mutation	Epidermolysis bullosa
Traumatic	Mechanical	Tongue bite
	Thermal	Pizza burn
	Chemical	Aspirin burn
	Factitious injury	Self-inflicted trauma
Infective	Bacterial	Necrotising ulcerative gingivitis Tuberculosis Syphilis
	Viral	Herpes simplex Varicella zoster Herpangina
	Fungal	Histoplasmosis
Idiopathic	Unknown	Recurrent aphthous stomatitis
Iatrogenic	Drug-induced	Nicorandil NSAIDs
	Radiation	Radiation mucositis
Associated with dermatological disease	Lichen planus	Erosive LP
	Lupus erythematosus	Discoid lupus erythematosus Systemic lupus erythematosus
	Vesiculobullous disease	Pemphigoid Pemphigus
Associated with systemic disease	Haematological disease	Anaemia Neutropenia Leukaemia
	Gastrointestinal tract disease	Crohn's disease Ulcerative collitis
	HIV infection	HIV-associated ulceration
	Behçet's disease	Behçet's disease
Neoplastic	Malignant neoplasia	Squamous cell carcinoma Mucoepidermoid carcinoma Melanoma Lymphoma, leukaemia Metastases

Inflammatory ulceration

Traumatic ulceration

Mechanical trauma arising from biting, the presence of sharp cusps, or ill-fitting dentures are common causes of oral ulceration (Fig. 2.42). Such ulcers do not usually present a problem in clinical diagnosis

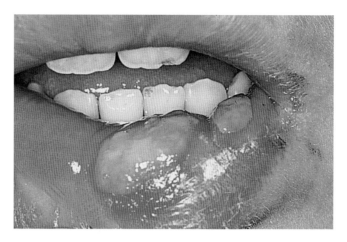

Fig. 2.42 Traumatic ulceration.

provided a cause of trauma is identified and the ulcer shows signs of healing in 7–10 days on removal of the cause. A biopsy is indicated when a presumed traumatic ulcer does not show signs of healing within 3 weeks (Box 3.18). Traumatic ulcerative granuloma with stromal eosinophils (TUGSE) is a distinctive oral ulcer that presents with malignant clinical features, but on biopsy shows crush injury to muscle and an inflammatory infiltrate rich in eosinophils. TUGSE is a self-limiting condition that usually heals within 2–3 weeks.

Chemical and thermal trauma may cause oral ulceration. Caustic agents used in dentistry may accidentally contact the mucosa and cause an iatrogenic chemical burn. Aspirin directly applied to the oral mucosa by a patient, in the erroneous belief that it will relieve toothache, also causes a chemical burn. Ulceration due to acute thermal trauma, for example from ingesting very hot food or drink, can occur on any part of the oral mucosa but most commonly affects the palate (Fig. 2.43).

Factitious ulcers are self-inflicted and may be a manifestation of anxiety or more severe emotional disturbance. Their appearances and distribution depend on how they have been induced. Patients

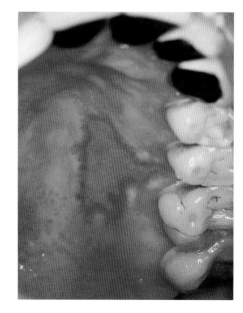

Fig. 2.43 Traumatic ulceration due to a thermal burn.

undergoing radiotherapy for head and neck cancer may suffer imme-diate mucosal damage due to the direct effects of radiation, but delayed effects are also encountered. The immediate effects include erythema and ulceration (radiation mucositis). Healing of these ulcers may be delayed.

Recurrent aphthous stomatitis

Recurrent aphthous stomatitis (RAS) is one of the most common oral mucosal conditions, with a reported lifetime prevalence of up to 60% of the population. There are three main clinical forms of the disease: minor, major, and herpetiform, with minor RAS, by far the most common. All have the characteristic of recurrence. The typical features of RAS are summarized in Table 2.9.

Minor aphthous ulceration accounts for 80% or more cases of RAS. The condition is characterized by the occurrence of from one to five, shallow, round, or oval ulcers that affect the non-keratinized areas of the oral mucosa (Fig. 2.44A). The ulcers are less than 10 mm in diam-eter (generally they are about 3–6 mm across), and have a grey/yellow base with an erythematous margin. They heal without scarring, usually within about 10 days.

Major aphthous ulcers are larger than minor aphthae, usually greater than 10 mm in dimension (Fig. 2.44B). They may occur anywhere in the mouth, including the keratinized oral mucosa, but the lips, soft palate, tonsillar areas, and oro-pharynx are common sites. The number of ulcers varies and they may take 4–6 weeks to heal, and may heal with scarring. Due to the chronic nature of the ulceration, they may have crater-like ulcers with rolled margins, which are indurated on palpation because of underlying fibrosis. Consequently, in the absence of a history of recur-rent ulceration, differentiation from a malignant ulcer requires a biopsy.

The least common form is *herpetiform ulceration*, which is character-ized by multiple, 1–2-mm sized ulcers that can occur on any part of the oral mucosa (Fig. 2.45). When several ulcers are clustered together,

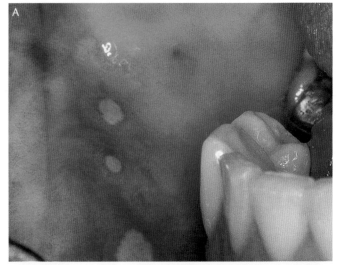
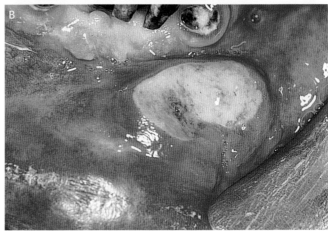

Fig. 2.44 Minor and major aphthous ulceration.

Table 2.9 Clinical features of the main types of RAS

	Minor	Major	Herpetiform
Age (years)	10–40	10–40	>20
Relative frequency	75–90%	10–15%	5–10%
Number	1–6	1–3	10–100s
Size	<10 mm, most 3–6 mm	>10 mm	<2 mm, but coalesce
Site	Non-keratinized mucosa of lips, cheeks, floor of mouth or ventral tongue	Predominantly soft palate and lips	Predominantly non-keratinized mucosa of lips, cheeks, floor of mouth or ventral tongue
Duration	7–10 days	>30 days	7–14 days
Incidence of scarring	None	Common	Uncommon

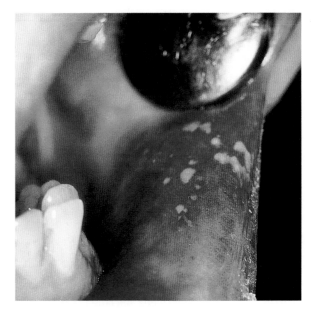

Fig. 2.45 Herpetiform aphthous ulceration.

confluence can result in larger areas of ulceration of irregular outline. The ulcers usually heal within 2–3 weeks. Large confluent ulcers may take longer and may heal with scarring. The ulcers may be associated with severe discomfort.

Aetiology and pathogenesis

The aetiology of RAS is far from clear, but there is increasing evidence that damaging immune responses are involved. In addition, a number of local and general factors have also been implicated (Table 2.10), and one or more of these may play a contributory role.

Local factors

Trauma may precipitate and influence the site of some ulcers but does not play an essential role in the aetiology of RAS. Changes in salivary composition, such as raised salivary cortisol, have also been associated with RAS.

Microorganisms

Various microorganisms have been isolated from recurrent oral ulcers but attempts to demonstrate a causal relationship have been unsuccessful. Hypersensitivity to cross-reacting *Steptococcus sanguis* antigens has been implicated in the pathogenesis of RAS, but studies of hypersensitivity to the organism in patients and control subjects have produced conflicting results. Other bacteria, such as *Helicobacter pylori*, have been suggested but no link has been proven.

Table 2.10 Suggested risk factors for RAS

Suggested factor	Detail/example
Local factors	Minor trauma may precipitate ulceration.
Microorganisms	*Streptococci, H. pylori*, and various viruses have been suggested with variable support.
Hereditary predisposition	40% have a family history: may be related to specific HLA haplotypes.
Psychological factors	Emotional stress may precipitate ulceration, but the mechanism is not clear.
Allergic disorders	Chocolate, coffee, certain nuts, tomatoes, and wheat (gluten) have been linked in some patients.
Hormonal disturbance	In some women, RAS may coincide with the menstrual cycle.
Tobacco	Exacerbations of RAS have been reported on cessation of smoking.
Systemic disease	RAS-type lesions have been reported in a number of systemic disorder such as Crohn's disease, HIV, Behçet's disease, and cyclic neutropenia.
Nutritional deficiency	Low serum levels of iron, folate, B vitamins.

A viral aetiology has been suggested but there is little evidence to support such a hypothesis. Adenoviruses and Epstein–Barr virus have been isolated from RAS but there is no evidence that they are causal. They are ubiquitous organisms and their presence may be purely coincidental. A rise in IgM antibody titres to varicella zoster virus and to cytomegalovirus has also been reported during recurrences, but the significance of this is unknown.

Aphthous-like ulceration can also be seen in patients infected with HIV (Chapter 10).

Hereditary predisposition

A family history is found in up to 40% of patients, but the mode and pattern of inheritance has not been established. Although some studies have suggested an increased prevalence associated with certain of the major histocompatibility (HLA) antigens, no consistent patterns have been established.

Psychological factors

Epidemiological studies have suggested that emotional stress may be a precipitating factor, but it is unlikely to be the direct cause of ulceration, and in any event is very difficult to quantify. Stress may also be associated with habits, such as cheek biting, which may precipitate and influence the pattern of ulceration in some cases.

Allergic disorders

Some patients with RAS associate the onset of ulceration with certain foods and this, together with the raised level of IgE found in some patients, has led to the claim that food allergies play a role in the aetiology of RAS. However, the evidence is often anecdotal, and results from studies in which patients were challenged with specific foods are inconclusive.

Nevertheless, the histological features seen in RAS are suggestive of a hypersensitivity reaction, either type III (immune complex-related) or type IV (cell mediated). In the pre-ulcer stage, the lamina propria is infiltrated by a lymphocyte-dominated infiltrate. As the ulcerative phase approaches there is increased infiltration of the tissues, especially of the epithelium, by lymphocytes, associated with oedema and damage to epithelial cells, leading eventually to their death and the formation of an ulcer. In the healing phase, the number of lymphocytes decreases. Immunological studies have shown that the infiltrate comprises different sub-populations of T lymphocytes at different stages of the ulceration cycle. In particular, as the ulcerative phase begins, the population of T lymphocytes capable of inducing cytotoxic effects (CD8+) increases dramatically, particularly within the epithelial infiltrate.

Current evidence suggests that RAS is due to immune-mediated cytotoxic damage to oral epithelial cells, through the activity of T lymphocytes (Box 2.3). The antigen, or antigens, that are responsible for triggering the immune response remain unknown. However, in both RAS and Behçet's disease, cross-reactivity between certain streptococcal antigens and oral epithelial antigens is thought to be an important pathogenic mechanism. Thus, in susceptible individuals, the host's immune response to streptococcal antigens may, inadvertently, also damage the oral epithelium.

Dietary allergens found in varied foods, such as benzoates (commonly used food preservatives), chocolate, coffee, various nuts, strawberries, cheese, and tomatoes have been implicated in the onset of ulceration in

There is extensive disruption of the immune response in RAS. Epithelial destruction is most likely the result of T cell-mediated cytotoxicity.

Alterations in CD4+/CD8+ T-cell ratio

- The pre-ulcerative lesion is characterized by infiltration of mainly CD4-positive (inducer/helper) T cells (CD4+/CD8+ ratio about 2:1).
- The ulcerative stage is characterized by an increase in CD8+ (suppressor/cytotoxic) T cells (CD4+/CD8+ ratio about 1:10).
- The healing phase is characterized by reversal of this ratio and CD4+ T cells predominate (CD4+/CD8+ ratio about 10:1).

γ-δ T cells and cross reactivity

- There is an increase in γ-δ T cells in patients with RAS. Their cytotoxic activity in response to streptococcal heat shock proteins (HSP) may cross-react with epithelial HSP (mitochondrial membrane HSP may be the target), leading to cell death.

Altered T helper cell populations

- Increased TH1 responses in the active phase of disease, which result in elevated IL-2, TNF-α, and IFN-γ production.

some patients. In a small number of patients, dietary exclusion may be a useful management strategy. Components of toothpaste, especially sodium lauryl sulphate (SLS), have also been implicated in precipitating ulceration in some patients.

Hormonal disturbance

In a small number of female patients, a relationship between RAS and the menstrual cycle has been reported. A hormonal association in some patients has also been suggested by observations that the onset of ulceration may coincide with puberty and that remissions may occur in pregnancy. However, no consistent association between RAS and the premenstrual period, pregnancy, or the menopause has been established.

Tobacco

Cigarette smoking has been reported to protect against RAS, and the onset of RAS in some patients has been associated with cessation of tobacco smoking. Whether the protective effect is related to increased keratinization of the mucosa or another mechanism is unknown.

Diagnosis

In most cases, the diagnosis can be established from the clinical history with due attention to possible underlying systemic disease. Biopsy is not useful, as the histological features are non-specific. One exception to this is to exclude malignancy in certain cases of major aphthous stomatitis.

Treatment

Before commencing treatment, any predisposing or provoking factors should be identified and, where possible, modified. No curative treatment is available. The aims of treatment are to palliate the symptoms, reduce ulcer number and size, and increase disease-free periods. A 'step-wise' approach of increasing therapeutic power, balanced against potential adverse effects, should be individualized according to the severity and impact of the disease on the patient.

Initial treatment with chlorhexidine mouthwash twice daily and benzydamine mouthwash, as needed, when ulcers are present, can be effective. If ulcer control is poor, topical corticosteroids can be used. These differ in their potency and the vehicle used to deliver them to the oral mucosa. Formulations include hydrocortisone in a muco-adhesive tablet, a betamethasone-soluble tablet dissolved in water and used as a mouthwash, and beclomethasone dipropionate sprayed directly on to the affected mucosa. They are most effective if applied in the 'prodromal' stage. Doxycycline mouthwash may also be of use in the treatment of RAS.

For severe RAS, systemic drugs can be used, including corticosteroids (prednisolone), colchicine, azathioprine, and thalidomide. Frequently, mixtures of topical and systemic drugs are used to control the most recalcitrant RAS.

Recurrent aphthous stomatitis-type ulceration in systemic disease

Aphthous-type oral ulceration occurs in various known systemic diseases (Chapter 10). This ulceration is frequently indistinguishable in appearance and natural history from RAS. It remains unclear whether the oral ulceration in RAS and RAS-type ulceration share a common pathogenesis.

Haematological/nutritional deficiency

Haematological abnormalities associated with deficiencies of haematinics may be found in up to 20% of patients with RAS assessed in secondary care. Iron deficiency, which may or may not be associated with anaemia, occurs most frequently, but in the majority of patients no underlying cause can be identified. Deficiencies of folate and/or vitamin B_{12} are also associated with RAS, but less frequently than iron. The role of haematological deficiency states in the aetiology of RAS is unclear, although it is known that deficiencies of iron, folate, and vitamin B_{12} can produce atrophic changes in the oral mucosa. However, the ulceration in some patients improves when the deficiency is corrected, suggesting a causal role. In some patients, haematological deficiency states are secondary to gastrointestinal disease.

Gastrointestinal diseases

RAS has been reported in patients with a variety of gastrointestinal diseases, some of which are associated with secondary haematological abnormalities as a result of malabsorption or chronic blood loss. An association with coeliac disease (gluten-sensitive enteropathy) is well recognized. RAS may also be seen in patients with ulcerative colitis and Crohn's disease.

Behçet's disease

Behçet's disease (also referred to as Behçet's syndrome) is characterized by recurrent aphthous stomatitis (RAS) and at least two of the following: recurrent genital ulcers, eye lesions (uveitis or retinoid vasculitis), or skin lesions (erythema nodosum, acniform lesions, or pseudo-folliculitis).

Lesions involving other body systems may also be seen. It is a rare disorder in Western countries and is seen mainly in countries from the eastern Mediterranean, extending to the Far East. There is a strong genetic link with the major histocompatibility antigen HLA-B51 in patients from these countries. In addition to a genetic predisposition, immune-mediated mucosal damage (as discussed previously for RAS) and vasculitis associated with the hyperactivity of neutrophils are involved in the pathogenesis of the lesions. Clinically, the oral ulcers are not distinguishable from the more common forms of aphthous stomatitis.

Medications causing oral ulceration

Medications associated with oral ulceration are described in Chapter 10.

Vesiculobullous diseases

Vesiculobullous diseases of the oral mucosa are characterized by the development of blisters, termed vesicles or bullae, which often rupture and present as oral ulceration. The distinction between a vesicle and a bulla is one of size: a vesicle is small and the term bulla is reserved for a lesion greater than 5 mm in diameter. Vesiculobullous diseases that affect the oral mucosa are outlined in Table 2.11. They are divided into two major groups, depending on the histological location of the lesions: intra-epithelial lesions that form within the epithelium and sub-epithelial lesions that form between the epithelium and the underlying lamina propria. Immunofluorescence studies are also important in diagnosis (Box 2.4). Just to note that viral infections of the oral mucosa also cause intra-epithelial vesicles, as described previously.

Pemphigus vulgaris

Pemphigus is a group of uncommon autoimmune diseases of which pemphigus vulgaris is the most common type (see Box 2.5 for rarer types). Pemphigus vulgaris usually presents in middle age and is more common in certain ethnic groups, e.g. Ashkenazi Jews. It is characterized by widespread bullous eruptions involving the skin and mucous membranes. The oral mucosa is involved in nearly all patients and in some patients the disease remains confined to the oral cavity. The bullae are fragile and readily rupture forming crusted or weeping areas of denudation on the skin and irregular, ragged superficial mucosal ulcers (Fig. 2.46A). Any part of the oral mucosa may be involved but the soft palate, buccal mucosa, and lips are most frequently affected. There may also be desquamative gingivitis. Gentle pressure to the mucosa in an involved area can lead to the formation of a bulla (Nikolsky sign).

Histological examination shows intra-epithelial cleft-like spaces produced by acantholysis, the process of breakdown of the specialized intercellular attachments (desmosomes) between epithelial cells. Typically, these changes occur between the prickle cells just above the basal cell layer (Fig. 2.46), with the basal cells forming the base of the lesion remaining attached to the lamina propria and projecting into the bulla. There is remarkably little inflammatory cell infiltration until the lesion ruptures. Acantholytic prickle cells occurring singly or in small clumps are found lying free within the blister fluid and are referred to as Tzanck cells.

Immunological studies are important in establishing the diagnosis and may be helpful in monitoring the progress of the disease. Circulating IgG autoantibodies to a constituent protein of the desmosome (desmoglein 3; DSG3) can be demonstrated in the serum of patients with pemphigus vulgaris using indirect immunofluorescence (Box 2.4). There is evidence that these IgG autoantibodies are responsible for inducing acantholysis, but the mechanisms by which this occurs are unclear. However, it is likely to involve the activity of proteases. The anti-DSG3 antibody titre is related to the severity of the disease, and monitoring this over time may be helpful in assessing the course of the disease and response to treatment. However, circulating antibodies may not be detectable in all patients, especially in the early stages of the disease, and biopsy of peri-lesional mucosa to demonstrate binding of autoantibodies to the inter-epithelial cell attachment is an essential diagnostic test. This is undertaken on fresh tissue when binding of IgG isotype autoantibodies can be demonstrated by direct immunofluorescence (Box 2.4), resulting in a 'net-like' appearance (Fig. 2.47).

Treatment

Pemphigus vulgaris usually requires early and active treatment with immunosuppressive therapy. In most cases, initial manifestations in the mouth herald a more widespread development of mucous membrane and skin lesions, and early effective intervention may prevent development. Rarely, the disease progresses very slowly and remains confined to the limited areas of the oral mucosa, and can be controlled with topical corticosteroids.

Prior to the discovery of synthetic corticosteroids, the disease was associated with significant levels of mortality when widespread infected skin lesions led to septicaemia. Treatment is usually commenced with high levels of corticosteroids (prednisolone). The immunosuppressive agents, azathioprine and mycophenolate mofetil, are used as steroid-sparing agents to allow reduction of prednisolone dosage without loss of disease control. Dosage levels are guided by the level of disease control achieved. For disease that is difficult to control, further possible treatments include intravenous immunoglobulin therapy, cyclophosphamide, and monoclonal antibody agents, including infliximab (anti-TNF α) and rituximab (anti-CD20).

Para-neoplastic pemphigus

This rare form of pemphigus is associated with certain neoplastic diseases, usually lymphoma or chronic lymphocytic leukaemia, and is associated with high morbidity and mortality.

Key points Pemphigus vulgaris

- Uncommon disease
- Oral lesions may be first presentation
- Widespread mucosal and skin lesions may develop
- Fragile intra-epithelial blisters that burst
- Sloughing of epithelium leaving ragged ulcers
- Desquamative gingivitis
- Autoantibodies to desmoglein 3 (component of desmosomes)
- Direct immunofluorescence shows 'net-like' pattern of staining
- Treatment systemic steroids and other immunosuppressive agents

Table 2.11 Immunologically mediated vesiculobullous disorders affecting the oral mucosa

Condition	Mean age	Male:female ratio	Oral lesions	Skin lesions	Bulla level	Autoantigen(s)	Immunofluorescence pattern
Pemphigus vulgaris	50	Equal	Bullae in 80% Bullae breakdown rapidly	Skin affected in almost all cases	Intra-epithelial	DSG1, DSG3	IgG and C3 inter-cellular
Erythema multiforme	30	M>F	Mucous membrane and lip lesions, often with crusting	Target lesions	Intra-epithelial	Unknown: may be cross-reacting with bacterial or viral antigens	Not specific: C3 and fibrin in basement membrane zone
Mucous membrane pemphgoid	60	F>M	Bullae in 100%. Desquamative gingivitis common	Bullae are rare	Sub-epithelial	BP180, laminin V, integrin β4. Also BP230	Linear IgG and C3 in basement membrane zone
Bullous pemphigoid	60	Equal	Bullae in 30–40%	Bullae in 100%	Sub-epithelial	BP180, BP230	IgG and C3 in basement membrane zone
Dermatitis herpetiformis	15–40	Equal	Small vesicles/bullae	Itchy, chronic papulovesicular rash	Sub-epithelial	Transglutaminase: may be associated with gluten-sensitive enteropathy	Granular deposits of IgA in basement membrane zone
Linear IgA disease	Bimodal	F>M (slight)	Small vesicles/bullae	Variable	Sub-epithelial	LAD1: may be associated with ulcerative colitis	Linear deposits of IgA and C3 in basement membrane zone
Epidermolysis bullosa aquista	Variable	Equal	Fragile blisters heal with extensive scarring	Bullae, scarring	Sub-epithelial	Collagen VII	Collagen VII in basement membrane zone
Bullous lichen planus	Variable	Not known	Fragile bullae, often of lip mucosa	Bullae, especially lower limbs	Sub-epithelial, but varies	Not known	Linear deposits of fibrin, maybe C3 in the basement membrane zone

Box 2.4 Immunofluorescence studies for vesiculobullous disorders

Direct immunofluorescence

- A fresh biopsy of peri-lesional mucosa is required for this test. Note that formalin-fixed biopsies are not suitable for direct immunofluorescence.
- The fresh mucosal biopsy is immersed in Michel's transport medium or snap frozen in liquid nitrogen and is then sent to the pathology laboratory.
- 5-μm frozen sections of the tissue are prepared and then each section is incubated with one of five fluorescein-labelled molecules: IgA, IgG, IgM, complement fragment C3, or fibrinogen.
- Each tissue section is viewed with an epifluorescence microscope with an ultraviolet light source to visualize the binding of the fluorescein-labelled molecules.
- Sections incubated with fluorescein-labelled IgG that show a net-like pattern of fluorescence in the epithelium is characteristic of pemphigus vulgaris (Fig. 2.47).
- Sections incubated with fluorescein-labelled IgG that show fluorescence of the basement membrane is characteristic of pemphigoid (Fig. 2.51).

Indirect immunofluorescence

- A clotted blood sample from the patient is required for this test.
- The serum from the clotted blood sample is incubated with 5-μm sections of fresh frozen human cadaveric skin.
- Any autoantibodies in the patient's serum sample bind to corresponding epitopes in the human cadaveric skin.
- The sections are then incubated with a fluorescein-labelled anti-human IgG antibody to detect the binding of IgG isotype autoantibodies.
- Each tissue section is viewed with an epifluorescence microscope with an ultraviolet light source to visualize the binding of the fluorescein-labelled anti-human IgG.
- Sections that show a net-like pattern of fluorescence is characteristic of pemphigus vulgaris.
- Sections that show fluorescence of the basement membrane is characteristic of pemphigoid.
- The technique can be refined by preparing serial dilutions of the patient's serum sample to estimate the titre of autoantibodies. An indirect immunofluorescence test that is positive, even after diluting the serum several times, is indicative of a high level of circulating autoantibodies. A technique called 'salt-split skin indirect immunofluorescence' can be also used to further classify vesiculobullous diseases.

Box 2.5 Subtypes of pemphigus

In addition to pemphigus vulgaris, oral lesions may also be seen in:

Pemphigus vegetans: a milder form of pemphigus vulgaris; exuberant granulation tissue (vegetative masses) develops following rupture of bullae

Drug-induced pemphigus: penicillamine, captopril, and others

Para-neoplastic pemphigus: associated with malignant disease, e.g. hematological malignancy

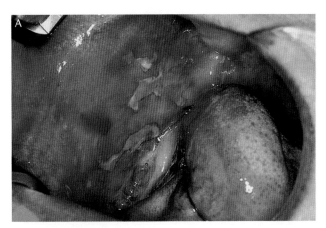
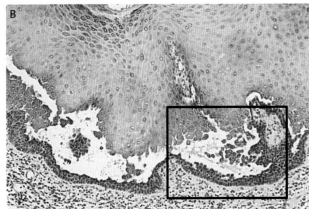
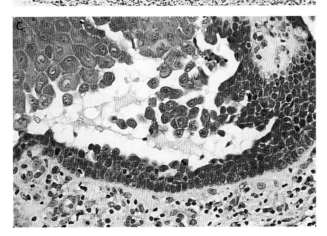

Fig. 2.46 Oral ulceration in pemphigus vulgaris. Histology shows intra-epithelial vesicle formation in the prickle cell layer due to acantholysis (loss of adhesion) of the keratinocytes.

Pemphigoid

Pemphigoid is a term applied to a group of immune-mediated blistering diseases characterized by the production of autoantibodies to various components of the hemi-desmosomes and epithelial basement

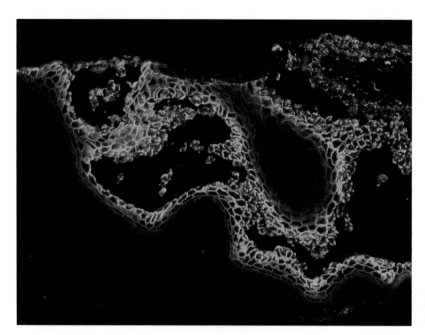

Fig. 2.47 Direct immunofluorescence in pemphigus vulgaris showing a net-like pattern of inter-cellular binding of IgG in the epithelium.

membrane (Fig. 2.2). Clinically, there are essentially two groups of patients: those with skin disease (mucosal involvement is very rare), called bullous pemphigoid, and those with mucosal disease that have minimal skin involvement, called mucous membrane pemphigoid or cicatricial pemphigoid.

Mucous membrane pemphigoid

Mucous membrane pemphigoid occurs most frequently in women in the sixth decade of life or older. The oral mucosa is almost always affected. Bullae occur anywhere on the oral mucosa and are relatively tough, so may remain intact for a few days (Fig. 2.48). They are occasionally haemorrhagic. Once ruptured, they give rise to erosions that heal slowly, sometimes with scarring, hence the alternative name for this disease: cicatricial pemphigoid. The most consistent oral lesions in dentate patients involve the gingiva, presenting as desquamative gingivitis (Fig. 2.49). In addition to the oral mucosa, the conjunctiva and mucosae of the nose, larynx, pharynx, oesophagus, and genitalia may be involved. Ocular involvement is the most serious complication with scarring leading to conjunctival adhesions, opacity of the cornea, and blindness (Fig. 2.50).

Histopathological examination shows separation of the full thickness of the epithelium from the lamina propria producing a sub-epithelial bulla (Fig. 2.51). Initially, there is little inflammatory reaction in the lamina propria, but as the vesicle develops, there is infiltration by variable numbers of neutrophils and eosinophils around and within the developing bulla. These changes are accompanied by a mainly lymphocytic infiltrate in the lamina propria, the intensity of which increases as the lesion develops.

Direct immunofluorescence studies of fresh biopsy material are essential to establish the diagnosis. In mucous membrane pemphigoid there is linear binding of immunoglobulin, predominantly IgG, and often also complement products, principally C3, in the basement membrane zone (Fig. 2.51). Circulating autoantibodies can be detected in the serum of well-established disease using indirect immunofluorescence. The autoantibody titre correlates with the severity of the disease.

Treatment

Mucous membrane pemphigoid can cause significant morbidity, most seriously when the eye is affected. Eye involvement can lead to blindness, so where both the mouth and eye are affected, the choice of treatment is guided to ensure sufficient suppression of eye disease.

Mild disease limited to small areas of the oral mucosa can sometimes be controlled by frequent application of topical corticosteroids. Various formulations, including dissolving tablets, mouthwash, and spray, are available. More widespread involvement of the oral cavity usually requires systemic treatment. Tetracycline, usually prescribed in the form of doxycycline, and dapsone can be used. Sulphamethoxypyridazine can also be of use. For unresponsive disease, more profound immunosuppressive therapy is frequently required. Initial control with systemic corticosteroid (prednisolone) is followed by addition of azathioprine or mycophenolate mofetil as a steroid-sparing agent. In recalcitrant disease, cyclophosphamide, intravenous immunoglobulin therapy, and monoclonal antibody agents, including rituximab, infliximab, and adalimumab, can be tried.

Key points Mucous membrane pemphigoid

- More common than pemphigus vulgaris
- Oral vesicles and bullae
- Desquamative gingivitis
- Ocular lesions may cause blindness
- Autoantibodies to components of hemi-desmosomes
- Direct immunofluorescence shows staining of the basement membrane zone
- Treatment with topical steroids and immunosuppressive medications

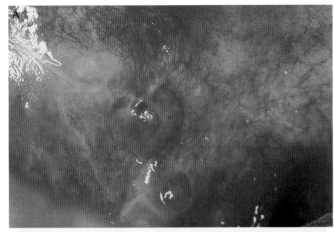

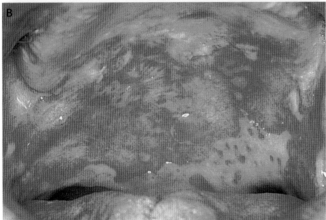

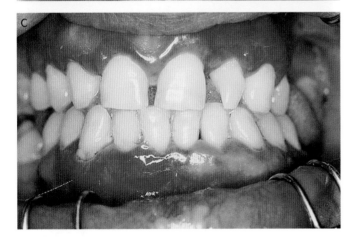

Fig. 2.48 Mucous membrane pemphigoid.

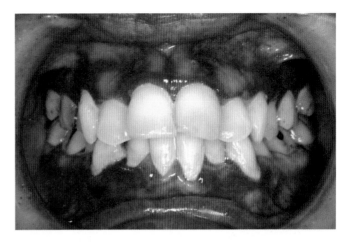

Fig. 2.49 Mucous membrane pemphigoid presenting with desquamative gingivitis.

immunofluorescence studies show granular deposits of IgA in the tips of the connective tissue papillae.

Linear IgA disease

Linear immunogloblin A (IgA) disease is a rare, heterogeneous auto-immune blistering disorder of mucous membranes and skin. It can be associated with ulcerative colitis. Oral manifestations include desquamative gingivitis, and mucosal blistering and erosions resembling the clinical manifestations of mucous membrane pemphigoid. Histologically it resembles the vesicles seen in mucous membrane pemphigoid, but immunofluorescence studies show continuous linear deposits of IgA at the basement membrane zone.

Erythema multiforme

Erythema multiforme is a muco-cutaneous disease of abrupt onset with a wide range of clinical presentations. Young adults, particularly males, are predominantly affected. The severity of the disease varies considerably. In its more severe form (Stevens–Johnson syndrome), there is widespread involvement of the skin and oral, ocular, and genital mucosae. Milder

Dermatitis herpetiformis

Dermatitis herpetiformis is a chronic, sub-epidermal, autoimmune blistering disease of skin, which may be associated with gluten hypersensitivity of jejunal mucosa. Oral manifestations are variable and range from small symptomless erythematous areas to extensive erosions. The blisters tend to be tiny vesicles that resemble those seen in herpes simplex infection, hence the term herpetiformis. Histologically, the vesicles resemble those seen in mucous membrane pemphigoid, but

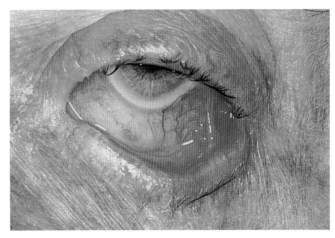

Fig. 2.50 Ocular lesion in mucous membrane pemphigoid.

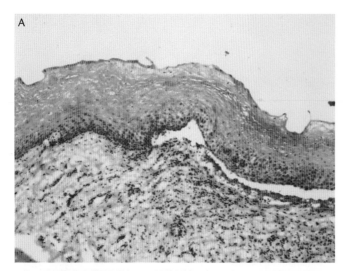

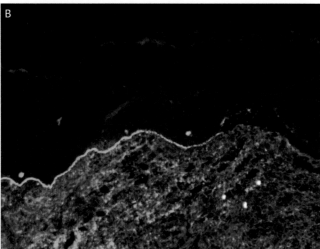

Fig. 2.51 A sub-epithelial vesicle in mucous membrane pemphigoid. There is separation of the squamous epithelium from the lamina propria at the basement membrane. Direct immunofluorescence shows deposition of IgG along the basement membrane (bright fluorescent line), there is some autofluorescence of the lamina propria, the squamous epithelium does not show any fluorescence.

forms may involve the oral mucosa, with or without skin lesions, or the skin alone may be involved. Generally, the disease tends to subside after 10–21 days but recurrences may occur.

The skin lesions have a variety of forms, including the virtually diagnostic target lesions (Fig. 2.52B). These consist of concentric rings of varying erythema and oedema, in the centre of which may be an intact or ruptured and crusted blister. The hands and feet are most commonly involved. Oral lesions may involve any part of the mucosa, although the lips and anterior parts of the mouth are most commonly affected (Fig. 2.52C). Initial erythematous patches are quickly followed by vesiculobullous eruptions that rapidly break down into erosions as the bullae disintegrate. The erosions on the lips are accompanied by bleeding and crusting. Circumoral crusting haemorrhagic lesions are an important characteristic sign in arriving at a clinical diagnosis (Fig. 2.52D).

The diagnosis of erythema multiforme is based primarily on the clinical findings. The histopathological features are variable and non-specific.

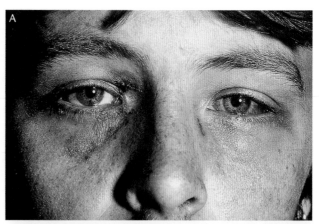

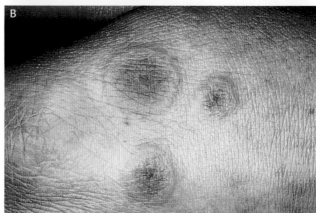

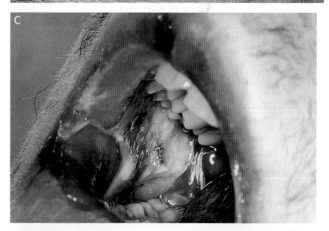

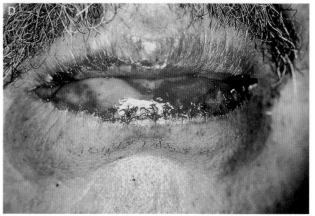

Fig. 2.52 Clinical presentation of erythema multiforme.

The pathogenesis of erythema multiforme is not fully understood but it is probably due to the formation of immune complexes and a subsequent type III hypersensitivity reaction. Deposition of immune complexes leads to complement activation and neutrophil chemotaxis, resulting in necrosis of epithelium. Circulating immune complexes have been detected in patients with erythema multiforme and in some cases they have been associated with herpes simplex viral antigens. Recurrent erythema multiforme is associated, in particular, with recurrent attacks of herpes simplex virus infection. Other precipitating factors have been implicated, including other infections (particularly *Mycoplasma pneumoniae*) and drugs (sulphonamides and barbiturates), but in many patients a cause is not identified.

Epidermolysis bullosa

The inherited forms of epidermolysis bullosa are a complex group of syndromes of which over 30 subtypes have been reported. They are due to mutation in genes coding either for specific keratins in the basal epithelial cells (resulting in intra-epithelial blister) or for various components of the basement membrane (resulting in sub-epithelial blisters). Some forms are lethal at birth. The less severe forms are characterized by the formation of skin blisters at birth or shortly afterwards. There is extreme fragility of the skin and blisters usually develop in response to minimal trauma or pressure. Oral and other mucosae may be involved. The blisters tend to heal slowly with severe scarring, which can result in claw-like deformity of the hands and other complications, such as difficulties in eating, speaking, and swallowing, as a result of involvement of the entire upper aero-digestive tract.

Epidermolysis bullosa acquisita

This is an uncommon autoimmune blistering disease acquired in adult life. Linear binding of IgG and C3 is seen in the basement membrane zone, resulting in the formation of sub-epithelial blisters. It is distinct from bullous pemphigoid and mucous membrane pemphigoid because the autoantibodies are directed against collagen VII fibrils that anchor the basement membrane complex to the lamina propria. It tends to affect the skin, but oral lesions may occur.

Angina bullosa haemorrhagica

This term is sometimes used to describe a blood-filled blister that develops on the oral mucosa. They are usually solitary, up to 2 cm in

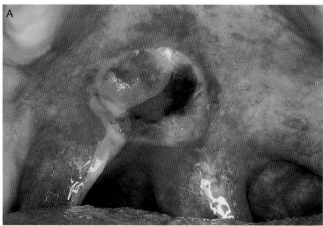

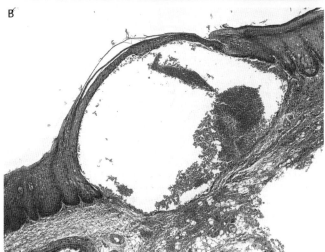

Fig. 2.53 Angina bullosa haemorrhagica (oral blood blister).

dimension, and present in middle-aged or elderly patients, most commonly on the soft palate (Fig. 2.53A). These bullae rapidly rupture leaving an ulcer that heals uneventfully. Histopathology shows a sub-epithelial bulla with separation within the basement membrane zone (Fig. 2.53B). Immunological findings are negative and no abnormalities in blood coagulation or in the tissues have been identified. The cause is unknown, but trauma and the use of steroid inhalers have been implicated.

Benign pigmented lesions of the oral mucosa

Oral pigmentation may result from exogenous substances on or within the mucosa, or may be due to deposition of endogenous pigments (i.e. substances produced by the body) in the tissues, of which melanin is the most common.

Exogenous pigmentation

Surface staining of the mucosa

This may be caused by a great variety of foods, drinks, and topical medicaments, as well as habits such as smoking, chewing tobacco, paan, or betel quid (Fig. 3.1A). Deposits of metallic sulphides in the marginal gingiva following absorption of bismuth, lead, or mercuric salts as a result of environmental exposure are now rarely seen.

Black hairy tongue

This is a condition in which there is marked hyperplasia of filiform papillae, sometimes up to about 1 cm in length, and discoloration associated with overgrowth of pigment-producing bacteria and fungi (Fig. 2.54). The aetiology is unknown but smoking may be a factor, and in some patients the disorder follows antibiotic therapy suggesting that disturbance of the normal oral flora is also involved. The condition is usually symptomless but 'tickling' of the soft palate may cause gagging and nausea.

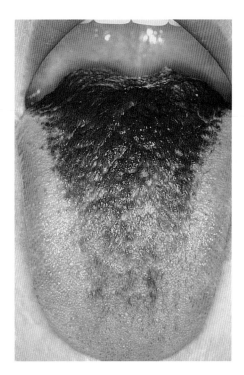

Fig. 2.54 Black hairy tongue.

Foreign bodies

A variety of foreign substances may be implanted in the oral mucosa giving rise to localized areas of pigmentation. Amalgam is the commonest and best-known example but other materials include road grit following road traffic accidents, tattooing of the labial mucosa (Fig. 2.55), and traumatic implantation of graphite in pencil chewers.

Amalgam tattoo

This is a relatively common, often incidental clinical finding, which rarely produces symptoms. It manifests as a localized blue or grey area (Fig. 2.56A) due to the introduction of amalgam into the soft tissues during dental procedures such as the insertion or removal of restorations, and the extraction

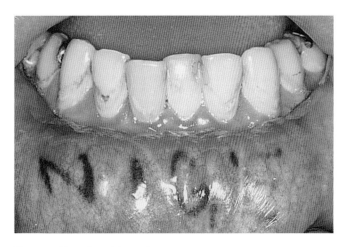

Fig. 2.55 Tattooing of the oral mucosa.

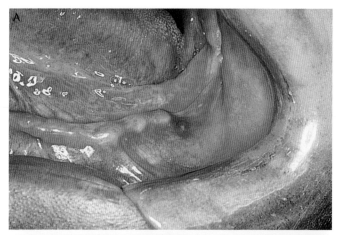

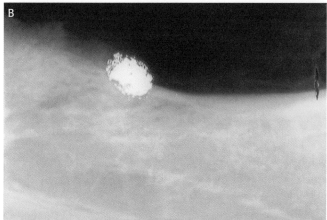

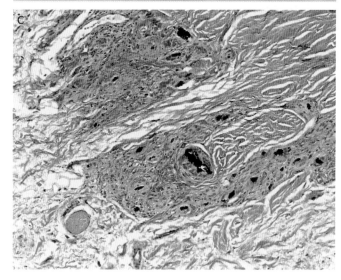

Fig. 2.56 Amalgam tattoo. The radiograph shows radio-dense material in the area of mucosal pigmentation. Histology shows extrinsic black deposits consistent with dental amalgam.

of teeth when portions of fractured restorations may fall into sockets. They are most common in mandibular gingiva or alveolar mucosa.

Histologically, amalgam debris is widely dispersed in the lamina propria as fine brown or black granules, or as solid fragments of varying size, which may be detected on radiographs (Fig. 2.56A). The pigment granules are often associated with collagen and elastic fibres and basement membranes and may be taken up by macrophages and foreign-body giant cells (Fig. 2.56). Apart from the phagocytic cells, there is little by way of an inflammatory response.

Endogenous pigmentation

Melanin is the commonest of the endogenous pigments in skin and oral mucosa, and is produced by melanocytes present in the basal layer of the epithelium. Melanin is formed in melanosomes within the cytoplasm of melanocytes, the melanin then passing into the dendritic processes to be transferred to neighbouring keratinocytes. Melanin pigment can also be taken up and retained by macrophages in the lamina propria.

There is no difference in the number of melanocytes between fair- and dark-skinned individuals, the variation in skin and mucosal pigmentation between racial groups being related to differences in melanocyte activity. The intensity and distribution of racial pigmentation of the oral mucosa is very variable not only between races, but also between different individuals of the same race and within different areas of the same mouth. Pigment may be found in any part of the mucosa, but the gingiva is the most common site (Fig. 2.57).

Hypermelanosis: developmental causes

Excessive melanin pigmentation of skin and/or oral mucosa is also associated with various developmental conditions that are not primarily disorders of the melanocyte system.

Peutz–Jeghers syndrome (OMIM 175200) is an autosomal dominant inherited disorder characterized by muco-cutaneous pigmentation and gastrointestinal polyposis. The melanin pigmentation resembles freckling and appears in infancy. Freckles occur around the mouth, nostrils, and eyes. The lips and buccal mucosa are usually affected (Fig. 8.4). There is a tendency for the skin pigmentation to fade in adult life but the mucosal pigmentation persists.

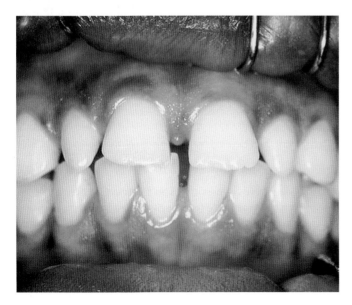

Fig. 2.57 Racial pigmentation.

Focal melanin pigmentation of skin, described as *café au lait* spots, is described in patients with neurofibromatosis and polyostotic fibrous dysplasia (McCune–Albright syndrome, OMIM 174800), but oral mucosal pigmentation is rarely observed.

Hypermelanosis: acquired causes

Acquired melanosis of the oral mucosa may be a manifestation of systemic disease, malignancy, or of a local disorder. It is an important sign indicating the need for careful investigation of the patient.

Melanin pigmentation is an occasional feature of some hyperkeratoses, giving the lesions a greyish hue, and also of some other chronic inflammatory mucosal diseases, including lichen planus. In many patients with pigmented hyperkeratosis, smoking appears to be an important aetiological factor. The pigmentation is presumably a reaction of melanocytes to chronic irritation and there may also be some associated dysfunction in the transfer of melanin from melanocytes to keratinocytes. Much of the melanin in these lesions is present in sub-epithelial macrophages, having apparently leaked out of melanocytes and/or basal cells (melanin drop-out).

The association of oral pigmentation with Addison's disease is well recognized and may be the initial manifestation of adrenal insufficiency. Adrenal insufficiency results in elevated secretion of adrenocorticotrophic hormone (ACTH) by the pituitary gland, with other cleavage products of pro-opiomelanocortin, such as α-melanocyte-stimulating hormone (αMSH), probably being responsible for the pigmentation. The pigmentation is most common in areas subjected to masticatory trauma, especially the cheeks, but can involve any part of the oral mucosa.

Laugier–Hunziker syndrome is an acquired disorder characterized by benign hyperpigmented macules of the lips and buccal mucosa, frequently associated with longitudinal nail pigmentation and other skin melanotic lesions. No underlying systemic abnormalities are associated.

Drug-induced hypermelanosis of the oral mucosa is rare, but may be seen in some patients taking various cytostatic agents or progestogens present in oral contraceptives. Oral hypermelanosis may also be seen in patients with HIV infection (Chapter 10).

Oral melanotic macule

Patients may present with single or, less frequently, multiple pigmented macules of the oral mucosa, which cannot be classified histologically into any of the recognized types of melanotic lesion and for which no local or systemic cause can be found. They occur more often in women than in men and frequently present around 40 years of age. The vermilion border of the lower lip, gingiva, and buccal mucosa are the commonest sites (Fig. 2.58A).

Histological examination shows a localized area of increased melanin pigment in the basal cell layer, with or without melanin drop-out (Fig. 2.58B). The term 'idiopathic oral melanotic macule' has been applied to this lesion but it is also referred to as an oral ephelis (freckle). The lesion is not associated with increase in the number of melanocytes or with melanocytic atypia.

Melanocytic naevi

Melanocytic naevi (often referred to as moles) are exceedingly common benign hamartomatous lesions, formed by proliferation of melanocytes.

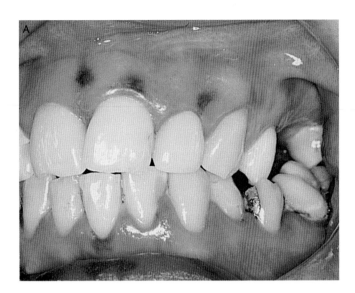
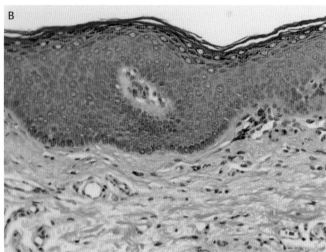

Fig. 2.58 Oral melanotic macules. Histology shows melanin pigmentation of the basal keratinocytes and melanin deposits in the lamina propria.

They are particularly seen in the skin of the head and neck (Chapter 8), but despite their abundance in skin, they are rare in the oral mucosa. Mucosal lesions may present as elevated, pigmented, or amelanotic lesions on the hard palate or buccal mucosa. In most oral melanocytic naevi, the naevus cells are located entirely within the lamina propria, i.e. they are of intra-mucosal type (equivalent to the intra-dermal melanocytic naevus of skin). Rarely, there is an associated intra-epithelial component. The amount of melanin pigment they contain is highly variable.

Malignant melanoma

See Chapter 3.

Other endogenous pigments

Oral pigmentation due to other endogenous substances is uncommon apart from transient discoloration caused by blood breakdown products in a haematoma and the yellowish hue produced by bilirubin in patients with jaundice (Fig. 10.5). Pigmentation associated with disturbances of iron metabolism can also be seen in haemochromatosis, where haemosiderin is deposited in many organs and tissues, including skin and oral mucosa.

White patches

An approach to the differential diagnosis of a white patch

White lesions of the oral mucosa are common with a wide differential diagnosis (Table 2.12). As with all oral diseases, it is important to take a careful history, including the duration of the lesion, initiating factors, symptomatology, and any changes that have been noted. A social history, with specific reference to habits such as smoking and alcohol intake, is also very important. This should be followed by thorough examination focusing on the site distribution of the lesion(s), consistency of the lesion, and its immediate surrounding soft tissue and surface appearance. Examination of the neck for lymphadenopathy is required. Identification of a potential cause allows for preliminary diagnosis. In addition, elimination of possible causes allows the clinician to see the effect on the lesion. If no change is seen, then the lesion should be biopsied. Similarly, if no possible cause can be identified or there are worrisome features, such as redness and ulceration, biopsy should be considered sooner. A patient with a red or red and white patch in the oral cavity consistent with erythroplakia or erythroleukoplakia should be urgently referred (for an appointment within 2 weeks) for assessment for possible oral cancer (Box 3.18).

Genodermatoses

A number of genetically based dermatological conditions can present with white lesions in the mouth (Box 2.6). These are rare, but of significance is dyskeratosis congenita (X-linked recessive OMIM 305000, autosomal dominant OMIM 127550, autosomal recessive OMIM 224230), in which patients may develop oral squamous cell carcinoma.

White sponge naevus

White sponge naevus is inherited as an autosomal dominant trait but with incomplete penetrance (i.e. not all affected individuals will show clinical lesions). Any part of the oral mucosa may be involved but, typically, there are white shaggy folds of mucosa bilaterally on the buccal mucosa (Fig. 2.59A). They may be apparent in early childhood, or may not become evident until adolescence. Clinically, the edges of the lesion are not well defined but gradually merge with the normal

Table 2.12 Differential diagnosis of white lesion of the oral mucosa

Cause	Lesion
Normal	Leukoedema
Hereditary	White sponge naevus
	Oral manifestation of genodermatoses
Traumatic	Mechanical (e.g. frictional keratosis)
	Chemical (e.g. aspirin burn)
	Thermal (e.g. smoker's keratosis)
Infective	Candidosis
	Hairy leukoplakia
	Syphilitic leukoplakia
Dermatological	Lichen planus
	Lupus erythematosus
Idiopathic	Leukoplakia
Neoplastic	Squamous cell carcinoma

Box 2.6 Genodermatoses with oral lesions
- Dyskeratosis congenita
- Pachyonychia congenita
- Tylosis
- Hereditary benign intra-epithelial dyskeratosis
- Follicular keratosis (Darier's disease)

Traumatic keratosis

Mechanical trauma

Chronic frictional trauma from varied sources, such as a sharp tooth, cheek biting, or the prolonged wearing of ill-fitting dentures, leads to epithelial thickening and hyperkeratinization. If the trauma continues, the lesions may become thick and white, with a roughened surface (Fig. 2.60A). To diagnose frictional keratosis, a source of chronic irritation must be identified that fits the size and shape of the lesion, and the lesion must resolve when the source of irritation is removed. Biopsy is necessary if the lesion does not resolve on removal of the presumed cause.

Histologically, frictional keratoses show hyperkeratosis, which may be accompanied by some acanthosis but there is no epithelial dysplasia (Fig. 2.60B). These lesions are not regarded as 'oral potentially malignant disorders' (Chapter 3).

Thermal and chemical trauma

Chemical insult to the oral mucosa may produce a variety of reactions, depending on the severity of the insult and its duration. A severe acute insult, such as that produced by the topical application of aspirin (aspirin burn) adjacent to a symptomatic tooth, will produce epithelial necrosis, sloughing, and ulceration (Fig. 2.61), while a low-grade, chronic insult, such as may be seen with excessive chlorhexidine mouthwash use, may result in hyperkeratosis. Chronic chemical insult to the mucosa is seen in patients who use tobacco, whether it is smoked, chewed, or used as snuff, and in those with other chewing habits, such as betel nut. These habits produce epithelial thickening and hyperkeratosis in a similar manner to chronic friction.

mucosa. Other mucosal surfaces, e.g. the nose, oesophagus, and anogenital region, may also be involved.

Histologically, the epithelium is acanthotic and the surface shows marked hyperparakeratosis (Fig. 2.59B). A characteristic feature is marked intra-cellular oedema of the prickle and parakeratinized cell layers. Only the cell walls and the pyknotic nuclei in the centres of the cells are visible, thus giving a so-called 'basket-weave' appearance. There are no inflammatory changes and there is no cellular atypia. White sponge naevus is not an oral potentially malignant disorder (Chapter 3).

This condition is caused by mutations in the genes coding for keratins 4 and 13 (*KRT4* OMIM 193900, *KRT13* OMIM 615785). The mutated proteins do not fit together properly, resulting in abnormal cytokeratin intermediate filaments. This may also result in abnormalities of the normal desquamation process.

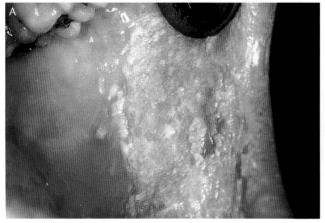
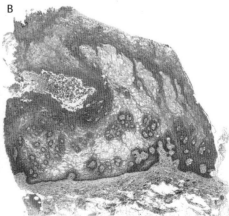

Fig. 2.59 White sponge nevus. Histology shows shaggy hyperkeratosis of the squamous epithelium.

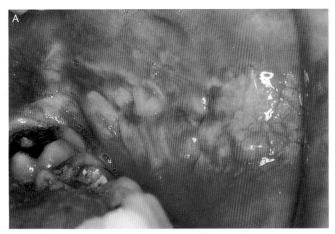

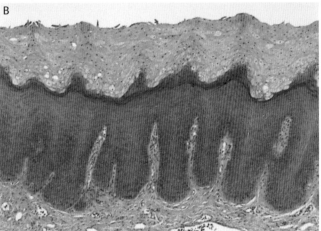

Fig. 2.60 Frictional keratosis. Histology shows marked hyperparakeratosis of the squamous epithelium.

Acute thermal insults, such as those caused by hot food, often result in epithelial necrosis and sloughing of the affected area. Regular smokers of tobacco may develop white plaques on their oral mucosa, particularly the anterior parts of the buccal mucosa, tongue, and

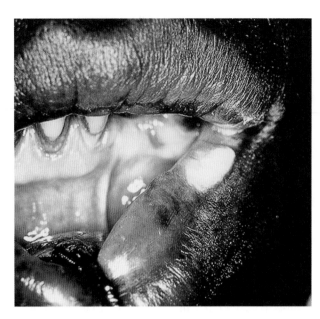

Fig. 2.62 Localized keratosis at the habitual position of a cigarette.

palate. It is likely that both thermal and chemical factors are involved in the development of these hyperkeratotic lesions. Smokers who place a cigarette or pipe in a favoured position may develop a localized keratosis at that site (Fig. 2.62).

Nicotinic stomatitis of the palate is a characteristic clinical condition, which may develop in association with any type of smoking, but particularly in pipe-smokers. In early lesions, the palatal mucosa is greyish-white with scattered red spots representing inflamed minor salivary gland duct orifices. In more advanced lesions, there are pavement-like swollen patches of rough white epithelium with central, red, duct orifices (Fig. 2.63). Areas covered by a denture are protected and spared.

Histological examination shows hyperkeratosis and acanthosis of the palatal epithelium. The surface keratosis extends up to the duct orifice where there is an associated inflammatory infiltrate. The condition is usually reversible if smoking is stopped and is not considered to be an oral potentially malignant disorder. However, the condition does

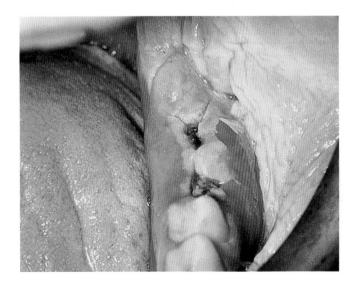

Fig. 2.61 Aspirin burn.

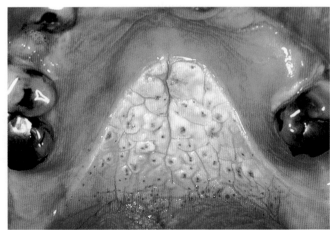

Fig. 2.63 Nicotinic stomatitis of the palate.

indicate that carcinogens are present in the mouth and the whole of the mucosa must be carefully examined for other lesions, given the risk of 'field cancerization' (Chapter 3).

Lichen planus and lichenoid-type lesions

Lichen planus

Lichen planus is a relatively common disease and has a prevalence of 0.5–2% in the general population. The majority of patients are over 40 years of age and at least 60% are women. Oral lesions can be detected in around half of patients with skin lesions, but the prevalence of skin lesions in patients who initially present with oral lichen planus is lower.

Oral lesions

Oral lichen planus pursues a chronic course, in some patients extending over several years. The buccal mucosa is the most commonly affected, while the tongue, gingiva, palate, and lips may also be affected. Lichen planus involving the gingiva often presents as desquamative gingivitis (Fig. 2.64A, Fig 2.65A). Lesions are generally bilateral (may be symmetrical) and a wide spectrum of clinical presentations occur, alone or in various combinations. The main clinical appearances are:

- *Reticular*: white lacy or web-like striae, often on a mildly erythematous background (Fig. 2.64B). This form is very common and usually symptom-free.
- *Plaque-like*: confluent white plaque, most often seen on the dorsum of tongue, usually symptom-free.
- *Papular*: small, white papules, usually symptom-free (Fig. 2.65B).
- *Atrophic/erosive/ulcerative*: the mucosa in the atrophic/erosive forms has a red and glazed appearance with areas of superficial ulceration of varying extent, which may take several weeks to heal (Fig. 2.66). Erosive lesions are often associated with typical areas of non-erosive lichen planus round the edges of the lesions. Pain and discomfort may be considerable and severe. Disagreement around nomenclature can occur. The term atrophic usually indicates a layer of epithelium is still present, but the mucosa thinned, whereas erosive usually indicates a superficial break in the epithelium (ulceration).
- *Bullous*: sub-epithelial blisters form in areas of basal cell damage. This form is very uncommon.

Genital and other mucosal lesions

Mucosal lesions of lichen planus can also occur at other sites. Genital lesions are not uncommon and a 'vulvo-vaginal-gingival syndrome' has

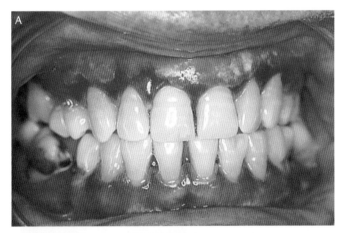

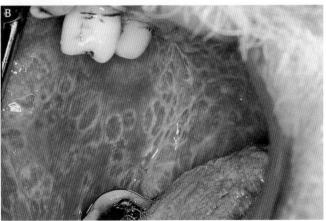

Fig. 2.64 Lichen planus presenting with desquamative gingivitis and reticular white striations on the buccal mucosa.

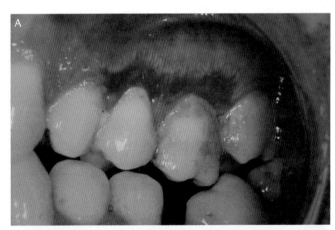

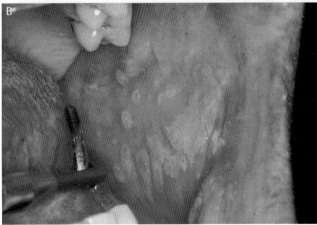

Fig. 2.65 Desquamative gingivitis and plaque-like lichen planus on the buccal mucosa.

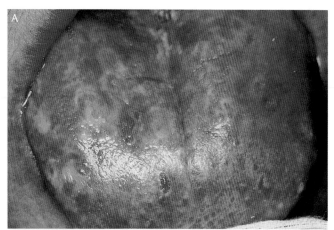

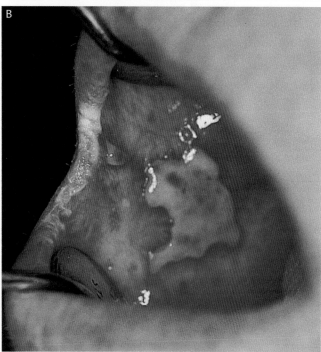

Fig. 2.66 Atrophic lichen planus affecting the dorsum of the tongue and erosive lichen planus affecting the buccal mucosa.

been described with lesions affecting the gingiva and vulvo-vaginal region at the same time. Oesophageal lesions can occur, causing strictures and difficulty in swallowing. Conjunctival lesions are rare.

Skin lesions

The characteristic skin lesion of lichen planus is an itchy violaceous (purple) papule, which may have distinctive white/silvery streaks on the surface, called Wickham's striae. The papules may have a variable pattern, discrete, linear, annular, or widespread rashes being described. Almost any area of skin may be involved, but the flexor surface of the wrist is the commonest site (Fig. 2.67). Fingernails are involved in up to 10% of patients, vertical ridges being the usual abnormality. The skin lesions develop slowly and the majority resolve within 18 months, although recurrences are not uncommon. Many patients with oral lichen planus never develop any clinically recognized skin lesions.

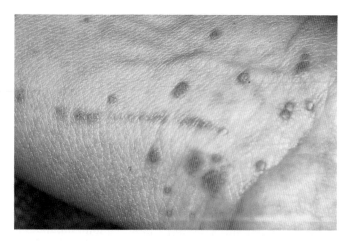

Fig. 2.67 Typical skin lesions in lichen planus. Macular and papular plaques on the flexor surface of the wrist.

Histopathological features

The histopathological features vary dependant on the clinical presentation. In general, the epithelium shows hyperparakeratosis or hyperorthokeratosis, and it varies considerably in thickness between cases. The epithelium may be atrophic or acanthotic, the latter usually resulting in irregular elongation and widening of the rete processes. There is a dense, well-defined, sub-epithelial band of inflammatory cells, consisting mainly of T lymphocytes in the lamina propria (Fig. 2.68). Lymphocytic infiltration of the basal compartment of the epithelium is associated with oedema, and degeneration of the basal epithelial cells. The degenerating cells appear as shrunken, condensed bodies (Civatte bodies) and are undergoing apoptosis (Fig. 2.68B). Once ulceration has occurred there is a non-specific mixed inflammatory response, which makes histological diagnosis problematic.

Aetiology and natural history

The aetiology and pathogenesis of lichen planus are not fully understood but it is widely accepted that cell-mediated immune responses to an external antigen, or to antigenic changes in the epithelial cells, are involved, producing a type IV hypersensitivity reaction (Box 2.7). This is borne out by the fact that the inflammatory infiltrate is dominated by lymphocytes and may contain a dominant population of CD8+ cytotoxic T lymphocytes. However, in most cases the precipitating factors are unknown and the disease is idiopathic. Lichen planus has also been associated with a variety of systemic diseases, although in many

---

Box 2.7 Immunological features of oral lichen planus

- T-cell mediated response to modified keratinocyte surface antigens
- Activation of CD8+ (cytotoxic) by CD4+ (helper) T lymphocytes
- Damage to the basal epithelial cells by induction of apoptosis
- Activation of mast cells and secretion of matrix metalloproteinases degrade the basement membrane may aid chronicity.

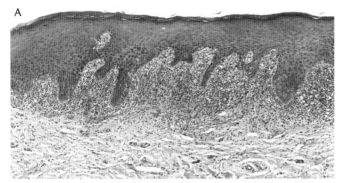

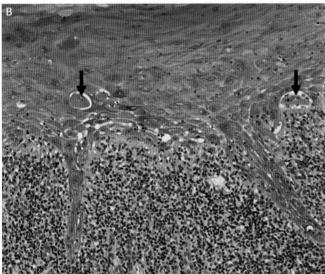

Fig. 2.68 Histological features of lichen planus. Low magnification showing hyperkeratosis and a band of lichenoid inflammation in the lamina propria. High magnification showing basal cell damage and a few apoptotic keratinocytes (arrows). The lichenoid inflammation is composed of lymphocytes and histiocytes.

a cause-and-effect relationship has not been established and the systemic disorder may merely exacerbate a pre-existing lesion. However, there is strong evidence of an association in some patients with chronic liver disease associated with hepatitis C virus infection. The presence of dental plaque can exacerbate lesions of oral lichen planus. This can be a particular problem around atrophic/erosive lesions and with desquamative gingivitis.

Almost all cases of oral lichen planus run a benign course, but malignant transformation has been described in a very small proportion. Some studies have suggested that the atrophic/erosive forms are more likely to undergo such change because of the decreased barrier presented to potential carcinogens. In contrast, others have found malignant transformation to be associated mainly with plaque lesions. This is a controversial area and there is considerable variation in the reported transformation rates, although in most studies it ranges from about 0.5 to 2.5% over a 5-year period.

Treatment

In general, treatments of oral lichen planus are aimed at alleviating symptoms. Where the accumulation of dental plaque causes irritation, regular gentle but effective oral hygiene procedures can help.

Medications are used to treat oral lichen planus in a 'step-wise' approach, according to the relief of symptoms and adverse effects. Initial treatment is usually with chlorhexidine mouthwash twice daily and benzydamine mouthwash, as needed. If further control is required, topical corticosteroids in the forms of adhesive tablets, mouthwash, ointment, and spray are used. The immunosuppressive agent, tacrolimus, is also effective as a topical agent, although concerns remain regarding possible promotion of malignant transformation. Topical retinoids have also been used.

In severe disease, where oral lichen planus significantly affects the patient's quality of life, systemic agents, including hydroxychloroquine, prednisolone, azathioprine, and mycophenolate mofetil, can be used. Systemic retinoids have also been tried.

Key points Oral lichen planus

Clinical

- May occur alone or in association with skin and genital lesions
- Buccal mucosa is the most common site
- Lesions are usually bilateral
- Reticular, plaque-like, papular, atrophic/erosive, bullous-types
- Desquamative gingivitis
- Classified as an 'oral potentially malignant disorder', but low rate of transformation
- Treatment usually with topical steroids

Histopathology

- Type IV hypersensitivity reaction
- Hyperkeratosis
- Acanthosis or atrophy of epithelium
- Basal cell degeneration (apoptotic basal keratinocytes)
- Intra-epithelial lymphocytes
- Band of lymphocytes and macrophages in superficial lamina propria
- Mainly T lymphocytes

Treatment

- Chlorhexidine and benzydamine mouthwash
- Topical steroids
- Systemic immunosuppressive medications in severe disease

Oral lichenoid reactions

In some patients, lesions very similar to those seen in lichen planus are triggered by adverse reactions to medication (Chapter 10) or contact hypersensitivity to dental materials, most often amalgam, particularly in older, corroded restorations (Fig. 2.69, Table 2.13).

Table 2.13 Potential causes of oral lichenoid reactions

Factor	Example
Dental restorative materials	Amalgam Gold Polymerized plastics
Medications	Anti-malarials Oral hypoglycaemics NSAIDs
Food and food additives	Flavourings: cinnamon and derivatives

These lesions are often referred to as lichenoid reactions to distinguish them from idiopathic lichen planus. In practice, it can be very difficult to distinguish these lesions from lichen planus, but features such as unilateral or unusual distribution, contact with a restoration, or a particular temporal association may be useful. In such cases the condition usually improves or resolves on withdrawal of the medication or use of an alternative dental material. In some cases idiopathic lichen planus is exacerbated by medication, most commonly, non-steroidal anti-inflammatory drugs (NSAIDs). Histologically, lichen planus and lichenoid reactions are indistinguishable.

Graft versus host disease

Oral and cutaneous lichenoid lesions are seen as part of a graft versus host disease in patients who have received bone marrow transplants. In such cases the transplanted T lymphocytes (graft-derived) react to antigens on the recipient (host) epithelial cells, which they regard as 'foreign', producing a type IV hypersensitivity reaction.

Lupus erythematosus

There are two main forms of lupus: chronic discoid lupus erythematosus (DLE), which is a localized disease, and systemic lupus erythematosus (SLE), which is a disseminated autoimmune disease, involving almost every organ of the body. Females are affected much more frequently than males. In either form, oral lesions may develop that are similar to the clinical spectrum of lichen planus.

The lesions in chronic DLE are often restricted to the skin and usually occur on the face. They present as scaly, red patches that heal with scar formation. Oral lesions have been reported in around half of cases, and, although any part of the mucosa may be involved, the buccal mucosa is most frequently affected. There is considerable variation in the type of oral lesion seen, but the most usual is a discoid area of erythema or ulceration surrounded by a white keratotic border, sometimes with radiating striae (Fig. 2.70A), which may be indistinguishable from lichen planus. Lesions on the lower lip are considered to be potentially malignant, although the risk of transformation to cancer is considered to be low.

The lesions in SLE include skin rashes that typically occur on the nose and cheeks, with symmetrical distribution—the so-called malar or butterfly rash. Oral lesions are very variable and occur in around

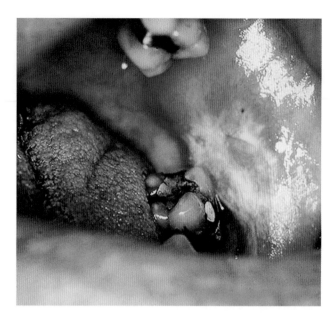

Fig. 2.69 Lichenoid reaction, associated with an amalgam restoration.

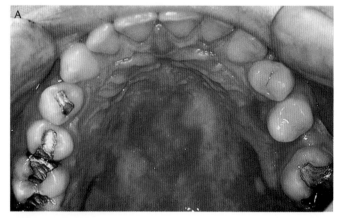

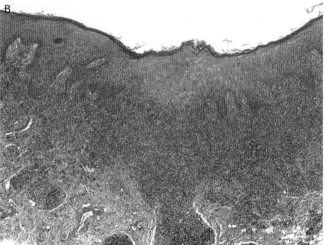

Fig. 2.70 Discoid lupus erythematosus affecting the palate. Histology shows hyperkeratosis and lichenoid inflammation. There is also perivascular inflammation in the deeper part of the lamina propria.

20% of patients. The most commonly described are superficial erosions and erythematous patches on the buccal mucosa, whilst keratotic areas are not so frequently seen as in the discoid type.

Histological examination of the oral lesions shows sub-epithelial and deeper peri-vascular foci of lymphocytes in the connective tissue and there may be liquefactive degeneration of basal cells (Fig. 2.70B). There may also be prominent thickening of the basement membrane, and immunofluorescent studies show deposits of immunoglobulin (mainly IgG) and complement in the basement membrane zone forming a prominent 'lupus band'.

Leukoplakia

Leukoplakia is defined as a predominantly white lesion of the oral mucosa that cannot be characterized as any other definable lesion. Leukoplakia is a clinical diagnosis and is one of the recognized 'oral potentially malignant disorders', described in detail in Chapter 3. Leukoplakia is an important differential diagnosis to be considered when dealing with any intra-oral white patch. Biopsy of persistent white lesions is important to assess epithelial dysplasia; occasionally, an unsuspected squamous cell carcinoma may be discovered.

3

Oral cancer

Chapter contents

Definitions

Oral cancer

The term 'oral cancer' encompasses all malignant neoplasms affecting the oral cavity. The majority, greater than 90%, are squamous cell carcinomas. The remainder are uncommon and comprise minor salivary gland adenocarcinomas, malignant melanoma, sarcomas, haematological malignancies, and metastases to the oral cavity from cancers at other sites.

Oral squamous cell carcinoma

Oral squamous cell carcinoma is a malignant epithelial neoplasm that arises from the lining mucosa of the oral cavity. The tumour shows varying degrees of squamous differentiation and is characterized by invasion of local structures and metastasis to regional lymph nodes, followed by metastasis to other organ systems (e.g. lungs and bones) later in the course of the disease.

Epidemiology of oral cancer

Epidemiological data pertaining to oral cancer can be difficult to evaluate because of variations in the methods of data collection (Box 3.1). Notwithstanding these confounding variables, a database produced by the International Agency for Research on Cancer (GLOBOCAN), estimated there were over 400,000 new cases of lip, oral, and pharyngeal cancer worldwide in 2012, placing the disease in ninth position with breast, prostate, lung, colorectal, cervical, stomach, liver, and uterine cancer being more common. These data suggest that oral cancer is uncommon, but there are enormous variations worldwide. Whereas oral cancer is relatively uncommon in the UK, accounting for 2% of all cancers, in India and parts of South-East Asia it is the most common malignant neoplasm and accounts for around a third of all cancers. Furthermore, the incidence rates for large countries, such as India and the USA, conceal regional and ethnic variations. For example, incidence rates tend to be higher in urban as opposed to rural communities, and in the USA are higher for blacks than whites. In the United Kingdom, incidence rates are slightly higher in Scotland than in England and Wales.

Cancer statistics

In the United Kingdom the incidence of oral cancer is 9 per 100,000 of the population, which represents around 6,800 new cases per annum. The disease is more common in men than in women; the male:female ratio is currently 2:1. Oral cancer incidence increases with age, and the majority of cases (greater than two-thirds) are diagnosed after the age of 50 years old; less than 5% occur in individuals below the age of 40 years old. The incidence of oral cancer has increased by around a third in the last decade. Interestingly, the rates of oro-pharyngeal cancer have more than doubled over a similar time frame, which is thought to be due to the recently recognized importance of oncogenic human papillomavirus (HPV) infection in the aetiology of the disease at this site. Despite this recently identified trend, the most common sites are still the tongue and oral cavity, which together account for around 60% of all oral cancers. Oral cancer has relatively high mortality rates, and in the UK, 2,100 people died of the disease in 2012, which is around six people every day. Mortality rates have not improved significantly over the last four decades despite advances in the management of the disease.

Box 3.1 Factors to be taken into consideration when assessing epidemiological data for oral cancer

Type of cancer

Does the information represent data from all oral malignant neoplasms or just the most common; oral squamous cell carcinoma?

Anatomical location

Which sites are included in the definition of 'oral cancer'?

Cancer Research UK data for oral cancer include the following anatomical sites: lip, tongue, mouth, oro-pharynx, piriform sinus, and hypo-pharynx. By contrast, the Oxford Cancer Intelligence Centre in the UK collects incidence data for oral cavity, palate, oro-pharynx, and hypo-pharynx separately. In some studies, oral cancer data are 'hidden' in data for head and neck cancers—a broader term that encompasses cancers of the oral cavity, oro-pharynx, sinonasal complex, naso-pharynx, hypo-pharynx, larynx, major salivary glands, and the neck.

Geographical region

Do the data represent estimates of global disease burden with variation between continents and countries?

Are the data derived from a National Cancer Registry producing relatively accurate incidence data for a specified population?

Are the data a hospital-based cancer registry producing data that reflect the clinical activity of a regional centre, but prone to underestimate the actual disease burden in the population.

Data collection

Are the data prospectively collected by a National Cancer Registry following standardized definitions and nomenclature, e.g. World Health Organization International Classification of Disease codes?

The Surveillance Epidemiology and End Results (SEERs) programme in the USA produces sufficiently reliable data for strategic healthcare planning.

Are the data a retrospective analysis of hospital records that is subject to data collection bias?

Risk factors for oral cancer

The International Agency for Research on Cancer (IARC) and the World Cancer Research Fund/American Institute for Cancer Research (WCRF/AIC) work together to evaluate the epidemiological evidence around the risk of developing various cancers. Oral cancer risk factors are shown in Table 3.1.

Tobacco and alcohol are the two most important risk factors for developing oral cancer in Western society. However, in India and South-East Asia, betel quid chewing is an important aetiological factor. The relatively recent increase in the incidence of oro-pharyngeal cancer documented in the USA and Western Europe is thought to be due to oncogenic HPV infection.

Tobacco

An abundance of epidemiological and experimental data implicate tobacco as an important factor in the aetiology of oral cancer, regardless of how it is used. However, the relative risks associated with different methods of consumption are still unresolved, and the relationship is complicated further by possible synergistic effects when tobacco is combined with other risk factors, such as alcohol and betel quid chewing.

Tobacco smoking

Tobacco smoke contains thousands of chemicals and many are known to be carcinogenic (Box 3.2). Two-thirds of oral cancers in the UK are associated with tobacco smoking. Patients can be broadly categorized as never-smoker, past-smoker, and current smoker. The risk of developing oral cancer increases with the amount of tobacco smoked. Tobacco exposure is usually estimated by calculating the number of packs of cigarettes an individual has consumed, called the 'pack years'. An individual that has smoked one packet of cigarettes (20 cigarettes per pack) each day for a period of 30 years would have accumulated 30 pack-years of exposure. For individuals who stop smoking, the relative risk falls to that of a never-smoker after about 20 years. There is evidence that second-hand or environmental tobacco smoke increases the risk of developing oral cancer, particularly with prolonged exposure in the home or the workplace.

Betel quid and other chewing habits

Betel quid or paan chewing is particularly common in Indian and South-East Asia, and is also prevalent within Asian communities in parts of the UK (Fig. 3.1). The composition of the quid varies but, typically, it consists of areca nut (*Areca catechu* palm seed, also referred to as 'betel nut') and slaked lime (calcium hydroxide) wrapped in a betel leaf (*Piper betel* is an evergreen perennial creeper that grows in South-East Asia) to which tobacco and various spices are often added. The quid is placed in the buccal sulcus and is frequently kept in the mouth for a long time (hours). As the quid is chewed, alkaloids are released from the nut and the tobacco, which act as a mild stimulant. Prolonged use of paan causes oral leukoplakia and where the paan is held in the mouth, malignant transformation is usually associated with development of a heterogeneous papilliferous, ulcerated mass. The contribution of the various constituents of paan to oral carcinogenesis is complex; however, several epidemiological studies have shown that the relative risk of oral cancer is greatly increased when tobacco is present in the paan. Chewing the areca nut alone is considered to be carcinogenic and it is the main aetiological factor in oral submucous fibrosis, an oral potentially malignant disorder.

Table 3.1 Oral cancer risk factors

Increases risk	May increase risk	May decrease risk	Decreases risk
Tobacco smoking	Solar radiation (lip)	Fruits	None identified
Tobacco smokeless	Tobacco smoke (passive)	Vegetables	
Betel quid with tobacco	Hot *maté* drinking		
Betel quid without tobacco	HPV-18		
Alcoholic beverages			
HPV-16			

Box 3.2 **Carcinogens in tobacco smoke**

- Acrolein
- Arsenic
- Benzene
- 1,3-Butadiene
- Cadmium
- Chromium
- Formaldehyde
- Polonium-210
- Polycyclic aromatic hydrocarbons
- Tar
- Tobacco specific nitrosoamines

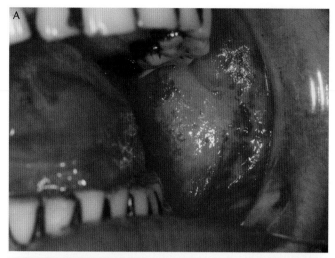

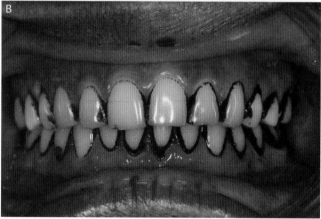

Fig. 3.1 Oral cavity of a paan user. Note the orange discoloration of the buccal mucosa and the black staining of the teeth.

Smokeless tobacco

Snuff is powdered tobacco, which, in addition to being inhaled, can also be placed in contact with the oral mucosa in the buccal and labial sulci (called 'snuff dipping'). It is practiced in the south-eastern USA and in some Scandinavian countries. Smokeless tobacco is also available in the USA and Scandinavian countries as small tobacco sachets, which resemble tea bags. The relative risk of oral cancer from the use of oral snuff is unclear.

Electronic cigarettes

These devices are commonly used as an alternative to smoking tobacco and deliver nicotine via the inhalation of a vaporized mixture of propylene glycol, glycerol, and water. Whilst there is general consensus that they are certainly less harmful than smoking, the devices are not currently regulated and there are health and safety risks that remain to be properly evaluated. There is controversy around the role of e-cigarettes in smoking-cessation programmes, as there are other proven efficacious methods and licensed products available.

Alcoholic beverages

Epidemiological studies from several countries have demonstrated an increased risk of oral cancer associated with alcohol consumption.

Although there is evidence to support a dose/time relationship, this is less striking than that seen with tobacco smoking. Pure ethanol has not been shown to be carcinogenic and it is thought that other chemicals in the beverage, called congeners, are responsible for the increased cancer risk. The consumption of unmatured home-distilled spirits containing carcinogenic by-products may be particularly important in certain parts of the world. All forms of alcoholic beverages, whether beer, wine, or spirits, have a similar magnitude of risk. The increasing incidence of oral cancer, especially in younger persons, may be linked to the rise in alcohol consumption over the past few decades.

Determining the role of alcohol in the aetiology of oral cancer has been complicated because of the close association between drinking and smoking habits. Although alcohol is an important factor independent of smoking, many studies have shown a marked increase in the relative risk when smoking and drinking are practiced concurrently, suggesting a synergistic or multiplicative effect.

The mechanisms by which alcohol consumption increases the risk of oral cancer are still unclear. Mention has already been made of possible carcinogenic contaminants and congeners that may be present in alcoholic beverages, and such drinks may also enhance the penetration of carcinogens across the mucosal barrier. Alcohol in the oral environment is partially metabolized to acetaldehyde, which causes DNA damage. It is also possible that nutritional deficiencies and impaired metabolism, which are common in heavy drinkers, could damage the ability of the oral mucosa to maintain its barrier function. Chronic alcohol intake may impair the ability of the liver to detoxify potential carcinogens, and can also suppress immune responses, increasing the risk of cancer.

A recent meta-analysis of epidemiological studies did not demonstrate any increased risk of oral cancer with use of alcohol-containing mouthwash, even at concentrations of 25% alcohol. Nevertheless many manufacturers have re-formulated brands as 'alcohol-free' against the background of uncertainty about the risk to oral health.

Although non-alcoholic, a South American beverage called 'hot *maté*' is associated with an increased risk of oral cancer and may be due to the very hot temperature at which it is consumed and/or carcinogenic constituents of the drink.

Key points Tobacco and alcohol

- Independent risk factors for oral cancer
- Effect together is synergistic
- Relative risk for tobacco increases with amount and duration of use
- Alcoholic drinks may include constituents (congeners) and/or contaminants that are carcinogenic
- Alcoholic drinks may enhance transport of carcinogens across the mucosal barrier
- Nutritional deficiencies in chronic alcohol abuse may impair the mucosal barrier
- Liver disease in chronic alcohol abuse may impair its ability to detoxify carcinogens
- Immunosuppression in chronic alcohol abuse may increase the risk of developing cancer

Microorganisms

Human papillomavirus

HPVs are double-stranded, circular DNA viruses that infect epithelial cells. There are over 170 different types. The majority are innocuous and cause transient infections with no detrimental effects or induce small papillomas on the surface of the skin and also at mucosal sites, including the oral mucosa (Chapters 2 and 8). In some circumstances, HPV infection can cause cancer, the most common being squamous cell carcinoma of the uterine cervix. The HPV types capable of causing cancer are termed 'high-risk' or oncogenic HPV. Whilst there are a number of high-risk HPVs, the most common type isolated from cervical cancers is HPV-16. Recently, the International Agency of Research of Cancer (IARC) indicated there is sufficient evidence that HPV-16 is causally associated with oral cancer. Specifically, the increased incidence of oro-pharyngeal squamous cell carcinomas in the USA and Western Europe is considered to be due to high-risk HPV infection. In Sweden, around 80% of oro-pharyngeal cancers are HPV-positive, in the USA the proportion is around 60%, and in the UK 50%. Epidemiological evidence from the USA suggests a link between HPV-related oro-pharyngeal cancer and sexual behaviour; risk factors include early age of first sexual intercourse, and increasing numbers of vaginal and oral sex partners. HPV-related oro-pharyngeal squamous cell carcinoma is defined by increased p16 expression by immunohistochemistry and evidence of high-risk HPV DNA by *in situ* hybridization or polymerase chain reaction (Fig 3.2). Significantly, patients with HPV-related oro-pharyngeal squamous cell carcinoma have improved survival when compared with individuals with HPV-negative disease at the same site. A smaller proportion of oral cavity squamous cell carcinomas harbour oncogenic HPV infection (less than 5%); however, there is evidence that these patients also have similarly favourable outcomes to those described in oro-pharyngeal disease.

Epstein–Barr virus

EBV has an aetiological role in the development of naso-pharyngeal carcinomas and some malignant lymphomas, but a similar role in oral carcinogenesis has not been established.

Candida

Candida is a common commensal in the oral cavity and is associated with a variety of oral lesions (Chapter 2). Fungal hyphae can often be identified in oral potentially malignant disorders.

Key points HPV-related oropharyngeal squamous cell carcinoma

- Incidence of OPSCC has doubled in last 15 years in the UK
- Around 50% show evidence of oncogenic HPV infection
- Most commonly HPV-16
- HPV-related OPSCC can be diagnosed using p16 immunohistochemistry and high-risk HPV *in situ* hybridization
- HPV-related OPSCC has better prognosis
- There is a dedicated staging system for p16 positive OPSCC
- Clinical trials are being carried out to evaluated less toxic treatments

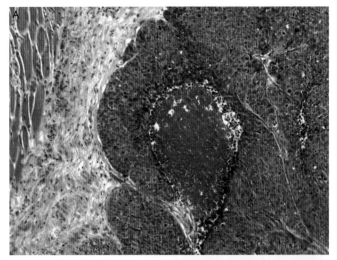
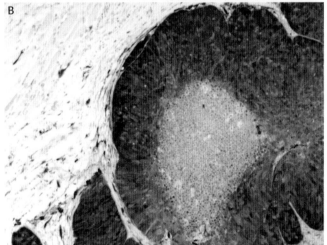
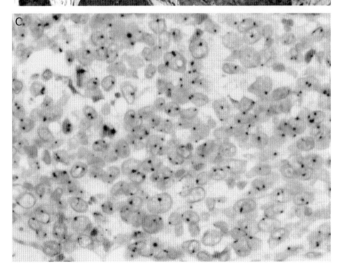

Fig. 3.2 HPV-related squamous cell carcinoma. The malignant cells contain abnormally high levels of p16 protein, which can be detected by immunohistochemistry (dark brown cells). There is also evidence of high-risk HPV DNA by *in situ* hybridization (blue dots).

Diet and nutrition

Sideropenic dysphagia (Plummer–Vinson or Patterson–Brown–Kelly syndrome), comprising difficulty swallowing, oesphageal webs, and iron-deficiency anaemia, has long been associated with increased risk of upper aerodigestive tract cancer, including oral cancer. Iron is essential for the maintenance of oral epithelium and it is possible that atrophic changes in iron-deficiency anaemia render the mucosa more susceptible to chemical carcinogens. A similar effect may be associated with other diseases showing epithelial atrophy, such as oral lichen planus. Vitamin A and related carotenoids (in particular β carotene) are also important in the maintenance of squamous epithelium, and several epidemiological studies have shown that individuals whose diets are high in the antioxidant vitamins A, C, and E have a decreased risk of oral cancer. The risk decreases with increasing consumption of fresh fruit and vegetables. The strongest protective effect is related, in particular, to a diet with a high fruit intake. The possibility of nutritional deficiencies associated with alcoholism has already been mentioned.

Genetic predisposition

A recent meta-analysis has shown that a family history of head and neck cancer in a first-degree relative is associated with a slight increased risk of developing the disease. Exposure to environmental risk factors are often shared between family members, so it is difficult to establish direct evidence of a genetic predisposition. Cancer syndromes, such as dyskeratosis congenita (OMIM 305000) and Fanconi anaemia (OMIM 227650), have an increased risk of developing oral cancer. Patients with these very rare conditions should be regularly screened for oral cancer as part of their multi-disciplinary care.

Solar radiation exposure

High ultraviolet light exposure is an important risk factor in squamous cell carcinoma of the lip. These cancers occur much more frequently on the lower than the upper lip, and are more common in men than women. It is less common in dark-skinned races because of the protection conferred by melanin pigmentation. Squamous cell carcinoma of the lip may be preceded by hyperkeratotic and dysplastic changes, termed actinic cheilitis or actinic keratosis.

Immunosuppression

There is an increased risk of carcinoma of the lip in patients following renal and other organ transplantation, which is likely to be related to the systemic effects of long-term immunosuppressive therapy.

Clinical presentation of oral squamous cell carcinoma

The clinical presentation of oral squamous cell carcinoma is variable. In most instances an accurate clinical assessment will identify 'red flag' signs and symptoms (Box 3.3) that should trigger an urgent referral to an appropriate specialist centre for further investigation. See Table 3.2 and Box 3.4 for further information on establishing an accurate history and the principles of assessment of a patient with oral cancer.

Early diagnosis of oral cancer, when lesions are small and localized, is the key to improving patient prognosis. Dental healthcare professionals have an obligation to screen patients for oral cancer as part of their routine dental examination. Patients with small oral cancers may not have noticed any abnormality, therefore a careful systematic examination of the entire oral cavity with optimal illumination, combined with inspection and palpation of the neck, is essential. Significantly, oral cancers are often located in areas that are overlooked during cursory examination of the oral cavity. Particular attention should be made to visualizing the postero-lateral aspects of the tongue, floor of the mouth, retromolar trigone, and pharyngeal tonsils.

Early lesions may present as a small ulcer, white patch (leukoplakia), red patch (erythroplakia), speckled leukoplakia, or as an exophytic growth (Fig. 3.3). Other clinical features include induration (hardening of the tissues) and tethering of tissue planes with fixation of the lesion to underlying structures. Small lesions on the alveolus may cause tooth mobility, mimicking periodontal disease. Extensive bone destruction is a feature of advanced disease. Carcinoma developing on the vermilion border of the lip is clearly visible and so may be noticed at an early stage as a slightly raised crusting lesion often resembling healing herpes labialis (Fig. 8.7).

An advanced lesion may present as a broad-based, exophytic mass with a rough, nodular, warty, haemorrhagic, or necrotic surface, or as a deeply destructive and crater-like ulcer with raised rolled margins (Fig. 3.4). Infiltration of the oral musculature may result in functional

---

Box 3.3 Red flag signs and symptoms for oral squamous cell carcinoma

Signs

- Non-healing ulcer (any ulcer that fails to resolve over a period of 3 weeks)
- Non-homogeneous leukoplakia
- Erythroplakia
- Exophytic growth
- Induration
- Tethering of tissue planes
- Tooth mobility
- Non-healing socket following exodontia
- Pathological fracture
- Cervical lymphadenopathy

Symptoms

- Discomfort and pain
- Loss of sensation over the distribution of the trigeminal nerve
- Difficulty eating, swallowing and speaking
- Loss of appetite, weight loss, and fatigue

Table 3.2 Establishing a history from a patient with suspected oral cancer

Feature	Questions
Site of lesion	Where is the lesion?
	Typically 'gutter areas': lateral border of tongue, floor of mouth, mandibular alveolus
	Buccal mucosa
	Oro-pharynx
	(Hard palate is an uncommon site for SCC)
Size	How big is the lesion?
	Estimate of size of lesion
	How fast is it growing?
	Slow or rapid; recently started to get larger?
Duration	How long have you had the lesion?
	Weeks to months
Associated features	Are there any other problems?
	Ulceration
	Pain
	Swelling
	Difficulty eating, swallowing, speaking
	Foul taste, halitosis
	Lumps in the neck
	Fatigue and weight loss
Risk factors	Do you smoke?
	Tobacco consumption (number per day, duration, pack years)
	Do you use paan?
	Constituents, number per day, duration
	Do you drink alcohol?
	Type of drink: beer, wine, spirits
	Alcohol consumption (units per week, duration)
	Frequency of binge drinking
	UK guidelines: maximum 14 units per week for men and women

disturbances, particularly if the tumour involves the tongue or floor of the mouth. Because of reduced mobility of the tongue, patients may complain of problems with eating, swallowing, and speaking. Pain may be a feature of an advanced lesion. Bone invasion may be detected by conventional radiography (Fig. 3.5). Occasionally, pathological fracture of the mandible and/or neural invasion may cause altered sensation over the distribution of the mandibular division of the trigeminal nerve.

Inspection and palpation of the neck is important to identify clinical signs of metastatic carcinoma in cervical lymph nodes (Chapters 1 and 9). A single enlarged lymph node on the same side as the primary tumour that is firm and fixed is highly likely to be metastatic carcinoma (Fig. 3.6). Tumours tend to metastasize initially to the lymph nodes in the superior drainage groups (levels I and II), with progressive involvement of the more inferior groups in the lymphatic chain as metastatic disease spreads. Metastasis to contralateral lymph nodes is a feature of advanced disease. Mid-line tumours, particularly in floor of the mouth, have a propensity to produce bilateral metastatic disease in the neck.

A common clinical scenario is the presentation of an enlarged cervical lymph node with no obvious sign of an intra-oral primary tumour. A fine-needle aspiration biopsy or a core biopsy can be used to establish the nature of the lymphadenopathy. If the material indicates metastatic squamous cell carcinoma, then a thorough search of the head and neck region is required to locate the primary tumour, usually by CT or PET–CT scanning combined with examination under general anaesthesia (Figs 3.7 and 3.8). Viral testing of the biopsy material can be used to direct the search. If the biopsy is positive for high-risk HPV, the primary tumour is most likely to be located in the oro-pharynx and if Epstein–Barr virus is detected, then naso-pharyngeal carcinoma is most likely.

The extent of the patient's disease is classified using the UICC (International Union Against Cancer) TNM classification of Malignant Tumours (Box 3.5). The T category describes the size and extent of the primary tumour. The N category describes the size, number, and distribution of metastases in the cervical lymph nodes and any extra-nodal extension of the disease. Clinical extra-nodal extension is classified

---

Box 3.4 Assessment of a patient with oral cancer

Clinical staging

Clinical examination

Primary tumour: anatomical site, laterality, size (maximum dimension, area), invasion of adjacent subsites

Check for second synchronous primary tumour

Metastatic tumour: number of enlarged lymph nodes, laterality, anatomical level in the neck, size of lymph node (maximum dimension), fixation to adjacent structures, fixation to skin, ulceration of skin surface

Investigations

Tissue biopsy of the oral lesion (incisional or punch biopsy)

Fine-needle aspiration biopsy or tissue core biopsy of a neck lump

Conventional radiography of jaws to assess bone invasion and aid dental health assessment prior to radiotherapy

Ultrasound to assess neck lumps

Computed tomography, magnetic resonance imaging, positron emission tomography-computed tomography of head, neck, and mediastinum to assess extent of the disease

These parameters are used to assign T (Tumour), N (Node), M (distant Metastasis) categories, described in the UICC TNM Staging system (Box 3.5)

Assessment of general health

Co-morbidities

Vital signs: pulse, blood pressure, breathing

Haematological investigations

Full blood count, liver function tests, urea, and electrolytes

Nutrition and weight

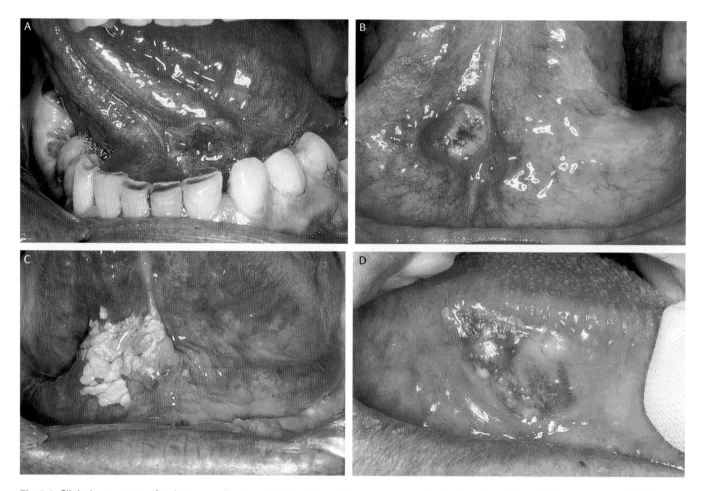

Fig. 3.3 Clinical appearance of early stage oral squamous cell carcinomas presenting as an ulcer (A), an ulcerated nodule (B), a white patch (C), and a red patch (D).

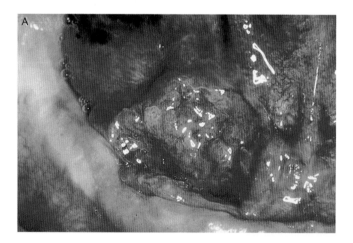
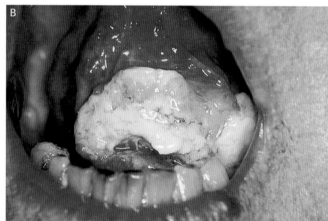
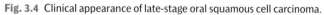

Fig. 3.4 Clinical appearance of late-stage oral squamous cell carcinoma.

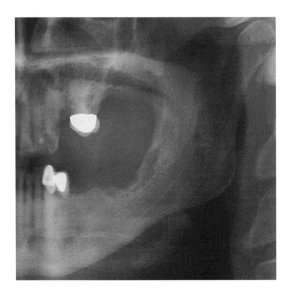

Fig. 3.5 DPT showing mandibular alveolar bone destruction in a patient with late-stage oral squamous cell carcinoma.

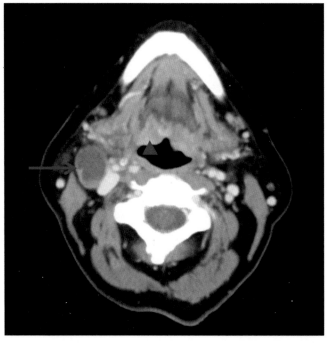

Fig. 3.7 CT scan showing an enlarged right cervical lymph node (arrow). There is a small clinically undetectable lesion in the right base of tongue (arrow head).

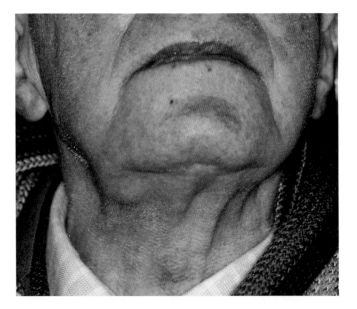

Fig. 3.6 Right submandibular lymph node enlargement in a patient with metastatic oral squamous cell carcinoma.

as the presence of skin involvement or soft-tissue invasion with deep fixation to underlying muscle or adjacent structures or clinical signs of nerve involvement. The M category pertains to the presence or absence of metastases in distant tissues or other organs.

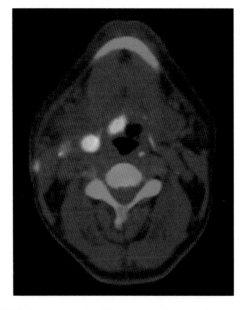

Fig. 3.8 PET–CT scan showing 'hot spots' at the base of tongue and within a cervical lymph node.

Box 3.5 Clinical staging of carcinomas of the lip and oral cavity

T—primary tumour

T1 Tumour 2 cm or less in greatest dimension and 5 mm or less depth of invasion.

T2 Tumour 2 cm or less in greatest dimension and more than 5 mm but no more than 10 mm depth of invasion or tumour more than 2 cm but not more than 4 cm in greatest dimension and depth of invasion no more than 10 mm.

T3 Tumour more than 4 cm in greatest dimension or more than 10 mm depth of invasion.

T4a (Lip) tumour invades through cortical bone, inferior alveolar nerve, floor of mouth, or skin (of the chin or the nose).

T4a (Oral cavity) tumour invades through cortical bone of the mandible or maxillary sinus, or invades the skin of face.

T4b (Lip and oral cavity) tumour invades masticator space, pterygoid plates, or skull base, or encases internal carotid artery.

N—regional lymph nodes

N0 No regional lymph node metastasis.

N1 Metastasis in a single ipsilateral lymph node, 3 cm or less in greatest dimension without extra-nodal extension.

N2a Metastasis in a single ipsilateral lymph node, more than 3 cm but not more than 6 cm in greatest dimension without extra-nodal extension.

N2b Metastasis in multiple ipsilateral lymph nodes, none more than 6 cm in greatest dimension without extra-nodal extension.

N2c Metastasis in bilateral or contralateral lymph nodes, none more than 6 cm in greatest dimension, without extra-nodal extension.

N3a Metastasis in a lymph node more than 6 cm in greatest dimension without extra-nodal extension.

N3b Metastasis in a single or multiple lymph nodes with clinical extra-nodal extension.

M—distant metastasis

M0 No distant metastases.

M1 Distant metastases.

Stage grouping

Stage I	T1	N0	M0
Stage II	T2	N0	M0
Stage III	T3	N0	M0
	T1, T2, T3	N1	M0
Stage IVA	T4a	N0, N1	M0
	T1, T2, T3, T4a	N2	M0
Stage IVB	Any T	N3	M0
	T4b	Any N	M0
Stage IVC	Any T	Any N	M1

Reproduced from TNM Classification of Malignant Tumours, 8th edition, Brierley J. D., Gospodarowicz M. K., Wittekind C. (Eds). Copyright (2017) with permission from John Wiley and Sons.

Pathology of oral squamous cell carcinoma

A tissue biopsy is required for a definitive diagnosis of oral squamous cell carcinoma. In the majority of cases, given an adequate tissue sample, the diagnosis will be straightforward for the pathologist (Figs. 3.9 and 3.10). The pathologist will grade the carcinoma using Broders' classification into well-differentiated, moderately differentiated, and poorly differentiated categories (Fig. 3.11). In well-differentiated tumours, the malignant cells are clearly recognizable as squamous cells and show distinct inter-cellular bridges representing the desmosomal attachments characteristic of keratinocytes. The cells are organized into islands and strands that have a peripheral layer of

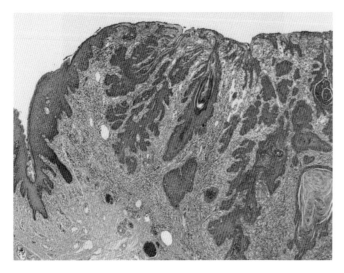

Fig. 3.9 Biopsy from the edge of an oral squamous cell carcinoma.

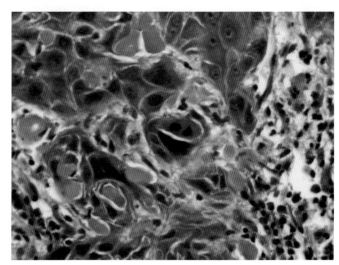

Fig. 3.10 The cytological features of squamous cell carcinoma.

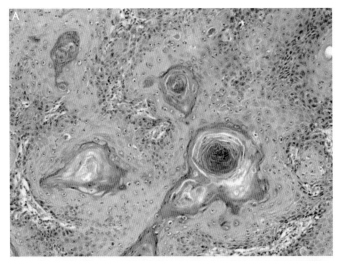

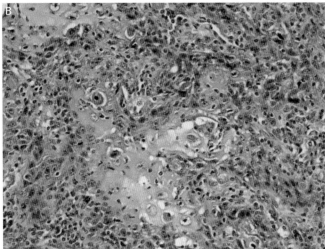

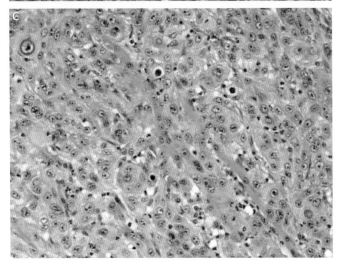

Fig. 3.11 Broders' grades of differentiation. Well-differentiated squamous cell carcinoma with abundant keratin formation (A). Moderately differentiated squamous cell carcinoma showing focal keratinization (B). Poorly differentiated squamous cell carcinoma with no keratinization (C).

basal-type cells, with centrally located cells showing a propensity to keratinization, forming keratin pearls. Nuclear and cellular pleomorphism is not prominent and there are relatively few mitotic figures. Moderately differentiated tumours show less keratinization and more nuclear and cellular pleomorphism, and increased numbers of mitotic figures, but are still readily identified as squamous cell carcinoma. By contrast, in poorly differentiated carcinoma, keratinization is absent and the cells show prominent nuclear and cellular pleomorphism and abundant, often abnormal mitoses. In some poorly differentiated neoplasms the cells may be so abnormal as to hardly be recognizable as epithelial cells. In such cases, immunohistochemical staining techniques are used to demonstrate the formation of cytokeratin intermediate filament proteins that characterize squamous epithelial cells, e.g. cytokeratins 5, 6, and 14. Expression of p63 and p40, nuclear transcription factors, can also be used as evidence of squamous differentiation (Fig. 3.12). There are also a few uncommon histological variants of oral squamous cell carcinoma, which are listed in Table 3.3 (Fig. 3.13). The malignant epithelial component is usually invested by inflamed fibro-vascular tissue, referred to as the tumour stroma. The inflammatory cells are predominantly a mixture of B and T lymphocytes, plasma cells, and macrophages. In areas of necrosis, neutrophils are abundant and foreign-body giant cells may accumulate around keratin debris. In recent years it has become increasingly apparent that the tumour stroma or tumour microenviroment plays an important role in carcinogenesis and disease progression.

Oral squamous cell carcinomas first invade the lamina propria and then the connective tissue of the submucosa, which contains structures such as striated muscle and minor salivary glands. The pattern of invasion can be categorized into cohesive and non-cohesive invasive patterns. The cohesive invasive pattern is composed of large islands and broad strands of carcinoma that present a 'pushing' invasive front. The non-cohesive pattern is more infiltrative with small islands, thin strands, and single malignant cells (Fig. 3.14A). Carcinoma may invade between muscle fibres or track down nerve bundles, usually in the perineural tissue investing the neurites. Neural invasion ahead of the invasive front is associated with local recurrence and persistence of disease following surgical treatment (Fig. 3.14B). Vascular invasion of either lymphatic channels or small blood vessels is associated with the development of metastasis (Fig. 3.15). Bone invasion of the mandible or maxilla is a feature of advanced disease. In the edentulous jaw, the main route of entry appears to be through the crest of the ridge, following the path of vessels communicating between the marrow and periosteum, rather than through the cortical plates. In the dentate patient, the periodontal ligament is also a conduit for tumour invasion of the bone. Within the jaws, the tumour spreads through the marrow spaces between the cancellous trabeculae and, particularly in the mandible, along the inferior alveolar neurovascular bundle (Fig. 3.16).

Oral squamous cell carcinoma metastasizes to the regional lymph nodes of the neck (Fig. 3.17). Significantly, even patients with smaller tumours (T1/T2 category) have a risk of lymph node metastasis. In this patient group, clinical assessment may fail to detect disease in the neck; however, around 25% harbour microscopic evidence

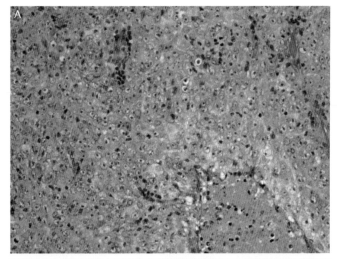
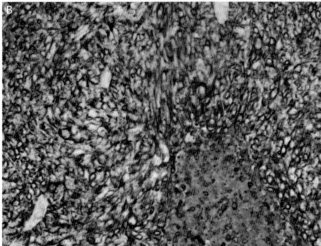
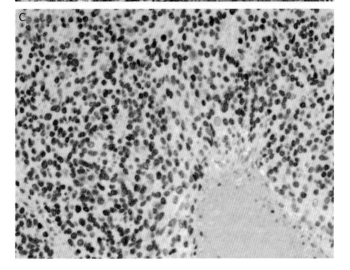

Fig. 3.12 Typical immunohistochemical profile of a poorly differentiated squamous cell carcinoma (A). There is strong cytoplasmic expression of cytokeratins 5/6 (B) and strong nuclear expression of p63 (C).

Table 3.3 Uncommon histological variants of squamous cell carcinoma

Name	Main features
Papillary squamous cell carcinoma	The name relates to a papillary excrescence, which often has a 'stalk'
	Minimal invasion and destruction
	Sometimes only shows invasion of the 'stalk'
	Metastasis uncommon
Verrucous carcinoma	The name relates to the verruciform (warty) surface
	Thickened squamous epithelium with minimal dysplasia
	Rete processes are broad and like 'elephant feet'
	'Pushing' invasive pattern sometimes difficult to establish invasion of lamina propria
	Metastasis uncommon
Basaloid squamous cell carcinoma	The name relates to the basaloid malignant epithelial cells
	High nuclear-to-cytoplasmic ratio makes the cells basaloid (purple) on H&E stain
	Tends to arise in the oro-pharynx
	Usually high stage at initial presentation (large primary tumour with extensive metastasis to regional lymph nodes)
	Poor prognosis
	HPV-related basaloid squamous cell carcinoma in the oro-pharynx has a better prognosis
Spindle cell carcinoma	The name relates to the spindle-shaped malignant epithelial cells
	Spindle cells are elongated cells with wisps of cytoplasm at each pole forming pointed projections
	Sometimes presents as a sessile polypoid nodule, with minimal invasion of underlying tissue
	May arise as a second metachronous primary tumour in a field of previous radiotherapy
Adenosquamous carcinoma	The name relates to a bi-phasic epithelial malignancy that has two components: adenocarcinoma and squamous cell carcinoma
	Usually high stage at initial presentation (large primary tumour with extensive metastasis to regional lymph nodes)
	Poor prognosis
Acanthoytic squamous cell carcinoma	The name relates to the malignant epithelial cells, which tend to 'fall apart' as they lose their desmosomal attachments (acantholytic)
	Typically occurs on lower lip and is associated with actinic damage (UV radiation exposure)
Carcinoma cuniculatum	The term 'cuniculatum' relates to the 'burrowing' pattern of invasion
	Usually a well-differentiated squamous cell carcinoma
	Sometimes not recognized as malignant on initial biopsies
	Extensive destructive of local structures particular bone
	Metastasis uncommon

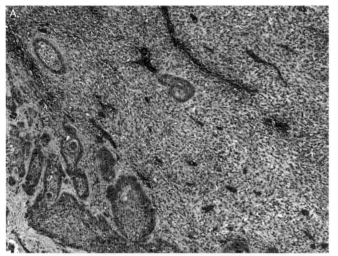

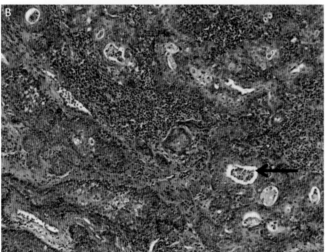

Fig. 3.13 Uncommon histological variants of squamous cell carcinoma. A spindle-cell carcinoma composed of sheets of malignant spindle cells alongside islands of conventional squamous cell carcinoma (A). An adenosquamous carcinoma comprising a mixture of squamous cell carcinoma and adenocarcinoma (B; arrow indicates ductal differentiation).

of carcinoma in cervical lymph nodes following a neck dissection. Elective neck dissection is often performed, even though no neck disease is evident, to eliminate the risk of failure to eradicate the disease. Alternatively, a technique called sentinel lymph node biopsy may be used to locate and remove the lymph nodes that are the first in the drainage pathway of the tumour (Box 3.6). If no metastatic disease is found in these sentinel nodes, then elective neck dissection can be avoided.

The clinical stage may require adjustment (up-stage or down-stage) following pathologic examination of a neck dissection. The new information is reported as the pN category (i.e. pathology N category); it is still formulated using the same parameters: size, number, and distribution of metastases in the cervical lymph nodes and any evidence of extra-nodal extension of the disease. Extra-nodal extension is defined as metastatic carcinoma invading through the capsule of the lymph node and into the parenchymal tissues of the neck; it may be microscopic (Figs. 3.18) or obvious on macroscopic examination of the surgical specimen (Figs. 3.19). Metastases to distant sites (most commonly lungs and bone) occur later in the clinical course of the disease and is usually associated with a failure to control loco-regional disease or in patients with extensive lymph node metastases. Previously, many patients died before distant metastases became apparent; however, improved patient survival has increased the likelihood of emergent distant disease, and highly sensitive imaging techniques, such as MRI and PET–CT, have improved the detection of what was previously occult disease.

Patients that survive oral cancer and have been smokers or continue to smoke have an increased risk of developing another cancer of the upper aerodigestive tract, called a metachronous second primary tumour (Fig. 3.20). The risk is underpinned by the biological theory of 'field cancerization', whereby chronic exposure of the mucosal surfaces of the upper aerodigestive tract to carcinogens leads to the accumulation of genetic damage in mucosal keratinocytes with the acquisition of the biological hallmarks of cancer. Around 10% of head and neck cancer survivors develop second primary tumours over time.

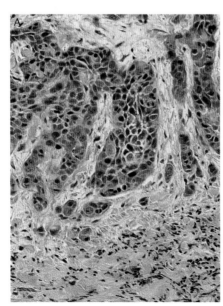

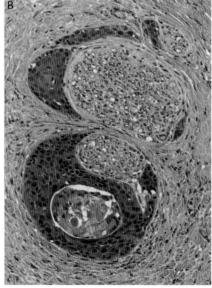

Fig. 3.14 The invasive front of a squamous cell carcinoma (A) and perineural invasion (B).

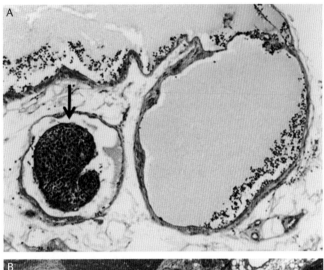

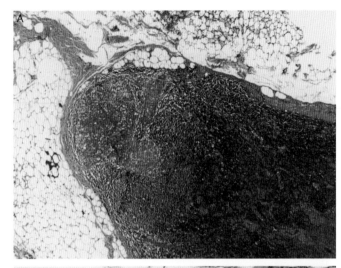

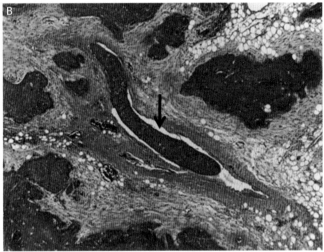

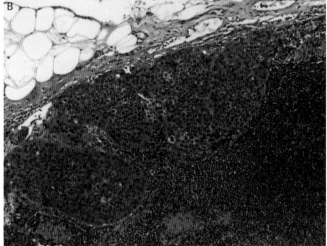

Fig. 3.15 Vascular invasion showing carcinoma in a lymphatic channel (A) and a blood vessel (B).

Fig. 3.17 Lymph node metastases.

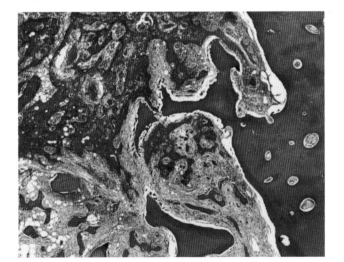

Fig. 3.16 Invasion of the medullary bone by squamous cell carcinoma.

Key points Pathology of oral squamous cell carcinoma
- Cytologically malignant squamous epithelium
- Keratinization varies with degree of differentiation
- Local invasion of adjacent tissues
- Vascular invasion
- Neural invasion
- Bone invasion
- Metastasis to cervical lymph nodes
- Extra-nodal extension
- Metastases to distant sites (lungs and bones)
- Second primary tumours

This technique is recommended for patients with early stage oral cavity squamous cell carcinoma; clinically T1/T2 N0.

Prior to, or at the time of, surgery, four sites around the oral carcinoma are injected with a radioactive-labelled colloid, sometimes mixed with a dye or fluorescent marker.

The radioactive colloid tracer enters the lymphatic system and drains to the first echelon lymph nodes, which are the most likely to harbour metastatic carcinoma.

The surgeon then uses a gamma radiation detection system to identify the most radioactive lymph nodes ('hot nodes') and harvests them using a small incision in the neck. Up to four sentinel nodes may be found in each side of the neck.

Each 'hot node' is then processed in the pathology laboratory using a detailed protocol that samples the entire lymph node at 125-μm intervals.

Immunohistochemical staining for cytokeratin molecules (AE1/AE3 cytokeratin cocktail) is used to increase the sensitivity of the test.

A negative sentinel lymph node biopsy has a high negative predictive value (95%) and the neck can be safely monitored, avoiding elective neck dissection.

A positive lymph node mandates a neck dissection, which is performed as a second operation.

Source data from *NICE guideline* [NG36], Cancer of the upper aerodigestive tract: assessment and management in people aged 16 and over, NICE, 2016.

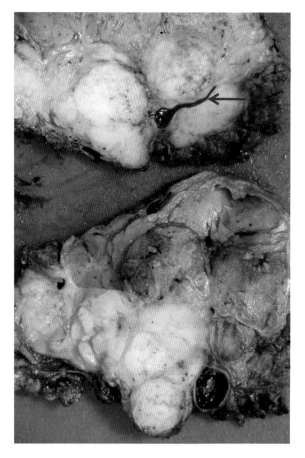

Fig. 3.19 Neck dissection showing metastatic carcinoma (white nodules) invading parenchymal fat (yellow tissue), the sternocleidomastoid muscle (brown tissue) and compressing the internal jugular vein (arrows).

Molecular pathology of oral squamous cell carcinoma

The general biological characteristics of cancer have been succinctly described by Hanahan and Weinberg (Hanahan D, Weinberg RA. The hallmarks of cancer. *Cell* 2000 100:57–70; Hanahan D, Weinberg RA. Hallmarks of cancer: the next generation. *Cell* 2011 144:645–647). They defined six

hallmarks of cancer: sustaining proliferative signalling; evading growth inhibition; resisting cell death (apoptosis); acquiring limitless replicative potential (immortality); developing an autonomous blood supply (angiogenesis); acquiring the ability to spread through the body (tissue invasion

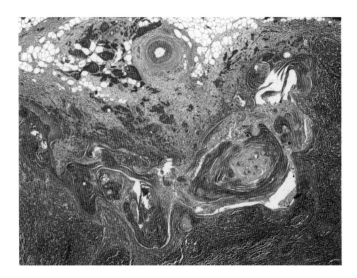

Fig. 3.18 Extra-nodal extension of carcinoma into the perinodal fat.

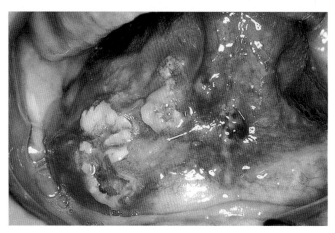

Fig. 3.20 Clinical appearance of multi-focal oral squamous cell carcinoma in an area of 'field cancerization'.

Table 3.4 Key oncogenes and tumour suppressor genes in oral carcinogenesis

Oncogenes	Chromosomal location	Function in normal cells	Hallmarks of cancer
EGFR Epidermal growth factor receptor	7p11	Cell cycle progression	Uncontrolled cell proliferation
MET Hepatocyte growth factor receptor	7q31	Cell cycle progression	Uncontrolled cell proliferation Angiogenesis Invasion and metastasis
CCND1 Cyclin D1	11q13	Cell cycle progression	Uncontrolled cell proliferation
Tumour suppressor genes			
TP53 Tumour protein 53	17p13	Cell cycle regulation Apoptosis DNA repair	Uncontrolled cell proliferation Escape apoptosis Genetic instability Angiogenesis

CDKN2A
Encodes two proteins:
  p16(INK4) cyclin dependent kinase
  inhibitor
  p14(ARF) involved in p53 pathway
	9p21	Cell cycle regulation
		Cell cycle regulation
		Apoptosis
			Uncontrolled cell proliferation
			Uncontrolled cell proliferation
			Escape apoptosis

PTEN Phosphatase and tensin homologue	10q23	Cell cycle regulation Apoptosis Cell adhesion Cell migration	Uncontrolled cell proliferation Escape apoptosis Invasion and metastasis

and metastasis). The acquisition of these capabilities is a multi-step process and the consequence of the accumulation of genetic damage, which may include changes to chromosomes (aneuploidy, translocations, amplifications), genes (mutations, deletions, amplifications), and epigenetic changes (chemical changes in DNA, such as methylation and modification of the histones that package DNA). In oral squamous cell carcinoma it is the mucosal keratinocytes that acquire these malignant characteristics. Some of the molecular changes that occur in oral squamous cell carcinoma are well known and a conceptual model of the molecular changes at different stages of oral carcinogenesis has been proposed. Whilst the model is far from complete, it helps researchers navigate the very complex changes that encode the process of oral carcinogenesis. The model has recently been reviewed and updated (Leemans C. R., Braakhuis B. J., Brakenhoff R. H.

The molecular biology of head and neck cancer. *Nature Reviews Cancer* 2011 11: 9–22). The best described genetic changes are abnormalities in two classes of genes, namely oncogenes and tumour suppressor genes. An oncogene is an amplified or mutated gene that promotes the development of cancer. In most cases, oncogenes encode cell cycle proteins that increase cell proliferation. Tumour suppressor genes encode proteins that are normally involved in inhibiting cell proliferation or promoting apoptosis. When tumour suppressor genes are mutated, deleted, or silenced (by methylation), the cell cycle 'brakes' fail and uncontrolled proliferation ensues. In addition, the cells may also escape apoptosis leading to the accumulation of cells that are genetically unstable and prone to further damage, called genetic instability. Key oncogenes and tumour suppressor genes described in oral carcinogenesis are shown in Table 3.4 and Fig. 3.21.

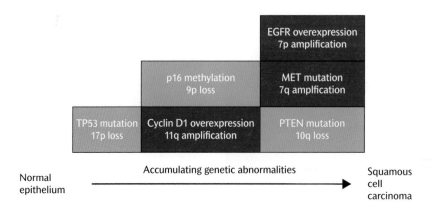

Fig. 3.21 Common genetic alterations during oral carcinogenesis.

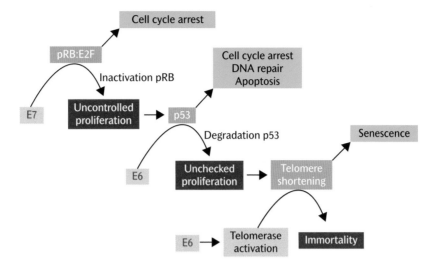

Fig. 3.22 Effects of HPV oncoproteins E6 and E7 on keratinocytes.

The paradigm for high-risk HPV causing cancer is based on the oncogenic actions of the HPV E6 and E7 proteins on mucosal keratinocytes. E7 binds and inactivates pRB, the product of the retinoblastoma gene, which is a tumour suppressor gene. Inactivation of pRB releases E2F, a transcription factor that induces cell cycle progression. E6 inactivates p53 by targeting it for degradation, blocking DNA repair and apoptosis.

E6 also activates telomerase expression producing an immortal cell with limitless replicative potential (Fig. 3.22).

The molecular differences between HPV-related squamous cell carcinoma and oral cancers caused by other aetiological agents are thought to explain the difference in prognosis between the two diseases.

Prognosis of oral cancer

The survival rate of patients with oral cancer depends on a number of factors, but early diagnosis is by far the most important. Loco-regional recurrences, either at the primary site within the oral cavity (local recurrence) or due to uncontrolled metastatic disease within the neck (regional recurrence), or both, are the major causes of death. The reduction in survival rates related to metastatic spread is well established. Several studies have shown 5-year survival rates of about 80% for patients without lymph node metastases compared to between 45 and 65% for those with metastases, depending on their extent. In particular, the presence of extra-nodal extension is an important indicator of poor prognosis, and for these patients the chances of surviving 5 years drops to around 20%. The main histopathological features that influence prognosis are listed in Box 3.7.

Oncogenic HPV and prognosis

More recently, evidence has emerged that the presence of oncogenic HPV in oro-pharyngeal squamous cell carcinoma influences patient survival. A patient who has an HPV-related squamous cell carcinoma of the oro-pharynx and is a non-smoker has an excellent prognosis; the majority of these patients (>90%) survive at least 3 years and many are cured of their disease. Significantly, second primary tumours in these patients are uncommon, which may account, in part, for the improved prognosis. By contrast, patients with HPV-negative oro-pharyngeal squamous cell carcinoma who are smokers have the worst prognosis; only around 45% survive the subsequent 3 years following treatment. These findings have led to the suggestion that HPV-related oro-pharyngeal squamous cell carcinoma should be considered a different disease to HPV-negative squamous cell carcinoma (Table 3.5). This has been recognized in the

Box 3.7 Histopathological features related to prognosis of oral squamous cell carcinoma

- Dimension of tumour
- Depth of invasion
- Bone invasion
- Non-cohesive invasion pattern
- Neural invasion
- Vascular invasion
- Metastatic spread to regional lymph nodes
- Extra-nodal extension
- Metastatic spread to distant sites

Table 3.5 Key differences between HPV-negative and HPV-positive squamous cell carcinoma

Feature	HPV-negative	HPV-positive
Incidence	Slight increase	Dramatic increase
Anatomical site	Oral cavity	Oro-pharynx
Age	Older	Younger
	Above 60 years	Under 60 years
Sex ratio (M:F)	2:1	3:1
Risk factors	Tobacco and alcohol	Sexual behaviour
Prognosis	Poor	Favourable

Box 3.8 Clinical staging of p16 positive carcinomas of the oropharynx

T—primary tumour

T1 Tumour 2 cm or less in greatest dimension.

T2 Tumour more than 2 cm but not more than 4 cm in greatest dimension.

T3 Tumour more than 4 cm in greatest dimension or extension to lingual surface of epiglottis.

T4 Tumour invades any of the following: larynx, deep/extrinsic muscle of tongue; medial pterygoid, hard palate, mandible, lateral pterygoid muscle, pterygoid plates, lateral nasopharynx, skull base, or encases carotid artery.

N—regional lymph nodes

N0 No regional lymph node metastasis.

N1 Unilateral metastasis, in lymph node(s), all 6 cm or less in greatest dimension.

N2 Contralateral or bilateral metastases in lymph node(s), all 6 cm or less in greatest dimension.

N3 Metastasis in lymph node(s) greater than 6 cm in dimension.

M—distant metastasis

M0 No distant metastases.

M1 Distant metastases.

Stage grouping

Stage I	T1, T2	N0, N1	M0
Stage II	T1, T2	N2	M0
	T3	N0, N1, N2	M0
Stage III	T1, T2, T3	N3	M0
	T4	Any N	M0
Stage IV	Any T	Any N	M1

Reproduced from TNM Classification of Malignant Tumours, 8th edition, Brierley J. D., Gospodarowicz M. K., Wittekind C. (Eds). Copyright (2017) with permission from John Wiley and Sons.

2017 UICC TNM Classification of Malignant Tumours (8th edition), where a new staging system for p16 positive oropharyngeal carcinomas is recommended (Box 3.8).

Whilst more patients are surviving HPV-related oro-pharyngeal cancer, there is growing concern that the survivors have a rather poor quality of life as a consequence of the side-effects of treatment. The majority of patients receive chemoradiotherapy (cis-platin and radiotherapy 70 Gy in 35 fractions over 7 weeks), which causes localized bystander tissue damage and functional difficulties with eating, drinking, swallowing, and speaking. The alternative treatment of surgery is also associated with functional deficits, depending on the extent of the operation, and many patients require post-operative radiotherapy with its associated side-effects (Box 3.9).

Box 3.9 Consequences of radiotherapy to the head and neck region

- Acute oral mucositis
- Acute dermatitis (skin of face and neck)
- Irreversible damage to the salivary glands, particularly parotid gland
- Xerostomia
- Dental caries
- Periodontal disease
- Acute pseudomembranous candidosis
- Angular cheilitis
- Difficulty eating, drinking, swallowing, and speaking
- Altered taste
- Risk of osteoradionecrosis particularly following exodontia

---

Oral potentially malignant disorders

It has long been recognized that a proportion of oral squamous cell carcinomas develop in pre-existing areas of morphologically altered mucosa. Variable terminology has been used over the years: oral precursor lesions, oral pre-cancers, oral pre-malignant lesions, oral pre-malignant conditions, and oral potentially malignant lesions; however, a working group convened by the World Health Organization (WHO) in 2005 recommended the term 'oral potentially malignant disorders'. The term suggests that not all the disorders listed in Box 3.10 will transform to cancer, at least not within the lifetime of the affected individual.

Genetic disorders

There are very rare genetic disorders that predispose to the development of oral cancer and they are included in the classification of oral potentially malignant disorders. Patients diagnosed with dyskeratosis congenita and Fanconi anaemia are screened for oral mucosal lesions as part of their multi-disciplinary care (Box 3.11).

Mucosal atrophy

A group of disorders is associated with a small increased risk of developing oral squamous cell carcinoma. All show epithelial atrophy and this may confer greater susceptibility to carcinogens. Also atrophic epithelium has altered cell turnover rates and permeability, which may allow carcinogens to reach the stem cells located in the basal layer. Patients with these conditions should be advised to eliminate tobacco and paan use, and to limit alcohol intake.

Oral submucous fibrosis

Oral submucous fibrosis is related to using paan, and it is an important aetiological factor for oral cancer. Paan is held in the mouth for long periods and stains the teeth and mucosa. In submucous fibrosis, the affected

Box 3.10 Oral potentially malignant disorders

Genetic disorders

- Dyskeratosis congenita
- Fanconi anaemia

Mucosal atrophy

- Oral submucous fibrosis
- Lichen planus
- Sideropenic dysphagia

Mucocutaneous lesions on the lip

- Actinic cheilitis (actinic keratosis)
- Discoid lupus erythematosus

Idiopathic

- Leukoplakia
- Erythroplakia

mucosa becomes pale in colour and feels firm on palpation. Fibrous bands develop in the buccal mucosa and a pale, constricting fibrosis typically involves the soft palate. With time, mouth opening becomes progressively restricted and swallowing may be difficult. The risk of developing oral carcinoma has been estimated at around 5%, although the risk of developing submucous fibrosis itself cannot be separated from the risks posed by carcinogenic substances in paan. Biopsy can help to confirm the clinical diagnosis and typically shows a sub-epithelial band of fine fibrillary collagen in the lamina propria. Atrophy of the oral epithelium often reduces the thickness to only a few cell layers. A thin layer of surface keratin may be present and lichenoid inflammation is often seen in the superficial lamina propria. Epithelial dysplasia, or even invasive squamous carcinoma, may be found, particularly in red or white areas of affected oral mucosa. Submucous fibrosis is difficult to treat and prevention is the best strategy.

Lichen planus

It is generally recognized that there is a link between lichen planus and oral cancer, particularly in the atrophic and erosive variants. The risk of

Box 3.11 Genetic disorders associated with oral cancer

Dyskeratosis congenita

- Skin pigmentation
- Nail dystrophy
- Oral leukoplakia
- Increased risk of oral cancer

Fanconi anaemia

- Haematological disorders, including bone marrow failure and leukaemia
- Oral leukoplakia
- High incidence of oral cancer and other head and neck cancers
- Cancer at very young age
- Surveillance for oral cancer is an important part of multi-disciplinary care for these patients

transformation to cancer is considered to be low and variably reported as being between 0.4% and 5%. The associations between oral non-erosive lichen planus or cutaneous lichen planus and malignant transformation is unclear. When patients first present with an oral mucosal disorder suspected to be lichen planus, biopsy examination is indicated to confirm the diagnosis and exclude other disorders, particularly dysplasia. It is good clinical practice to offer long-term follow-up to patients with erosive lichen planus. Cessation of the risk factors for oral cancer should be advised.

Sideropenic dysphagia

Sideropenic dysphagia (Plummer–Vinson or Patterson–Kelly–Brown syndrome) is an association of iron-deficiency anaemia and difficulty in swallowing because of formation of an oesophageal web. Chronic iron deficiency results in generalized mucosal atrophy because iron is an essential requirement for the maintenance of oral epithelium. Cytological atypia may be seen in biopsies from the atrophic epithelium. Squamous carcinoma can develop in the oesophagus and, less commonly, in the oral cavity or oro-pharynx.

Muco-cutaneous lesions on the lip

Actinic cheilitis (actinic keratosis)

Patients with excessive UV exposure, such as outdoor workers, fair-skinned individuals living in sunny climes, and sun-bed abusers are prone to develop actinic cheilitis. Predominately the lower lip on the vermillion border is affected. Degeneration of the superficial dermis leads to solar elastosis and the lip appears pale. There is variable hyperkeratosis and evidence of epithelial dysplasia. Not all lesions transform to cancer, but squamous cell carcinoma may develop, particularly on the lateral aspects of the lower lip and rarely on the upper lip.

Discoid lupus erythematosus

Discoid lupus erythematosus is a chronic autoimmune disease and squamous cell carcinoma of the lower lip has been documented in these patients.

Leukoplakia

Leukoplakia is a predominantly white lesion of the oral mucosa that cannot be characterized as any other definable lesion. The current WHO definition is provided in Box 3.12. Leukoplakia is a clinical diagnosis, has a variable histology, and the diagnosis, therefore, can only be made after biopsy. Sampling of a suspected leukoplakia is an important consideration in order to obtain representative pathological material. Areas showing the most abnormal appearance should be chosen, and sometimes multiple biopsies are taken to map the field of abnormal changes. Rarely, an incisional biopsy of a white patch will reveal an invasive squamous carcinoma that was not suspected clinically. Patients with leukoplakia can be stratified for risk of malignant transformation on the basis of the clinical appearance of the lesion. Multi-focal or very extensive leukoplakia carries a higher risk than small, solitary lesions.

Homogeneous leukoplakias are plaque-like lesions with a uniform smooth or wrinkled surface; there is a low risk of malignant transformation. *Non-homogeneous leukoplakias* tend to be less circumscribed, show a greater range of appearances, and have a higher risk of malignant transformation (Fig. 3.23). *Verrucous leukoplakia* has a

Box 3.12 Definition of leukoplakia

A white plaque of questionable risk having excluded (other) known diseases or disorders that carry no increased risk for cancer.

Reproduced from *Journal of Oral Pathology & Medicine*, 36, Warnakulasuriya, S., Johnson, Newell. W. and Van Der Waal, I, Nomenclature and classification of potentially malignant disorders of the oral mucosa, pp. 575–580. Copyright (2007) with permission from John Wiley and Sons

warty appearance and *speckled leukoplakia* has interspersed red areas. Heaping up of keratin, nodularity, and ulceration may be present.

The diagnosis can only be made after careful clinical examination and with representative mucosal biopsy, as these procedures are essential for exclusion of other defined disorders. Sometimes special fluorescent lights (e.g. VELscope) and tissue stains (e.g. toluidine blue) are used during examination, but their added value remains unclear. A semantic problem exists with the current practice of diagnosis by exclusion: it is imprecise because there are many other diseases that present with a white lesion (Box 3.13 and Chapter 2). Also, the diagnosis depends on which diseases are recognized in current classifications. The global prevalence of leukoplakia is 2–3%, but varies by geographical region and prevalence of risk factors, which are the same as those for oral cancer.

The risk of malignant transformation is difficult to estimate in any individual case, but is considered to be low and around 1–2%. Lesions in the floor of the mouth and ventral tongue, and those showing evidence of epithelial dysplasia, are at high risk. Paradoxically, the risk of malignant transformation is greater in non-smokers than in smokers. Leukoplakia is uncommon in non-smokers. The regression of leukoplakia in smokers following cessation suggests that a proportion of lesions are, in fact, simple keratoses, whereas leukoplakia in non-smokers more often represents a local cellular genetic abnormality that drives carcinogenesis.

Sublingual keratosis

This term is applied to leukoplakia affecting the floor of the mouth and ventral tongue. In the past it was originally thought that over 30% of these lesions underwent malignant transformation, but more recent evidence suggests that the data were flawed. Consequently, the term is not generally used except as a descriptor, because of lack of evidence supporting it as a distinct clinical entity.

Candidal leukoplakia

The term candidal leukoplakia should be used if *Candida* hyphae invade the keratin on the surface of leukoplakia. The presence of epithelial dysplasia in this situation should flag the risk of malignant transformation. Candidal leukoplakia should be distinguished from chronic hyperplastic candidiasis. Chronic hyperplastic candidosis occurs most commonly on the dorsal tongue and buccal commisures. Staining with diastase periodic acid–Schiff stain (DPAS) shows hyphae of *Candida* species growing

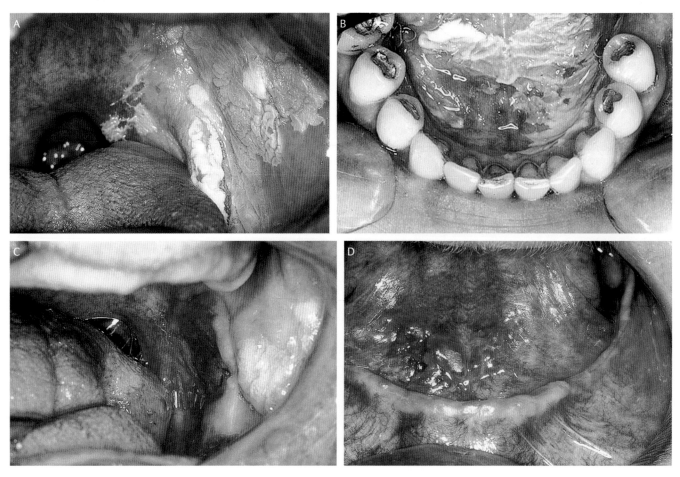

Fig. 3.23 Clinical appearance of non-homogeneous leukoplakia (A, B) and erythroplakia (C, D).

Box 3.13 Disorders that should be excluded for a diagnosis of leukoplakia

- Leukoedema
- White sponge nevus
- Frictional keratosis
- Chemical injury
- Acute pseudomembraneous candidosis
- Hairy leukoplakia
- Lichen planus (plaque-like variant)
- Lichenoid reaction (local factors and medications)
- Discoid lupus erythematosus

into the keratin layer, where they are typically associated with the formation of neutrophil microabscesses. There is marked epithelial hyperplasia with formation of elongated and blunted (test-tube shaped) rete processes. A dense chronic inflammatory infiltrate is typically present in the lamina propria. Elimination of predisposing factors, such as smoking, poor denture hygiene, and haematinic deficiency, combined with systemic anti-fungal therapy, may cause resolution of the white plaque. Whilst some cellular atypia may be observed in chronic hyperplastic candidosis, if dysplasia is present, then the lesion should be termed a candidal leukoplakia to indicate the risk of malignant transformation.

Syphilitic leukoplakia

This is not relevant to contemporary practice but carried a high risk of malignant transformation when it was prevalent. It was a complication of tertiary syphilis and tended to affect the dorsum of the tongue. Some cases may have been caused by medications containing arsenic.

Proliferative verrucous leukoplakia

The WHO classification of oral potentially malignant disorders recognizes this condition as a high-risk oral potentially malignant disorder, with up to 85% of cases undergoing malignant transformation in some published series. Accurate diagnosis requires careful clinicopathological correlation. Clinically, proliferative verruous leukoplakia (PVL) has a warty surface and is white, yellow, or brown in colour. Lesions are most often present on the palate and gingiva, and after careful examination, lesions are often found elsewhere in the oral cavity. Over time, the leukoplakia enlarges and new lesions may appear. Biopsy frequently shows minimal evidence of epithelial dysplasia; many of the typical features are absent. Consequently, if the clinical diagnosis raises the possibility of PVL, the pathologist places greater emphasis on the abnormal verruciform epithelial architecture when considering the diagnosis. Frequently, PVL is too extensive to remove and careful follow-up with elimination of risk factors is then recommended. Biopsy of suspicious areas is undertaken to detect the development of squamous cell carcinoma at the earliest possible stage.

Erythroplakia

Erythroplakia has been defined by the WHO as a 'fiery red patch that cannot be characterized clinically or pathologically as any other definable lesion'. Erthroplakia is uncommon, but there is a high risk of

transformation to cancer. Histopathologically, erythroplakia tends to show dysplasia, often in a distinctive pattern with drop-shaped rete processes, marked nuclear and cellular pleomorphism, and minimal keratinization. Erythoplakia and leukoplakia (red and white areas) may be present in an individual lesion or may co-exist in the oral cavity, indicating that there is considerable overlap between the two conditions.

Epithelial dysplasia

The term 'dysplasia' is used in a variety of contexts in descriptive pathology and means literally 'abnormal growth'. In the context of oral potentially malignant disorders, dysplasia is used to describe the accumulation of abnormal epithelial cells with disturbances of the cellular arrangements (abnormal architecture), features characteristically seen during the process of malignant transformation. A recent meta-analysis of oral epithelial dysplasia indicates that around 12% of cases undergo malignant transformation and the mean time from diagnosis to development of cancer is around 4 years. The histopathological features currently recognized as features of dysplasia are listed in Box 3.14 and illustrated in Figs 3.24 and 3.25. Epithelial dysplasia is usually graded and forms part of the risk-assessment of the lesion. The WHO classification (2017) recommends a three-point grading system: mild dysplasia, moderate dysplasia, and severe dysplasia. An alternative scheme uses a binary system of 'low-grade' and 'high-grade' epithelial dysplasia. Low-grade lesions comprise mild epithelial dysplasia, the high-grade lesions severe epithelial dysplasia Moderate dysplasia is split between low- and high-grade groups, depending on the architectural and cytological features. The use of the term 'carcinoma in *situ*'

Box 3.14 Architectural and cellular features of epithelial dysplasia

Architectural features

- Irregular epithelial stratification
- Loss of polarity of basal cells
- Drop-shaped rete processes
- Increased number of mitotic figures
- Abnormally superficial mitotic figures
- Premature keratinization in single cells (dyskeratosis)
- Keratin pearls within rete processes
- Loss of epithelial cell cohesion

Cellular features

- Abnormal variation in nuclear size (anisonucleosis)
- Abnormal variation in nuclear shape (nuclear pleomorphism)
- Abnormal variation in cell size (anisocytosis)
- Abnormal variation in cell shape (cellular pleomorphism)
- Increased nuclear to cytoplasmic ratio
- Atypical mitotic figures
- Increased number and size of nucleoli
- Nuclear hyperchromasia

Adapted from *WHO Classification of Tumours. Pathology and Genetics of Head and Neck Tumours*. Eds. Barnes L, Eveson JW, Reichart P, Sidransky D (2005).

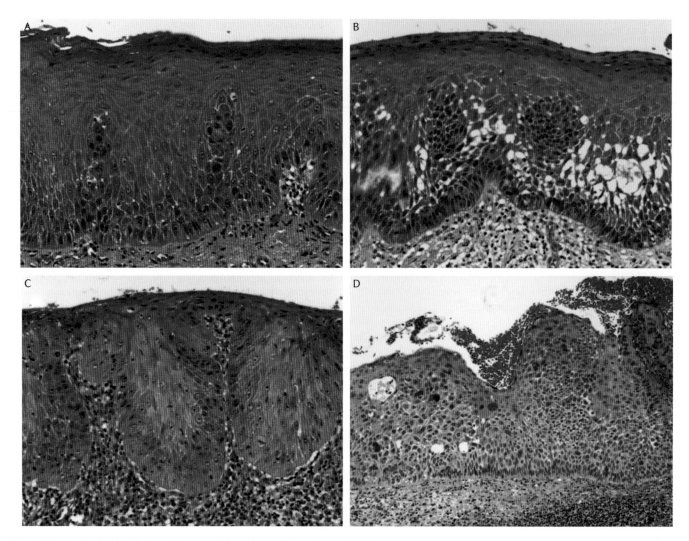

Fig. 3.24 Grades of epithelial dysplasia: mild (A), moderate (B), and severe (C, D).

has been discontinued. The term was used to indicate the worst grade of dysplasia, when abnormalities occupied the full thickness of the epithelium. Such changes are now reported as severe or high-grade dysplasia.

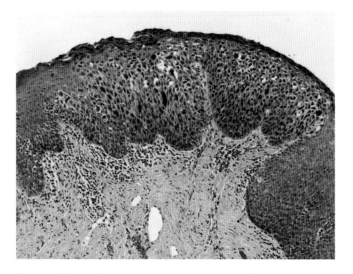

Fig. 3.25 The architectural and cytological abnormalities in severe epithelial dysplasia.

Grading of epithelial dysplasia

Studies on histopathological grading show poor inter-observer and intra-observer agreement, even between specialist pathologists. This problem arises partly because of lack of scientific evidence for weighting the various features of dysplasia. For example, drop-shaped rete processes are generally accepted as a sinister feature, whereas increased mitotic rate may be seen in reactive processes. Not only are there marked observer variabilities but also the biological behaviour of an individual lesion does not always correlate with its grading. Sometimes patients in a surveillance programme develop squamous cell carcinoma at other sites in the upper aerodigestive tract, implying that the molecular changes conferring malignant potential may extend beyond the clinically recognized lesion. Problems may also arise because of non-representative sampling at the time of biopsy. Although histopathological grading is intrinsically unreliable, it provides essential information in the risk-assessment of oral potentially malignant disorders. A case can be made for using a simplified binary dysplasia grading system, assigning lesions into either 'high-grade' or 'low-grade' categories. This results in better inter-observer agreement, as might be anticipated with fewer categories, but further research that defines the positive and negative predictive value of a grade system is awaited. Numerous studies have aimed to identify molecular markers that might predict malignant transformation; for example, determination of loss of hetrozygosity (LOH) at

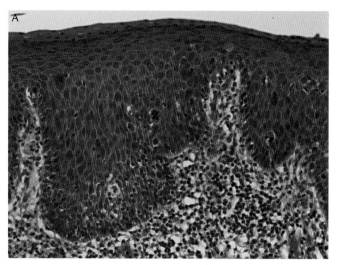

chromosomal loci (chromosomes 3p, 9q and 17p) and gross assessment of chromosome number (called ploidy analysis). However, there is no widespread acceptance of which tests have sufficient utility to be incorporated into routine clinical practice.

Cytological techniques (scrapes and brushes) have been employed to assess oral potentially malignant disorders, but have not been widely adopted in clinical practice (Box 3.15). The cytological features of dysplasia used for assessment of lesions in cell smears and liquid based cytological preparations are listed in Box 3.16.

HPV-related dysplasia

High-risk HPV has been identified in a proportion of lesions clinically diagnosed as leukoplakia or erythroplakia. HPV-related dysplasia appears to occur most frequently in the floor of the mouth and ventral tongue, though it may occur at other oral sites. Microscopically, there is typically severe epithelial dysplasia and distinctive features such as mitosoid bodies, spindle-shaped keratinocytes, and viral cytopathic (koilocyte-like) changes may be seen (Fig. 3.26). These morphological changes were known before HPV testing became readily available and the lesions were described as showing 'koilocytic atypia'. The natural history of HPV-related dysplasia is not yet understood, but malignant transformation to oral squamous carcinoma has been reported.

Management of oral potentially malignant disorders

Known risk factors for malignant change include tobacco, paan chewing habit, high alcohol intake, HPV infection, *Candida* infection, poor

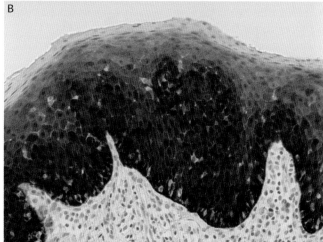

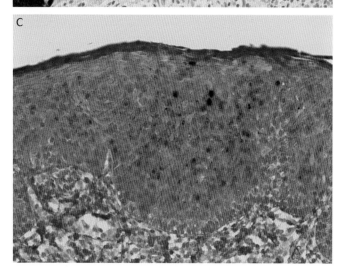

Fig. 3.26 HPV-related epithelial dysplasia with increased expression of p16 by immunohistochemistry (dark brown cells) and evidence of high-risk HPV DNA by *in situ* hybridization (blue dots).

diet, and genetic susceptibility. When assessing a patient with an oral potentially malignant disorder, clinical factors that are associated with higher levels of risk are:

- Female, particularly non-smoker
- Extensive or spreading lesions

Box 3.16 Morphological features of epithelial dysplasia in cytology preparations

- Nuclear hyperchromasia
- Anisonucleosis
- Nuclear pleomorphism
- Increased nuclear to cytoplasmic ratio
- Irregularities of nuclear membrane
- Nuclear crowding
- Nuclear moulding
- Clumping and irregular distribution of chromatin

- Lesions in the floor of the mouth/ventral tongue, retromolar area, or pillar of fauces
- Red, speckled, verrucous, or nodular appearance
- Presence of epithelial dysplasia, particularly severe dysplasia; high-grade dysplasia
- Previous history of head and neck cancer

The evidence-base for management of oral potentially malignant disorders is weak, with no appropriately powered randomized controlled trials of interventions. There is general consensus that the management should include the following:

- Clear information and explanation of the significance of the disorder to the patient
- Intervention for cessation of tobacco smoking or chewing habits, and to limit alcohol intake (Box 3.17)

- Elimination of any underlying causes such as anaemia or *Candida* infection
- Surgical or laser excision may be considered for discrete lesions but is not always feasible for extensive lesions
- Regular follow-up and observation; immediate investigation if signs of malignant transformation such as ulceration, bleeding, pain, paraesthesia, or anaesthesia develop
- Regular dental care to secure and maintain oral health

Referral to a specialist centre is advisable for patients presenting with suspicious white or red mucosal patches (Box 3.18). Biopsy is required for definitive diagnosis and to determine the presence of epithelial dysplasia. Some patients with oral potentially malignant disorders may be followed-up in primary care settings following assessment by a specialist.

Malignant salivary gland neoplasms

Salivary gland malignancies are presented in Chapter 4.

Malignant melanoma

Malignant melanoma of the skin is common and mainly due to excessive UV exposure (Chapter 8). Oral mucosal melanoma is rare, but slightly more common in men than women, and over 70% of cases involve the posterior maxillary alveolar ridge and hard palate (Fig. 3.27). Most are advanced and extensively invasive lesions at presentation, but in about a third of cases there is a history of previous pigmentation in the area. Pigmented lesions of the oral mucosa should be carefully assessed and suspicious lesions require a biopsy for definitive diagnosis. Most oral mucosal malignant melanomas present as dark-brown or bluish-black, slightly raised lesions with an uneven nodular or papillary surface. Histologically, they are highly pleomorphic neoplasms. The amount of melanin pigment is variable and in some may be absent. Immunohistochemistry is often required to make a definitive diagnosis and melanomas are positive for S100, MelanA, HMB45, and SOX10. Melanomas are difficult to eradicate and are characterized by failure of loco-regional control and distant metastasis. The prognosis for most patients is poor; however, early detection when the melanoma is in 'radial growth phase' is associated with better prognosis.

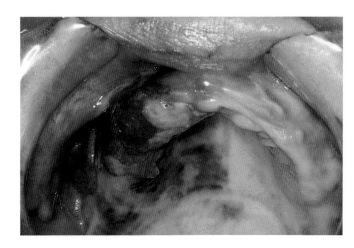

Fig. 3.27 Malignant melanoma.

Malignant bone and soft-tissue tumours

Malignant bone tumours are presented in Chapter 7. Malignant soft-tissue tumours are rare in the oro-facial complex (Table 3.6). The majority occur in adults, but children are also affected and some are related to genetic syndromes (e.g. Li-Fraumeni syndrome). Most present with local disease and around 10–20% show evidence of regional lymph node metastasis and distant metastasis (lung, liver, and bone). The management of these rare diseases is complex and usually involves multi-modal therapy: chemotherapy, radiation, and surgery.

Table 3.6 Malignant bone and soft-tissue tumours

Tissue	Malignant tumour
Fibrous tissue	Fibrosarcoma
	Low-grade myofibroblastic sarcoma
Adipose tissue	Atypical lipomatous tumour
	Liposarcoma
Vessels	Angiosarcoma
	Haemangioendothelioma
	Kaposi sarcoma
Perivascular	Malignant solitary fibrous tumour
Nerve	Malignant peripheral nerve sheath tumour
Smooth muscle	Leiomyosarcoma
Striated muscle	Rhabdomyosarcoma
Malignant cells (not otherwise specified)	Alveolar soft part sarcoma
	Synovial sarcoma
	Hyalinizing clear cell sarcoma
Cartilage	Chondrosarcoma
Bone	Osteosarcoma

Haematological malignancy

Lymphomas

Lymphomas are a diverse group of malignant neoplasms characterized by the proliferation and accumulation of malignant lymphoid cells within lymph nodes. Consequently, the majority of lymphomas in the head and neck region present as cervical lymphadenopathy (Chapter 9). Oral mucosal deposits and jaw lesions are uncommon and are referred to as 'extra-nodal' disease (i.e. disease outside the lymph nodes). Lymphomas are traditionally classified into Hodgkin and non-Hodgkin lymphomas. Hodgkin lymphoma presents with lymphadenopathy in young adults and extra-nodal disease is very rare. Non-Hodgkin lymphomas are most commonly derived from the B lymphocyte lineage and are either high-grade B cell lymphomas (e.g. diffuse large B cell lymphoma and Burkitt lymphoma) or low-grade B cell lymphomas (e.g. small lymphocytic lymphoma, follicular lymphoma, marginal zone lymphoma, and mantle cell lymphoma). T cell lymphomas are uncommon, but nasal-type NK/T cell lymphoma has a predilection for head and neck sites, and may present with a mucosal lesion in the mid-line of the palate that also destroys the sinonasal complex.

Burkitt lymphoma is an endemic childhood malignancy in tropical equatorial Africa and typically presents with jaw lesions. The lesions arise more frequently in the maxilla than the mandible, but multiple quadrants may be involved. The tumours are rapidly growing and may produce gross facial disfigurement. Teeth in the area are loosened, displaced, and may be exfoliated. Burkitt lymphoma is a B cell lymphoma and consists of sheets of small, darkly staining, malignant lymphoid cells, scattered amongst which are numerous pale-staining macrophages producing a 'starry sky' pattern. Epstein–Barr virus (EBV) infection is a causal factor and malaria is a co-factor. Without treatment, Burkitt lymphoma is rapidly fatal; however, chemotherapy has dramatically increased survival.

There are two other conditions that produce bone lesions: myeloma, which is a plasma cell neoplasm, and Langerhans cell histiocytosis. These conditions are discussed in Chapter 7.

Leukaemias

Leukaemias are the most common malignancy in children, usually acute lymphoblastic leukaemia. However, overall, the majority of leukaemias occur in adults—acute myeloid leukaemia and chronic lymphocytic leukaemia are the most frequent (Table 3.7). Patients with leukaemia may present with general pallor (due to anaemia), abnormal bleeding

Table 3.7 Basic leukaemia classification

Acute leukaemia is characterized by primitive undifferentiated white cells in the blood (suffix -*blastic*).

Chronic leukaemia is characterized by abnormal white cells in the blood, they have the morphological features of normal counterparts (suffix -*cytic*).

Lymphoid leukaemia is derived from the lymphocyte lineage.

Myeloid leukaemia is derived from the granulocyte/monocyte lineage.

	Lymphoid	Myeloid
Acute	Acute lymphoblastic leukaemia (ALL)	Acute myeloid leukaemia (AML)
Chronic	Chronic lymphocytic leukaemia (CLL)	Chronic myeloid leukaemia (CML)

Box 3.19 Oral manifestations of leukaemia

- Mucosal pallor
- Oral petechiae, ecchymosis, purpura
- Gingival bleeding
- Gingival swelling
- Loose teeth
- Oral ulceration
- Viral infection (herpes simplex, varicella zoster)
- Fungal infection (candidosis)
- Lymphadenopathy
- Parotid swelling

(petechiae, ecchymosis, and purpura; due to thrombocytopenia), inter-current infection (due to leukopenia), lymphadenopathy, and spleno-megaly. Patients with chronic leukaemias tend to have skin lesions.

Metastasis to the oral cavity

Metastasis to the oral cavity from a cancer at another anatomical site is uncommon and accounts for less than 1% of all oral malignan-cies. The majority of patients are elderly and have one of the more common cancers: lung, colorectal, breast, or prostate. Tumours of the kidney also tend to metastasize to the jaws. The retromolar region of the mandible is the most frequent location for the meta-static deposit. Patients may present with pain and swelling, paraes-thesia or anaesthesia over the distribution of the trigeminal nerve, loose teeth, a non-healing socket or pathological fracture (Fig. 3.29). Radiology may demonstrate an ill-defined radiolucency or, occa-sionally, a radio-dense abnormality (breast and prostate cancer). In around a third of cases, the oral lesion leads to discovery of a previ-ously undiscovered primary tumour. On further investigation, the patient may have disseminated metastatic disease will require multi-disciplinary oncology care.

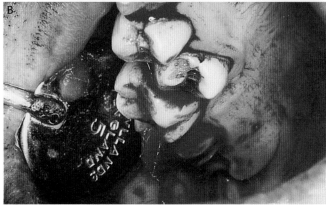

Fig. 3.28 Buccal and lingual gingival enlargement (A) and spontaneous gingival haemorrhage (B) in acute leukaemia.

Nevertheless, oral features may be the first sign of leukaemia (Box 3.19 and Fig. 3.28). Dental healthcare professions may be involved in sup-portive care, such as the management of oral symptoms from ulcera-tion and infection. Patients with leukaemia or undergoing treatment for leukaemia are at risk of excessive haemorrhage following exodontia. Patients may be taking cytotoxic drugs and systemic steroids, which can exacerbate the associated oral problems.

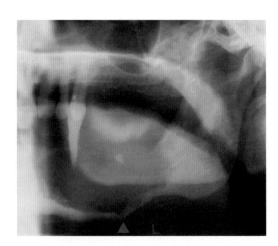

Fig. 3.29 Metastatic lung adenocarcinoma causing extensive destruction of the left body of the mandible and a pathological fracture (arrow head).

4
Salivary gland diseases

Introduction

The salivary glands consist of three paired major glands—parotid, submandibular, and sublingual—and the countless minor salivary glands found in almost every part of the oral cavity, except the gingiva and anterior regions of the hard palate. The secretion of saliva is essential for the normal function and health of the mouth, and disorders of salivary gland function predispose to oral disease. Functional disorders in salivary secretion may be associated with primary salivary gland disease but in other cases are a consequence of systemic factors, such as medications, endocrine disturbances, and neurological disease, which are discussed in Chapter 10.

Developmental anomalies

Developmental anomalies of the salivary glands are rare. Aplasia of one or more major glands and atresia of one or more major salivary gland ducts have been reported. Congenital aplasia of the parotid gland may be associated with other facial abnormalities, e.g. ectodermal dysplasia, mandibulofacial dysostosis, and hemifacial microsomia.

Heterotopic salivary tissue has been reported from a variety of sites in the head and neck region, the most frequent being its inclusion at the angle, or within the body, of the mandible, called a Stafne bone cavity. It is usually an incidental radiological finding and appears as a round or oval, well-demarcated radiolucency between the premolar region and angle of the jaw, and is typically located beneath the inferior dental canal (Fig. 4.1). The radiographic appearances are due to a saucer-shaped depression or concavity of varying depth on the lingual aspect of the mandible, which contains salivary tissue in continuity with the submandibular gland.

Accessory parotid tissue within the cheek or masseter muscle is relatively common and is subject to the same diseases that may affect the main gland.

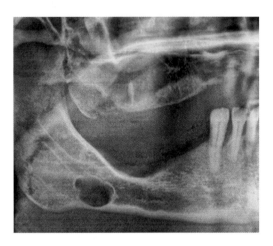

Fig. 4.1 Stafne bone cavity.

Age changes

Age changes can be detected in both major and minor salivary glands. Reduction in the weights of submandibular and parotid glands has been reported with increasing age, associated in the submandibular gland with an age-dependent reduction in flow rates. By contrast, several studies have demonstrated that there is no significant reduction in parotid flow rates in the elderly. In both glands the reduction in weight is related to atrophy of secretory tissue and replacement by fibro-adipose tissue. The accumulation of fat tends to increase linearly with age and there is a reduction in the volume of acinar tissue of about 30–35% from approximately 20 years to 75 years of age. Similar changes, amounting to about 45% loss of acinar tissue, have been reported in minor glands in the lower lip. Oncocytic change in ductal epithelium is also a common age change.

Sialadenitis

Inflammatory disorders of the major salivary glands are usually the result of bacterial or viral infection. Occasionally, sialadenitis is due to other causes, such as irradiation or trauma. Pneumoparotitis is a rare cause of parotid gland swelling caused by air being forced into the parotid ductal system; it has been reported in wind instrument players.

Bacterial sialadenitis

Inflammatory disorders of the salivary glands may mimic soft-tissue infections and can present as acute or chronic conditions.

Acute suppurative bacterial sialadenitis

This uncommon disorder principally involves the parotid gland. Acute parotitis is an ascending infection, where the bacteria reach the gland from the oral cavity by ascending the ductal system. The main microorganisms are *Streptococcus pyogenes* and *Staphylococcus aureus*. In the past, acute bacterial sialadenitis was a common postoperative complication in debilitated and dehydrated patients, particularly following abdominal surgery, but it is now a rare occurrence in such patients. Reduced salivary flow is the major predisposing factor and acute parotitis may occur in patients with Sjögren's syndrome or

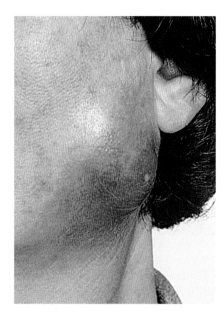

Fig. 4.2 Acute bacterial sialadenitis of the parotid gland showing redness and swelling of the skin overlying the gland.

following the use of drugs that cause a dry mouth (Chapter 10). Acute infection may also arise in immunocompromised patients or as a result of acute exacerbation in a previously chronic sialadenitis. The onset of acute sialadenitis is rapid. Clinically, it presents as swelling of the involved gland accompanied by pain, fever, malaise, and redness of the overlying skin. Pus may be expressed from the duct of the affected gland (Figs 4.2 and 4.3).

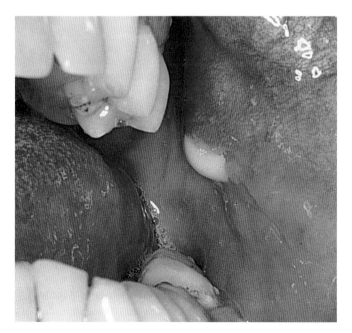

Fig. 4.3 Purulent saliva being expressed from the parotid papilla in acute supurative bacterial parotitis.

Chronic bacterial sialadenitis

Chronic sialadenitis of the major salivary glands is usually a non-specific inflammatory disease associated with duct obstruction, most often due to salivary calculi and low-grade ascending infection. The submandibular gland is much more commonly involved than the parotid gland. In cases where no cause of obstruction can be identified, the predisposing factor may be a disorder of secretion resulting in decreased salivary flow. The sialadenitis is usually unilateral, and the symptoms of recurrent tender swelling of the affected gland are mainly related to the associated obstruction. The duct orifice may appear inflamed, and in acute exacerbations there may be a purulent or salty-tasting discharge. Histopathological examination shows varying degrees of dilatation of the ductal system, mucous metaplasia of duct epithelium, periductal fibrosis, acinar atrophy with replacement fibrosis and elastosis, and chronic inflammatory cell infiltration (Fig. 4.4). Ductal obstruction, destruction of glandular tissue, and duct dilatation (sialectasia) may be demonstrated by sialography. Ultrasound examination may be used to distinguish between cystic and solid salivary lesions, and is sometimes helpful in this context. In the submandibular gland, progressive chronic inflammation may result eventually in almost complete replacement of the parenchyma by fibrous tissue, producing a firm mass that may be mistaken clinically for a neoplasm. This type of inflammatory reaction may be referred to as chronic sclerosing sialadenitis and is sometimes a feature of IgG4-related disease, which is a systemic chronic inflammatory disease characterized by tumour-like swellings that typically affect the pancreas, salivary glands, thyroid gland, and liver, although other organ systems may also be involved. The tumour-like swellings have three components: dense fibrous tissue that has a storiform pattern (like a woven mat); dense lymphoplasmacytic inflammatory infiltrate that contains numerous IgG4 positive plasma cells (>100 per high-power field in salivary gland disease); and obliterative phlebitis. Treatment is based on damping down the immune system with corticosteroids and other immunosuppressive drugs. It should be noted that IgG4-related

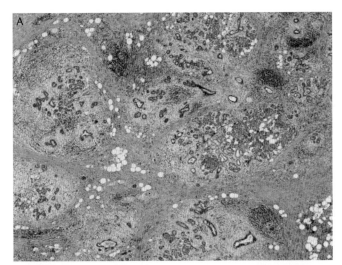

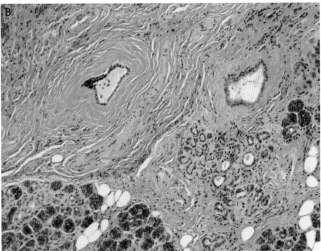

Fig. 4.4 Chronic bacterial sialadenitis showing patchy chronic inflammation, interlobular fibrosis, acinar atrophy, and peri-ductal fibrosis.

disease affecting the salivary glands may cause xerostomia and mimic Sjögren's syndrome.

Recurrent parotitis of childhood

The aetiology of recurrent parotitis of childhood is unclear but an abnormally low secretion rate predisposing to ascending infection and immaturity of the immune response in infants may be involved. Congenital abnormalities of the ductal system have also been suggested and almost all cases show sialectasia or some other duct abnormality on sialography. The condition may be unilateral or bilateral and is associated with recurrent painful swelling of the gland. Pus may be expressed from the duct orifice. In most cases the condition resolves spontaneously by the time the patient reaches early adult life, but repeated infection may result in irreversible damage to the main duct, predisposing to duct obstruction and recurrent parotitis in adult life. Treatment is supportive and includes adequate hydration, gland massage, and antibiotic management of active infection. Surgery is rarely required.

Viral sialadenitis

Mumps (epidemic parotitis)

Mumps is an acute, contagious infection that occurs in minor epidemics and is caused by a paramyxovirus. Before the introduction of the MMR (measles, mumps, rubella) vaccine in 1988, mumps was a common childhood infection. Whilst mumps is now uncommon in children, young adults who have not received the vaccine are the most likely to contract the disease. The virus is transmitted by direct contact with infected saliva and by droplet spread, and has an incubation period of 2–3 weeks. Non-specific prodromal symptoms of fever and malaise are followed by painful swelling of sudden onset, involving one or more salivary glands. The parotid glands are almost always involved, bilaterally in about 70% of cases, and, occasionally, the submandibular and sublingual glands may be affected, but rarely without parotid involvement. The salivary gland enlargement gradually subsides over a period of about 7 days. The virus is present in the saliva 2–3 days before the onset of sialadenitis and for about 6 days afterwards.

Occasionally in adults, other internal organs are involved, such as testes, ovaries, central nervous system, and pancreas.

The diagnosis of mumps is usually made on clinical grounds, but in atypical cases can be confirmed using molecular tests such as real time polymerase chain reaction for viral RNA in a saliva sample or by testing for IgM class antibodies in serum. After an attack, immunity is long-lasting and so recurrent infection is rare.

Other viral infections affecting the salivary glands

Human immunodeficiency virus (HIV) infection is associated with xerostomia and salivary gland enlargement (usually the parotid gland) and may mimic Sjögren's syndrome (Chapter 10). Similar features are seen in other viral infections such as hepatitis C virus (HCV), Epstein–Barr virus (EBV), and cytomegalovirus (CMV).

Radiation-induced sialadenitis

Radiation-induced sialadenitis is a common complication of radiotherapy and can also occur after radioactive iodine therapy for thyroid cancer. There is a direct correlation between the dose of irradiation and the severity of the damage. The damage is often irreversible, leading to fibrous replacement of the damaged acini and squamous metaplasia of ducts; but, with less severe damage, some degree of function may return after several months. Serous acini are more sensitive to radiation damage than mucous acini. Advances in the targeting of radiotherapy, such as intensity modulated radiotherapy (IMRT), can be used to minimize unwanted damage to the salivary glands.

Sarcoidosis

Sarcoidosis is a chronic granulomatous inflammatory disorder that may affect the salivary glands, particularly the parotid gland (Chapter 10). Parotid gland involvement presents as persistent, often painless, enlargement and may be associated with involvement of the lacrimal glands. Heerfordt's syndrome is a rare presentation of sarcoidosis that includes parotitis, uveitis (inflammation of the eye), and facial palsy (lower motor neuron palsy of the facial nerve).

Sialadenitis of minor glands

Sialadenitis of minor glands can be an incidental and insignificant finding, although it may be of diagnostic significance, e.g. in Sjögren's syndrome and sarcoidosis. Labial gland biopsy is sometimes performed to allow histopathological examination of a representative salivary gland because it can be readily accessed for biopsy with minimal morbidity. Minor gland sialadenitis is seen most frequently in association with mucus extravasation cysts and nicotinic stomatitis of the palate.

Very rarely, sialadenitis of minor glands may present with multiple mucosal swellings associated with cystic dilatation of ducts and chronic suppuration. This condition may be referred to as stomatitis glandularis or cheilitis glandularis when it occurs on the lips. The ductal cells often undergo oncocytic changes, where the cytoplasm becomes filled by mitochondria, imparting a granular eosinophilic appearance on H&E stained sections.

Obstructive and traumatic lesions

Duct obstruction and trauma are important factors in the aetiology of a number of salivary gland diseases, such as chronic sialadenitis in major glands and mucocoele in minor glands. Duct obstruction may be due to a blockage within the lumen or result from disease in or around the duct wall, such as fibrosis or neoplasia. It can involve any part of the ductal tree. Obstruction to the duct orifice is usually due to chronic trauma, e.g. from sharp cusps or overextended dentures, resulting in fibrosis and stenosis.

Salivary calculi (sialoliths)

Salivary calculi or stones cause obstruction within the duct lumen and can occur at any age, but are most common in middle-aged adults. Calculi may form in ducts within the gland or in the main excretory duct. Data on their distribution vary considerably but the submandibular gland is most frequently involved, accounting for about 70–90% of cases (Fig. 4.5). The parotid gland is the next most commonly involved, whereas sialolithiasis in sublingual and minor glands is uncommon and generally accounts for less than 2% of cases. Calculi are usually unilateral, although multiple stones in the same gland are not uncommon. The typical symptoms and signs of calculi associated with major glands are pain and sudden enlargement of the gland, especially at meal times when salivary secretion is stimulated. The reduction in salivary flow predisposes to ascending infection and chronic sialadenitis. The calculi

may be detected by palpation, but imaging is usually required and ultrasound examination is the first-line modality, if available. Calcified stones may be detected by radiography (Fig. 4.6). The stones may be round or ovoid, rough or smooth, and vary considerably in size. They are usually yellowish in colour and comprise mainly calcium phosphates with smaller amounts of carbonates (Fig. 4.7). On section, they may be homogeneous but many have a lamellated structure (Fig. 4.8). The aetiology and pathogenesis of salivary calculi are largely unknown. It is generally thought that they form by deposition of calcium salts around an initial organic nidus, which might consist of altered salivary mucins together with desquamated epithelial cells and microorganisms. Successive deposition of inorganic and organic material would produce a lamellated calculus. Ultrastructural studies have also shown that microcalculi form in acinar cells and stagnant secretions of the submandibular gland, especially during periods of secretory inactivity. Although in the normal gland these microcalculi are eliminated, if there is disturbed secretion, they could accumulate and lead to the formation of sialoliths. There is no evidence that sialolithiasis is associated with gallstones or kidney stones. The treatment of sialolithiasis is outlined in Box 4.1.

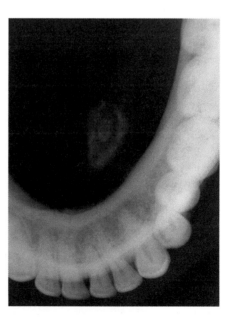

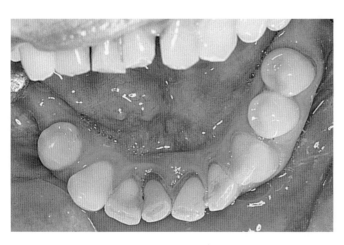

Fig. 4.5 Swelling of the floor of the mouth associated with a calculus in the submandibular duct (mirror view).

Fig. 4.6 Salivary calculus in the left submandibular duct (lower occlusal).

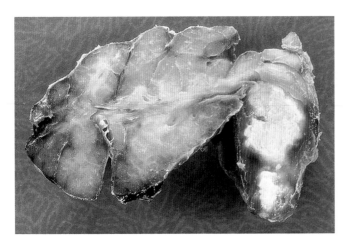

Fig. 4.7 Calculus in the intra-glandular portion of the submandibular duct.

Key points Duct obstruction and salivary calculi

- Duct obstruction may be due to: blockage of the lumen, disease in/around the duct wall, stenosis of the orifice
- Salivary calculi are commonest cause of duct obstruction
- Salivary calculi occur mainly in the submandibular duct
- Recurrent swelling related to gustation
- Duct obstruction predisposes to ascending infection and sialadenitis
- Turbid saliva may be expressed from the main duct on bimanual palpation

Salivary mucocoele

Cysts arising in connection with minor salivary glands are common and usually a consequence of trauma. The majority (90%) are of the mucous extravasation type, the remaining are mucous retention cysts. Treatment is surgical removal of the mucocoele and the associated damaged salivary gland.

Extravasation mucocoele

Over 70% of all mucous extravasation cysts arise in the lower lip, followed by the buccal mucosa and floor of the mouth. They are uncommon in the upper lip. By contrast, salivary tumours occur much more frequently in the upper lip than in the lower lip. The cyst occurs over a wide age-range but most affected patients are under 30 years of age and there is a peak incidence in the second decade.

Clinically, the lesion presents as a bluish or translucent submucosal swelling (Fig. 4.9) and there may be a history of rupture, collapse, and refilling, which may be repeated. It arises as a result of extravasation of mucus from a ruptured duct and a history of trauma can often be elicited from the patient.

Microscopically, the lesion typically consists of a mucin-filled cystic cavity or cavities lined by inflamed granulation tissue (Fig. 4.10). There is no epithelial lining, but a remnant of ruptured collecting duct lining may be present. The extravasated mucus evokes a chronic inflammatory reaction and the wall of the cyst is infiltrated by large numbers of macrophages with vacuolated cytoplasm containing phagocytosed mucin, called foamy macrophages (Fig. 4.10). Similar cells are seen within the extravasated mucus. In some cases the mucus is present as diffuse pools, rather than being contained within a more or less discrete cyst-like space.

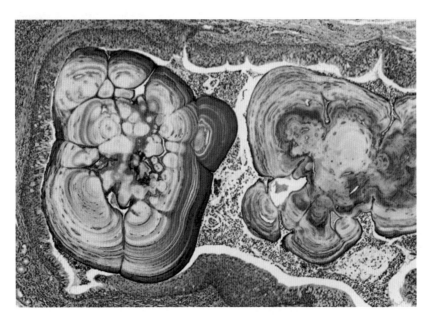

Fig. 4.8 Decalcified section showing a lamellated calculus in a dilated submandibular duct.

Retention mucocoele

By contrast to mucous extravasation cysts, retention mucocoeles occur most frequently in patients over 50 years of age and are most common in the upper lip. Most are derived from cystic dilatation of a minor gland duct and are lined by epithelium of ductal-type (Fig. 4.11). Retention cysts rarely form in the major glands. Because the mucus is still contained within the duct, there is no surrounding chronic inflammatory reaction. Occasionally, micro-sialoliths form in the inspissated mucus.

Ranula

Ranula is a clinical term used to describe a swelling of the floor of the mouth that is said to resemble a frog's belly (Fig. 4.12). Histologically, most ranulae are mucous extravasation cysts. Occasionally, a ranula may extend through the mylohyoid muscle and present as a swelling in the submandibular triangle of the neck, referred to clinically as a plunging ranula.

Necrotizing sialometaplasia

Necrotizing sialometaplasia is an uncommon disorder that clinically, and on histological examination, may be mistaken for malignant disease. It occurs most frequently at the junction of the hard and soft

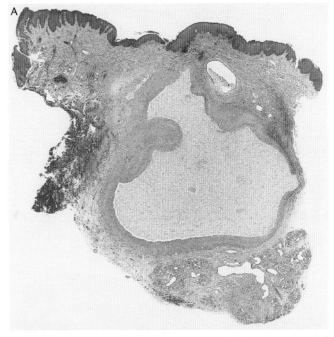
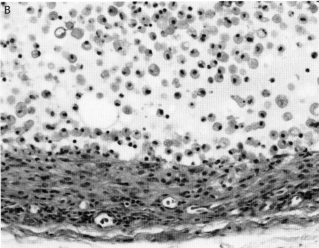

Fig. 4.10 Histology of a mucous extravasation cyst showing a pool of mucus. The cyst lining is composed of inflamed granulation tissue and there are numerous foamy macrophages floating in the pool of mucus.

palate in middle-aged patients, and is about twice as common in men as women. It typically presents as a deep crater-like ulcer that looks malignant (Fig. 4.13A).

Histopathological examination shows lobular necrosis of salivary glands, squamous metaplasia of ducts and acini, mucus extravasation, and inflammatory cell infiltration (Fig. 4.13B). The overlying palatal mucosa shows pseudo-epitheliomatous hyperplasia and the histopathological features may be mistaken for either squamous cell carcinoma or muco-epidermoid carcinoma.

Necrotizing sialometaplasia is thought to result from ischaemia leading to infarction of salivary lobules. In some patients there may be a history of trauma or embolism, but usually no cause is identified. Surgical excision is not required, but healing may take up to 10–12 weeks, producing a fibrous scar.

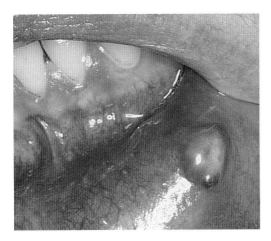

Fig. 4.9 Mucocoele.

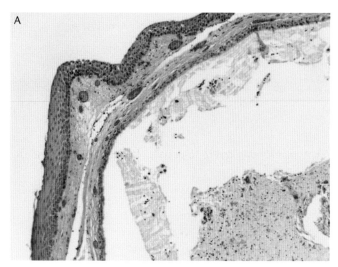

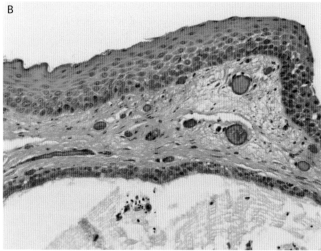

Fig. 4.11 Histology of a mucous retention cyst lined by ductal epithelium.

Sjögren's syndrome

Sjögren's syndrome is a chronic autoimmune disease characterized by lymphocytic infiltration and acinar destruction of lacrimal and salivary glands, leading to dry eyes and dry mouth. In about half of the cases

the syndrome occurs in association with another autoimmune disease, most frequently rheumatoid arthritis or systemic lupus erythematosis. On this basis the syndrome is divided into:

Primary Sjögren's syndrome. The combination of dry mouth (xerostomia) and dry eyes (xerophthalmia or keratoconjunctivitis sicca).

Secondary Sjögren's syndrome. The triad of xerostomia, xerophthalmia, and an autoimmune connective tissue disease (usually rheumatoid arthritis).

Unless otherwise specified, the general term 'Sjögren's syndrome' is used to encompass both types. In addition to xerostomia and xerophthalmia, Sjögren's syndrome can present with a wide spectrum of clinical features involving abnormalities of other exocrine glands and a variety of extra-glandular manifestations (Table 4.1). Criteria for the diagnosis of Sjögren's syndrome are given in Box 4.2. The investigations for Sjögren's syndrome are outlined in Box 4.3.

Clinical features

Sjögren's syndrome predominantly affects middle-aged females (female:male ratio 9:1), and symptoms related to dryness and soreness of the mouth and eyes are common presentations. Xerostomia may be associated with difficulty in swallowing and speaking, increased

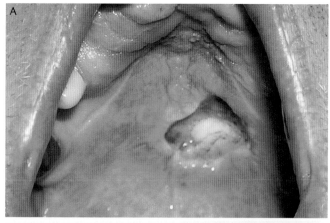

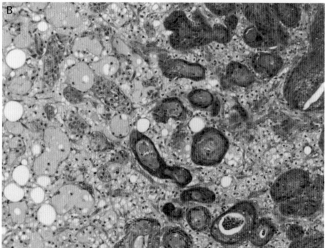

Fig. 4.13 Necrotizing sialometaplasia. Histology shows necrosis of salivary tissue (left) and squamous metaplasia of ducts (right).

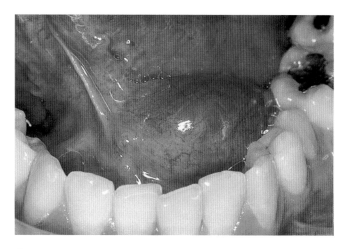

Fig. 4.12 Ranula.

Table 4.1 Sjögren's syndrome: features and associated systemic effects

Glandular (exocrine glands)	Features
Salivary	Xerostomia
Lacrimal	Xerophthalmia
Skin	Xeroderma
Respiratory tract	Nasal dryness, sinusitis, tracheitis
Pharynx and GI tract	Dysphagia, atrophic gastritis, pancreatitis
Genito-urinary tract	Vaginal dryness
Extra-glandular	
General	Chronic fatigue
Joints	Arthritis
Skin	Systemic sclerosis, Raynaud's phenomenon
Liver	Primary biliary cirrhosis
Renal	Renal tubular defects
Endocrine	Thyroiditis
Neurological	Central and peripheral neuropathies
Haematological	Anaemia, leucopenia, thrombocytopenia
Immunological	Autoantibodies, hypergammaglobulinaemia

fluid intake, and disturbances of taste. In addition, dry mouth predisposes to bacterial sialadenitis, dental caries, and oral candidosis. The oral mucosa appears dry, smooth, and glazed; lingual changes may be prominent, the dorsum of the tongue often appearing red and atrophic, and showing varying degrees of fissuring and lobulation (Fig. 4.14). Keratoconjuctivitis sicca manifests as dryness of the eyes

Box 4.2 American European Consensus Group Revised International Criteria for Sjögren's syndrome

- Ocular symptoms
- Oral symptoms
- Ocular signs
- Salivary gland function
- Ro and La autoantibodies
- Labial salivary gland histology
- Four of the six criteria need to be fulfilled for a diagnosis of Sjögren's syndrome

Source data from *Annals of the Rheumatic Diseases*, 61, Vitali C, Bombardieri S, Jonsson R et al., Classification criteria for Sjögren's syndrome: a revised version of the European criteria proposed by the American-European Consensus Group, pp. 554–558, 2002, BMJ Publishing Group Ltd.

Box 4.3 Investigations for Sjögren's syndrome

- Ophthalmic opinion to assess ocular signs resulting from reduced tear flow
- Assessment of salivary gland function: salivary flow rates, sialochemical studies
- Assessment of salivary gland involvement: ultrasound, sialography, scintigraphy
- Autoantibody screen, especially for anti-Ro and anti-La antibodies
- Labial gland biopsy to assess focal lymphocytic sialadenitis (Focus score)

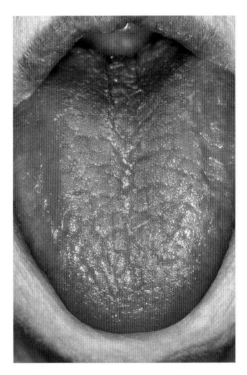

Fig. 4.14 Secondary Sjögren's syndrome showing changes to the tongue associated with xerostomia.

with conjunctivitis, and causes a gritty, burning sensation (Fig. 4.15). Salivary gland enlargement is very variable. Although approximately 30% of patients may give a history of such enlargement, it is only clinically apparent in about half that number. The enlargement is usually bilateral, predominantly affects the parotid glands and is seldom painful. Lacrimal gland enlargement is uncommon.

Histopathology

Histopathological examination of involved major glands shows lymphocytic infiltration, initially around intra-lobular ducts, which eventually replaces the whole of the affected lobules. The infiltration is accompanied by acinar atrophy, but in contrast, the ductal epithelium may show proliferation. The hyperplasia of ductal epithelium eventually obliterates the duct lumen leading to islands of epithelial tissue surrounded by sheets of lymphocytes, replacing entire salivary lobules. These

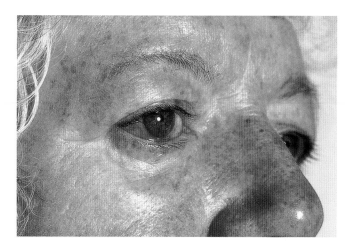

Fig. 4.15 Xerophthalmia in Sjögren's syndrome.

appearances are described by the term, 'salivary lympho-epithelial lesion' (Fig. 4.16). The salivary lympho-epithelial lesion is characteristic, but not pathognomic, of Sjögren's syndrome, as it also develops in the sialadenitis associated with hepatitis C virus infection and in HIV-associated salivary gland disease.

Clinical involvement of the minor salivary glands is uncommon, but they are involved at a microscopic level. The glands show focal collections of lymphoid cells, initially around the intra-lobular ducts, and the number of such foci reflects the overall severity of the disease. The semi-quantitative assessment of this focal lymphocytic sialadenitis in biopsies of labial minor salivary glands is an important investigation in establishing a diagnosis of Sjögren's syndrome and forms one of the internationally agreed diagnostic criteria (for Focus score, Box 4.4).

Other investigations

Other investigations useful in assessing the degree of salivary gland involvement include estimation of parotid salivary flow rates, which are usually reduced, and sialography, with or without CT, which shows varying degrees of sialectasis, often producing a 'snowstorm' or 'cherry tree in blossom'-like appearance (Fig. 4.17). Salivary scintigraphy using

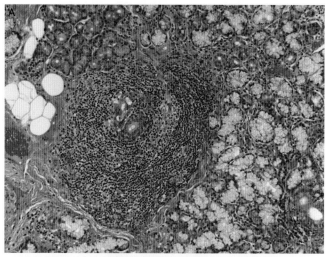

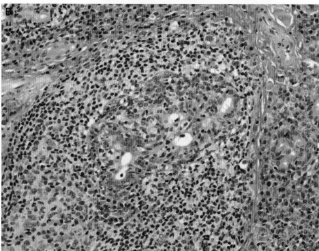

Fig. 4.16 Focal lymphocytic sialadenitis in a minor salivary gland biopsy from a patient with Sjögren's syndrome (A). High magnification showing a lympho-epithelial lesion with an epimyoepithelial island in the centre of the field (B).

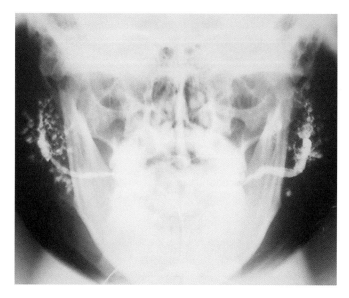

Fig. 4.17 Sialogram showing sialectasia in Sjögren's syndrome.

Box 4.5 Pathogenesis of Sjögren's syndrome

Pathogenic mechanisms in Sjögren's syndrome are complex and multifaceted, involving the interplay of T lymphocyte subsets, cell-mediated cytotoxicity, cytokine production, B cell hyperactivity, and autoantibody effects.

---

technetium-99m pertechnetate is also of value. The radioisotope is concentrated in salivary glands and its uptake is reduced in patients with Sjögren's syndrome. Characteristic changes on ultrasound examination are increasingly being recognized and this imaging investigation has the advantage of reducing patient exposure to ionizing radiation.

A variety of circulating autoantibodies can also be detected, of which antibodies to the extractable nuclear antigens known as Ro and La (also referred to as SS-A and SS-B, respectively) are the most important diagnostically. Anti-Ro antibodies are found in about 75% of patients with primary Sjögren's syndrome and are also found in patients with secondary Sjögren's syndrome. Anti-La can also be detected in 40% of patients with Sjögren's syndrome.

Although the immunological and histopathological findings in Sjögren's syndrome support an autoimmune pathogenesis (Box 4.5), little is known about either the aetiological factors underlying the disturbance in immunoregulation or the mechanisms involved in the destruction of the salivary and lacrimal glands. However, genetic factors are thought to be important in increasing the susceptibility of an individual to external environmental factors, which then trigger the disease. Sjögren's syndrome occurs with increased frequency in patients with particular combinations of the HLA class II major histocompatibility genes, supporting a genetic role, and several viruses, especially EBV, have been suggested as potential trigger factors. Immunological mechanisms leading to destruction of glandular tissue probably involve mainly T cells and their associated cytokines. The pathogenic significance of the range of autoantibodies that can be detected is uncertain but experimental studies suggest that some may be associated with functional disturbances in salivary secretion, exacerbating the xerostomia.

Risk of malignancy in Sjögren's syndrome

A recent meta-analysis indicates that patients with Sjögren's syndrome have an increased risk of developing any cancer (relative risk 1.53), a much higher risk of developing non-Hodgkin lymphoma (relative risk 13.76), and also have an increased risk of thyroid cancer (relative risk 2.58). The most common type of malignancy is a marginal zone B cell lymphoma (a type of non-Hodgkin lymphoma). The development of lymphoma is associated with proliferation of atypical lymphoid cells around existing 'salivary lympho-epithelial lesions'. As the malignant population expands, it destroys and replaces the gland. Marginal zone cell lymphomas tend to pursue an indolent course and remain localized to the salivary gland until late in their natural history.

Key points Oral problems associated with Sjögren's syndrome

- Xerostomia
- Stringy saliva
- Oral discomfort
- Change or loss of taste sensation
- Difficulty eating, swallowing, talking
- Salivary gland swelling
- Bacterial sialadenitis
- Dental caries
- Gingivitis
- Oral candidosis
- Angular cheilitis

Sialadenosis

Sialadenosis (or sialosis) is a condition characterized by non-inflammatory, non-neoplastic, recurrent bilateral swelling of salivary glands. The parotid glands are most commonly affected. It is probably due to abnormalities of neurosecretory control and has been reported in association with diverse conditions such as malnutrition, eating disorders, diabetes mellitus, chronic alcoholism, liver cirrhosis, and following the administration of various drugs. The histology of sialadenosis is characterized by hypertrophy of serous acinar cells to about twice their normal size.

Salivary gland tumours

Salivary gland tumours are uncommon with an annual incidence in the Western world of about 3 per 100,000 population; salivary gland malignancies are even rarer. Tumours of the major glands are far more frequent than those of the minor glands, which account for only about 15–20% of all salivary tumours. Of the tumours in major glands, 90% occur in the parotid gland and about 10% in the submandibular gland, sublingual gland tumours being rare (Table 4.2). Just over 50% of all minor salivary gland tumours arise in the palate and 20% in the upper lip, with the remainder scattered throughout the oral cavity. Tumours of the lower lip are rare. Although only a small fraction of salivary tumours occur in the minor glands, around 50% are malignant. Exceptionally rare examples of

Table 4.2 Salivary gland tumours in the major salivary glands

Site	Proportion of salivary gland tumours	Proportion that are malignant
Parotid gland	90%	15%
Submandibular gland	10%	30%
Sublingual gland	<1%	80%

salivary neoplasms, arising as central intra-osseous lesions of the jaws (mainly the mandible), have also been reported. These may be derived from ectopic entrapped salivary glands or from mucous metaplasia in the lining of odontogenic cysts.

Classification

About 40 different types of salivary gland tumours are recognized, although some of them are very rare. The classification and nomenclature used in this chapter are based on that proposed by the World Health Organization (2017). The tumours listed in Box 4.6 are all primary neoplasms of epithelial origin and account for the majority of salivary gland tumours. In addition to the primary tumours of epithelial origin, other neoplasms, such as soft-tissue tumours, malignant lymphomas, and metastatic deposits, may occasionally involve the salivary glands.

Box 4.6 Basic classification of salivary tumours

Adenomas

- Pleomorphic adenoma
- Warthin tumour
- Canalicular adenoma
- Basal cell adenoma
- Oncocytoma

Carcinomas

- Muco-epidermoid carcinoma
- Acinic cell carcinoma
- Adenoid cystic carcinoma
- Polymorphous adenocarcinoma
- Epithelial-myoepithelial carcinoma
- Salivary duct carcinoma
- Basal cell adenocarcinoma
- Carcinoma ex-pleomorphic adenoma
- Adenocarcinoma NOS

Adenomas

Pleomorphic adenoma

Pleomorphic adenoma is by far the commonest type of salivary gland tumour and accounts for 60–65% of all tumours of the parotid gland (Fig. 4.18) and for about 45% of all tumours of the minor glands, the most common sites being palate and upper lip (Figs 4.19 and 4.20). The tumour can occur at all ages but the majority of patients are in the fifth and sixth decades of life, and there is a preponderance of women (about 60% of cases). The tumour is usually solitary, although recurrences may be multi-focal, and presents as a slowly growing, painless, rubbery swelling that the patient may have been aware of for several years. The overlying skin or mucosa is usually intact. Neurological disturbance of the facial nerve or trigeminal nerve is not a feature of pleomorphic adenoma.

Pleomorphic adenomas show a great variety of histological appearances with complex intermingling of epithelial components and mesenchymal-like areas (Fig. 4.21). The diversity and complexity of appearances account for the term pleomorphic; the term does not imply cellular pleomorphism. The pleomorphic adenoma is a benign tumour, although a connective tissue pseudo-capsule does not always envelop the lesion completely. The pseudo-capsule may also show variation in thickness and density, but regardless of its completeness or not, the tumour is clearly demarcated (Fig. 4.22). Apparently, isolated nodules of tumour may also be seen within or even outside the capsule in histological sections, giving the impression of invasive growth, but these are in reality pseudopod-like outgrowths of the main mass (Fig. 4.23). Tumour may also be seen within vessels around the pseudo-capsule. Neither extra-capsular extension nor intra-vascular invasion should be taken as indicators of malignancy, or of malignant potential. An important aspect of the deficient encapsulation, and of intra- and extra-capsular nodules, is that they influence the surgical management of the tumour. Simple enucleation could establish a plane of cleavage within or just below the pseudo-capsule, leaving behind islands of neoplastic tissues in the tumour bed that could give rise to recurrence. For these reasons, pleomorphic adenoma is usually excised by extra-capsular dissection, including a margin of surrounding normal tissue.

There is considerable variation in the arrangement of the epithelial and stromal components between different tumours and within different areas of the same tumour. The epithelial component may be arranged in duct-like structures or as sheets, clumps, and interlacing strands (Figs 4.22 and 4.23). Both epithelial-duct luminal cells and myoepithelial-type cells are present. Duct-like structures in the tumour may vary in size, shape, number, and distribution, and are lined by epithelial luminal cells (Fig. 4.24). They often contain brightly eosinophilic mucin. Myoepithelial cells may be polygonal, spindle, or stellate-shaped. Occasionally, groups of ovoid cells with eccentric nuclei and abundant hyaline cytoplasm are seen. These plasmacytoid or hyaline cells are thought to represent modified myoepithelial cells and are considered to be a diagnostic feature of pleomorphic adenoma (Fig 4.24). Areas of squamous differentiation and epithelial keratin pearl formations may also be present.

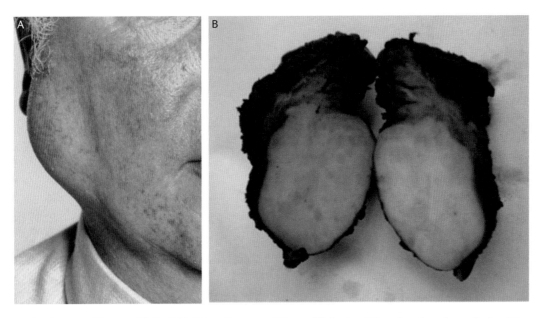

Fig. 4.18 Pleomorphic adenoma of the parotid gland. Facial swelling over right parotid gland and the cut surface of a surgical excision specimen (the surgical margins have been painted with black ink).

Some pleomorphic adenomas are highly cellular, whilst others contain abundant extracellular matrix. The matrix material varies in quantity and quality. It may be predominantly fibrous, but the most characteristic feature is the presence of myxoid and/or chondroid areas. These appearances are associated with the accumulation of abundant connective tissue mucins. In myxoid areas, tumour cells are widely separated and surrounded by mucoid material. In chondroid areas, isolated tumour cells appear as rounded cells lying in lacunae within the mucoid material, so that the tissue comes to resemble hyaline cartilage (Figs 4.21). These components are usually referred to as myxochondroid or chondromyxoid. They are composed of glycosaminoglycans and consist mainly of chondroitin sulphates produced by tumour cells showing myoepithelial differentiation. At operation, pleomorphic adenomas rich in mucoid material have the consistency of a fluid-filled sac and can easily rupture during surgical removal, allowing spillage and implantation of tumour cells into surrounding tissues, giving rise to multi-focal recurrences.

Malignant transformation is well recognized in pleomorphic adenoma, usually in tumours that have been present for many years. Sudden growth, neurological disturbance, such as facial nerve palsy, pain, or ulceration are all features that suggest malignant change in a longstanding salivary swelling.

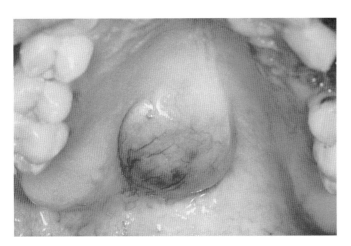

Fig. 4.19 Pleomorphic adenoma of the palate with prominent superficial blood vessels stretched over the tumour surface.

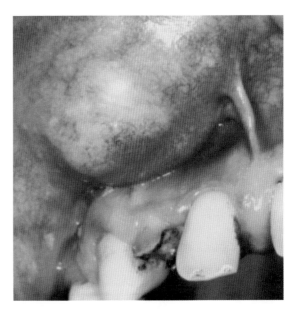

Fig. 4.20 Pleomorphic adenoma of the upper lip.

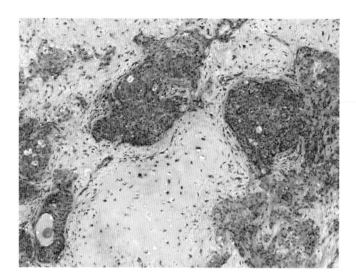

Fig. 4.21 Pleomorphic adenoma is characterized by a mixture of epithelial and mesenchymal components.

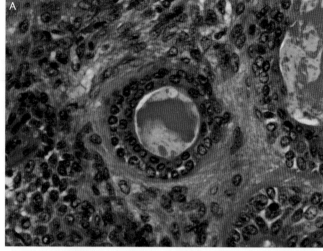

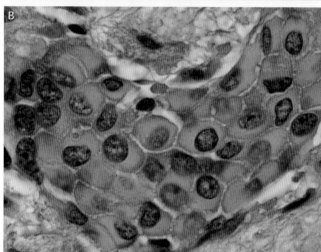

Fig. 4.24 Pleomorphic adenoma showing a double-layered duct structure with secretory material in the lumen (A). High magnification showing a nest of distinctive plasmacytoid hyaline cells (B).

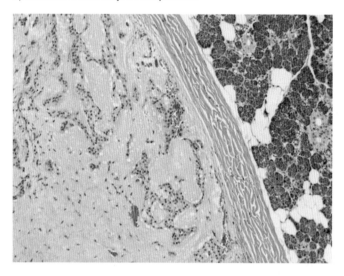

Fig. 4.22 An encapsulated pleomorphic adenoma clearly demarcated from the adjacent parotid gland (right) by a thick fibrous capsule (pink band).

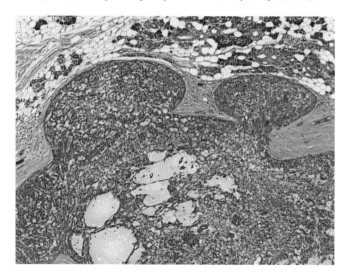

Fig. 4.23 Pleomorphic adenoma showing two pseudopodial-like extensions of tumour into the capsule.

Key points Pleomorphic adenoma
- Commonest of the salivary tumours
- Benign neoplasm
- Circumscribed tumour, but encapsulation variable
- Architectural diversity of epithelial and stromal components
- Epithelial and myoepithelial cells forming ductal structures, sheets, and reticular networks of cells
- Chondromyxoid stroma, connective tissue mucins produced by myoepithelial cells
- Requires complete surgical removal by extra-capsular dissection
- Recurrences tend to be multi-focal
- Longstanding pleomorphic adenomas may undergo malignant change

Warthin tumour

Warthin tumour occurs in the parotid gland and is a slow-growing lesion that may be multi-focal. Bilateral parotid tumours occur in 5–10% of cases and most patients are over 50 years of age. Occasionally, Warthin tumour may be discovered as an incidental finding on PET–CT imaging being performed for other reasons.

Warthin tumour is well circumscribed and has a brown cut surface (Fig 4.25A). The tumour has a characteristic papillary cystic structure and has multiple, irregular cystic spaces containing mucoid material separated by papillary projections of tumour tissue. Microscopically, the tumour consists of epithelial and lymphoid elements (Fig. 4.25B). The epithelial component, which covers the papillary processes, is double-layered and comprises cuboidal basal cells surmounted by columnar luminal cells. The epithelial cells have markedly eosinophilic granular cytoplasm rich in abnormal mitochondria, termed oncocytes (Fig 4.25C). The stroma contains a variable amount of lymphoid tissue that often includes numerous lymphoid follicles with sharply defined germinal centres. Warthin tumour is found mainly in tobacco smokers and is often regarded as a reactive rather than truly neoplastic disorder. Diagnosis can be made by fine-needle aspiration cytology (FNAC) that often collapses or reduces the lesion in size (Fig 4.26). Surgical removal is not always required once the diagnosis is established, as the lesion has a limited growth potential and does not undergo malignant transformation.

Canalicular adenoma

Canalicular adenoma occurs mainly in patients over 50 years of age and almost all cases are located in the upper lip. It consists of anastomosing strands of cytologically bland basaloid epithelial cells and may be partly or grossly cystic due to degeneration of its loose vascular stroma (Fig 4.27). Multiple canalicular adenomas may be encountered in some patients. In some cases, multiple microscopic foci of adenomatous change may be seen in surrounding minor salivary glands. They do not appear to be of clinical significance and should not be interpreted as invasive growth. Recurrence following surgical removal probably reflects the multi-focal nature of the disease, rather than any propensity to recur.

Basal cell adenoma

Basal cell adenoma accounts for about 1–2% of all salivary tumours, of which about 70% occur in the parotid gland and 20% in the upper lip. The peak incidence is in the seventh decade of life. The tumour is well encapsulated and consists of cytologically uniform basaloid cells typically arranged in a tubulo-tabecular pattern. Recurrence following surgical removal is uncommon.

Oncocytoma

Oncocytoma is a rare tumour usually arising in the parotid gland and occurring in patients over 60 years old. It is usually surrounded by a thin capsule and consists of sheets of oncocytes. Oncocytes are enlarged cells that are packed with mitochondria, imparting a granular eosinophilic appearance on H&E stained sections. Oncocytoma sometimes arises in a background of multi-focal oncocytic hyperplasia, which may affect the whole gland. Oncocytoma requires surgical removal and recurrence is uncommon.

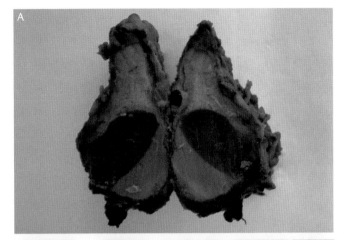
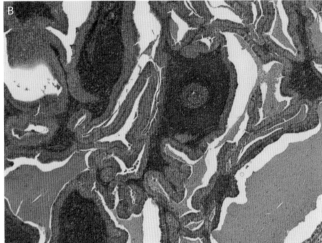
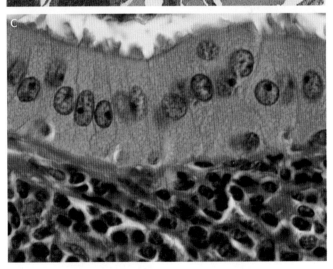

Fig. 4.25 Warthin tumour showing the cut surface of a surgical excision specimen (A). Histology shows the characteristic papillary cystic architecture with a lymphoid stroma (B) and high magnification of oncocytic ductal-type epithelium (C).

Carcinomas

Malignant tumours of the salivary glands are uncommon, accounting for less than 1% of all malignancies and about 5% of malignant tumours in the head and neck region. Although carcinomas of

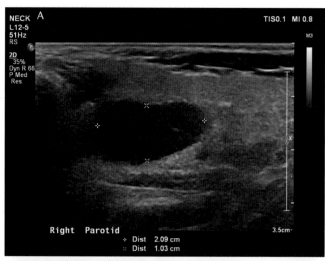

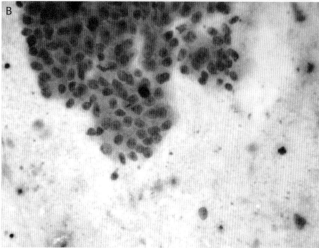

Fig. 4.26 Ultrasound image of a Warthin tumour in the parotid gland. A cytology preparation showing a papillary epithelial structure and proteinaceous fluid.

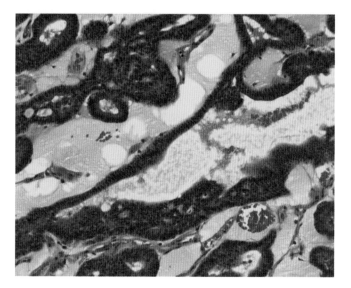

Fig. 4.27 Canalicular adenoma showing anastomosing strands of basaloid cells and a degenerate mucoid stoma.

salivary glands arise most frequently in the major glands, especially the parotid, the proportion of malignant to benign tumours is higher in minor glands. There are also differences in the incidence of the various types of carcinomas between major and minor glands. For example, the adenoid cystic carcinoma accounts for between 10% and 15% of tumours of the minor salivary glands, but only for about 3% of parotid gland neoplasms. The prognosis of salivary carcinomas depends on the histological type, histological grade (low, intermediate, or high grade), and tumour stage. High-grade tumours tend to present with advanced stage disease and have a poorer prognosis. For malignancies of the minor salivary glands, the staging system described in Chapter 3 is used (see Box 3.5). Major salivary gland cancers have a separate TNM classification, the T category reflecting the extent of tumour invasion of anatomical structures in the region of the major salivary glands (Box 4.7). Curative treatment is based around complete surgical removal +/− regional lymph node dissection +/− postoperative radiotherapy/chemoradiotherapy.

Muco-epidermoid carcinoma

Muco-epidermoid carcinoma is the commonest malignant salivary gland tumour, accounting for about 10% of all salivary tumours. Most occur in the parotid gland; in the minor glands, the palate is the most frequent site and very rare intra-osseous tumours occur.

Muco-epidermoid carcinoma may occur at any age but the highest incidence is during the fourth and fifth decades of life. There is a slight female predominance. The tumour often presents clinically in a similar manner to a pleomorphic adenoma, but grossly cystic tumours may be fluctuant and the more aggressive ones may be accompanied by pain and ulceration.

Microscopically, the tumours are characterized by the presence of squamous (epidermoid) cells, mucocytes, and cells of intermediate types that have the potential for further differentiation towards mucous or squamous cells (Fig. 4.28). The relative proportions of individual cell types and their arrangements vary from lesion to lesion. Muco-epidermoid carcinoma is graded into low, intermediate, and high grades using histological criteria, and these have been shown to be useful in predicting clinical outcomes (Table 4.3). Muco-epidermoid carcinomas are non-encapsulated and invasive. Some (mainly low- and intermediate-grade types) may appear to advance on a broad 'pushing' front, whilst others (mainly high-grade types) are ill-defined, highly infiltrative growths.

In low-grade muco-epidermiod carcinomas, mucus-secreting and epidermoid cells predominate, and there is minimal cellular pleomorphism. Such tumours are often cystic, either wholly or in part, the cysts being lined mainly by mucus-secreting cells (Fig. 4.28). The epidermoid cells are usually present in the form of clumps or strands that do not typically show keratinization but may also partially line the cysts. Discharge of mucus into the cysts can lead to their distension, coalescence, or rupture, in which case the release of mucus into the stroma is accompanied by inflammation.

In high-grade muco-epidermoid carcinomas, epidermoid and intermediate cells predominate, and there is nuclear and cellular pleomorphism, and nuclear hyperchromatism. Cystic spaces are not prominent and may be absent. In some cases separation of muco-epidermoid

Box 4.7 Clinical staging of carcinomas of the major salivary glands

T—primary tumour

T1 Tumour 2 cm or less in greatest dimension without extra-parenchymal extension.*

T2 Tumour more than 2 cm but not more than 4 cm in greatest dimension, without extra-parenchymal extension.*

T3 Tumour more than 4 cm and/or tumour with extra-parenchymal extension.*

T4a Tumour invades skin, mandible, ear canal, and/or facial nerve.

T4b Tumour invades base of skull and/or pterygoid plates, and/or encases carotid artery.

N—regional lymph nodes

N0 No regional lymph node metastasis.

N1 Metastasis in a single ipsilateral lymph node, 3 cm or less in greatest dimension, without extra-nodal extension.

N2a Metastasis in a single ipsilateral node, more than 3 cm not more than 6 cm in greatest dimension, without extra-nodal extension.

N2b Metastasis in multiple ipsilateral lymph nodes, none more than 6 cm in greatest dimension, without extra-nodal extension.

N2c Metastasis in bilateral or contralateral lymph nodes, none more than 6 cm in greatest dimension, without extra-nodal extension.

N3a Metastasis in a lymph node more than 6 cm in greatest dimension, without extra-nodal extension.

N3b Metastasis in a single or multiple lymph nodes with clinical extra-nodal extension.

M—distant metastasis

M0 No distant metastases.

M1 Distant metastases.

Stage grouping

Stage I	T1	N0	M0
Stage II	T2	N0	M0
Stage III	T3	N0	M0
	T1, T2, T3	N1	M0
Stage IVA	T1, T2, T3	N2	M0
	T4a	N0, N1, N2	M0
Stage IVB	T4b	Any N	M0
	Any T	N3	M0
Stage IVC	Any T	Any N	M1

*Extra-parenchymal extension is clinical or macroscopic evidence of invasion of soft tissue or nerve.

Reproduced from *TNM Classification of Malignant Tumours*, 8th Edn, Brierley J. D, Gospodarowicz M.K., Wittekind C. (Eds). Copyright (2017) with permission from John Wiley and Sons.

carcinoma from squamous cell carcinoma is problematic. The characteristic fusion oncogenes (Table 4.4) that are present in low- and intermediate-grade muco-epidermoid carcinomas may be absent in high-grade carcinomas.

The overall 5-year survival rate is about 70%. However, low-grade muco-epidermoid carcinomas have a local recurrence rate of less than 10% and a 5-year survival of about 95%. By contrast, high-grade tumours have been reported to have local recurrence rates of 80% and 5-year survival rates of only 30–40%. Figures vary for intermediate-grade muco-epidermoid carcinomas, falling somewhere between the two extremes.

Key points Muco-epidermoid carcinoma

- Commonest salivary malignancy
- Comprises mucous, epidermoid, and intermediate cells in varying proportions
- Low-grade tumour: mucous cells predominate; mucin-filled cysts common; good prognosis
- High-grade tumour: epidermoid and intermediate cells predominate; solid rather than cystic pattern; usually poor prognosis

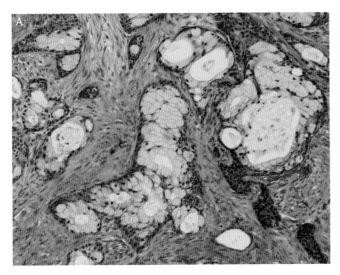
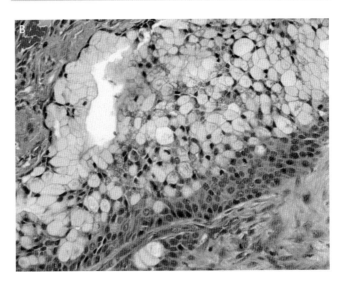

Fig. 4.28 Muco-epidermoid carcinoma showing mucus-filled cysts. High magnification showing a mixture of mucus-secreting cells (large pale cells) and epidermoid cells (smaller eosinophilic cells).

Table 4.3 Histopathologic features, point values, and scores used to grade muco-epidermoid carcinoma

Histopathological feature	Point value
Cystic component <20%	2
Neural invasion	2
Necrosis	3
4 or more mitoses/10^{HPF}	3
Anaplasia	4
Tumour grade	**Total score**
Low	0–4
Intermediate	5–6
High	7 or more

Reproduced from WHO Classification of Tumours. Pathology and Genetics of Head and Neck Tumours. Eds. Barnes L, Eveson JW, Reichart P, Sidransky D (2005).
HPF = high power fields

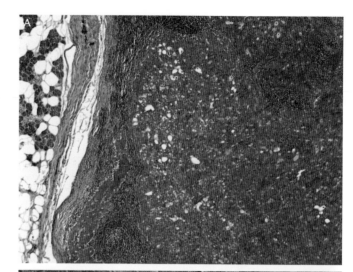

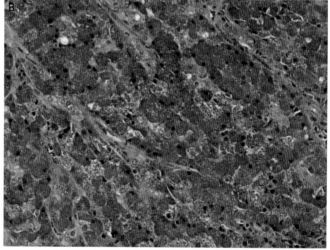

Fig. 4.29 Acinic cell carcinoma with a lobular outline (A). The tumour is composed of serous acinar cells that are packed with zymogen granules (B).

Acinic cell carcinoma

The acinic cell carcinoma is less common than muco-epidermoid carcinoma and the great majority arise in the parotid gland. Acinic cell carcinoma accounts for around 20% of malignant parotid neoplasms.

It presents a spectrum of histological appearances, but typically consists of sheets or acinar groupings of large, polyhedral cells that have basophilic, granular cytoplasm, similar in appearance to the serous acinar cells of salivary glands (Fig. 4.29). DPAS staining can be useful to identify the zymogen-like cytoplasmic granules. Other tumours may show a papillary cystic pattern, follicular or microcystic pattern, and contain other cell types, including intercalated duct cells and clear cells. A small number show obvious cytological features of malignancy and are termed de-differentiated acinic cell carcinomas.

It is not possible to predict the behaviour of acinic cell carcinomas on the histological features and no prognostic grading system has been validated. However, with the exception of de-differentiated types, acinic cell carcinoma is generally regarded as a low-grade malignancy and 5-year survival rates of 80–100% have been reported.

Adenoid cystic carcinoma

Adenoid cystic carcinomas usually arise in middle-aged or elderly patients. They account for up to 30% of minor salivary gland tumours, but only for about 6% of parotid tumours. Clinically, they may present as slowly enlarging tumours indistinguishable from pleomorphic adenoma, but pain and ulceration of the overlying skin or mucosa are much more common than in pleomorphic adenoma (Fig. 4.30). Parotid tumours may also present with facial palsy or unexplained facial pain. The neurological manifestations are a reflection of the predilection of the tumour to infiltrate and spread along peripheral nerves.

The tumour has a wide spectrum of histological appearances but, most commonly, the neoplastic epithelium is arranged as ovoid and irregularly shaped islands or as anastomosing strands lying in a connective tissue stroma. The characteristic feature of the tumour is the

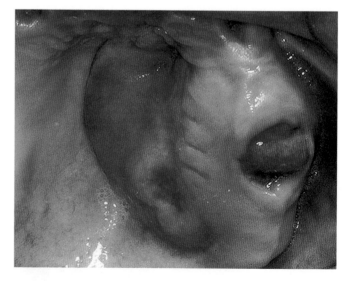

Fig. 4.30 Ulcerated adenoid cystic carcinoma of the palate.

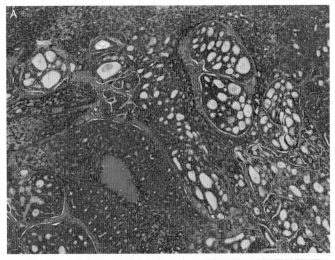

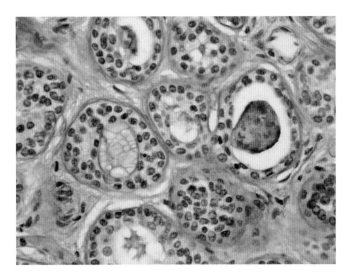

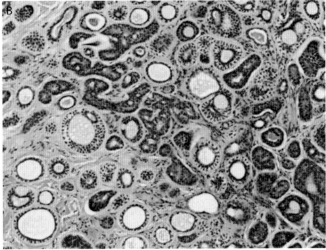

Fig. 4.31 Adenoid cystic carcinoma showing characteristic cribriform (A) and ductal arrangements (B).

Fig. 4.32 Adenoid cystic carcinoma stained with an Alcian blue (AB) and diastase periodic acid Schiff (DPAS). AB stains stromal mucin blue in a 'pseudo-ductal structure' (left). DPAS stains epithelial mucin purple in a tumour duct (right).

adenoid cystic carcinoma. Radiotherapy may be used to obtain palliation in inoperable cases, but is not curative. The disease runs a prolonged clinical course and metastases, usually via the bloodstream to the lungs, are a late feature. The long-term prognosis is poor and patients must be followed for much longer than 5 years before assuming that a permanent cure has been obtained. For example, survival rates for adenoid cystic carcinoma of the parotid are about 75% at 5 years, about 40% at 10 years, but less than 15% at 20 years. Cribriform and tubular types have a better prognosis than the solid type. The prognostic outcome for patients with primary tumours of the minor salivary glands appears less favourable than those arising in the major glands.

presence of numerous microscopic cyst-like spaces within the epithelial islands, producing a cribriform, lace-like or 'Swiss-cheese' pattern (Fig 4.31A). The spaces are formed by partial enclavement of areas of stroma or of mucoid materials produced by the tumour cells and deposited adjacent to the stroma. They contain acellular basophilic or, occasionally, hyaline substances rich in glycosaminoglycans and basement membrane-like material (Fig 4.32).

In adenoid cystic carcinomas showing the characteristic cribriform pattern, the epithelial component consists predominantly of small, rather uniform polygonal cells with angular hyperchromatic nuclei and basophilic cytoplasm. Mitoses are rarely seen. Less frequently, the tumour shows a tubular or solid pattern. Adenoid cystic carcinoma has a characteristic fusion oncogene, *MYB-NFIB*, which is present in 80–90% of tumours (Table 4.4).

Infiltration of adjacent tissues and spread along and around nerves are often prominent features and may be extensive (Fig. 4.33). In addition, in the maxilla, the tumour may infiltrate extensively along marrow spaces with little or no evidence of bone destruction, and these factors must be borne in mind in the surgical treatment of

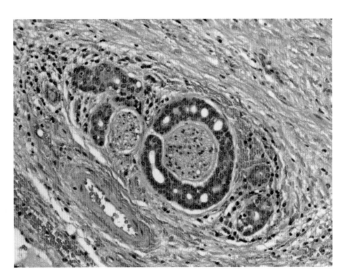

Fig. 4.33 Adenoid cystic carcinoma showing peri-neural spread.

Key points Adenoid cystic carcinoma

- Proportionally more common in minor glands
- Cribriform (Swiss-cheese pattern) is the commonest histological type
- Peri-neural invasion is characteristic
- Metastatic spread tends to be via the bloodstream to the lungs
- Poor long-term prognosis

Polymorphous adenocarcinoma

Polymorphous adenocarcinoma occurs almost exclusively in minor salivary glands and most present in the palate. The term 'polymorphous' refers to the morphological diversity of the growth patterns, which include solid, tubular, and cribriform areas that may mimic adenoid cystic carcinoma. The tumour cells appear cytologically bland; mitoses are infrequent, and nuclear atypia and hyperchromatism are lacking. Nevertheless, the tumour has an infiltrative pattern of growth and may show peri-neural whorling. Generally, the tumour has a good prognosis, although it has an unpredictable potential to metastasize in about 15% of cases. Recent molecular analysis has demonstrated that polymorphous adenocarcinomas have consistent abnormalities of the *PRKD1* gene (Table 4.4).

Epithelial-myoepithelial carcinoma

Epithelial-myoepithelial carcinoma is essentially confined to major glands and occurs mainly in the parotid gland. The neoplasm is characterized by double-layered ductal differentiation. Typically, the neoplastic ducts are comprised of a luminal layer of cuboidal or columnar epithelial cells and a myoepithelial layer of larger cells with cytoplasmic clearing. Often extensive sheets of clear myoepithelial cells are present. Generally, epithelial-myoepithelial carcinoma shows low-grade biological behaviour and the majority are cured by complete surgical excision, though metastatic disease sometimes occurs. No grading system has been validated that predicts outcome, and rare de-differentiated high-grade tumours have been described.

Salivary duct carcinoma

Salivary duct carcinoma is a rare tumour accounting for 1–3% of all malignant salivary gland tumours. The carcinomas are characterized by ductal formations and central necrosis, and often show a histological feature described as 'Roman bridging'. Salivary duct carcinoma resembles its counterpart in the breast, known as ductal carcinoma not otherwise specified. Salivary duct carcinoma is a highly aggressive neoplasm with less than 50% 5-year survival in most published series.

Basal cell adenocarcinoma

This is a generally low-grade adenocarcinoma that occurs mostly in the major glands. Histologically, the basal cell adenocarcinoma closely resembles basal cell adenoma and in some cases the two tumours cannot be distinguished in a core biopsy. The basal cell adenocarcinoma is identified by invasive growth at its boundary with normal salivary

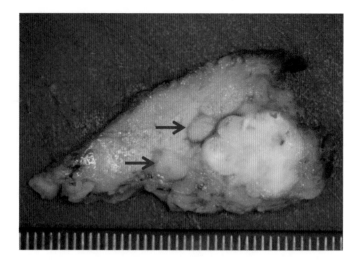

Fig. 4.34 Carcinoma arising in pleomorphic adenoma. The residual pleomorphic adenoma is the large heterogeneous yellowish nodule (right). Smaller areas of white, glistening carcinoma are seen outside the adenoma indicating an invasive pattern (arrows).

parenchyma and, therefore, the diagnosis is sometimes only made after excision of the entire tumour.

Carcinoma arising in pleomorphic adenoma

Carcinoma arising in pleomorphic adenoma is relatively uncommon and accounts for about 3% of salivary tumours, although the true incidence may be higher because the diagnosis is not always recognized. Almost all arise in pleomorphic adenomas of the parotid or submandibular gland that have usually been present for many years. The diagnosis requires evidence of a pre-existing pleomorphic adenoma remnant (Fig 4.34), but the adenoma may be overrun by the malignant tumour and all that remains is hyaline scar tissue. The malignant component is usually an adenocarcinoma or undifferentiated carcinoma but may assume the features of any of the types of salivary carcinomas (Fig 4.35). In some

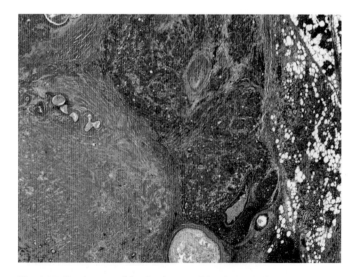

Fig. 4.35 Carcinoma arising in pleomorphic adenoma showing three components: scarred pleomorphic adenoma (left), high-grade ademocarcinoma (centre), and normal parotid gland (right).

Box 4.8 Risk stratification of salivary gland malignancy

- WHO classification is complex and includes 24 different carcinomas, some of which are exceptionally rare.
- Tumours can be classified into low-, intermediate-, and high-grade types for management purposes, but the clinical behavior of some tumour types remain unpredictable.
- Anaplasia, invasive growth, and necrosis are seen in high-grade carcinomas.
- Stage is a better prognostic indicator than grade.
- The 4-cm rule. Tumours less than 4 cm (T1/T2) generally have good prognosis, regardless of grade.
- Advances in molecular pathology may be the key to accurate diagnosis of salivary gland tumours and more effective treatment.

Table 4.4 Molecular pathology of key salivary gland tumours

Salivary tumour	Fusion oncogene	Diagnostic utility
Pleomorphic adenoma	*PLAG-1* fused to *CTNNB1*, *TCEA1* or others	Present in 30%
Muco-epidermoid carcinoma	*CRTC1-MAML2* (>80%) *CRTC3-MAML2* (<7%)	Present in most low and intermediate grades
Adenoid cystic carcinoma	*MYB-NFIB*	Present 80–90%
Polymorphous adenocarcinoma	*PRKD1* fusions to *ARID1A* or *DDX3X*; other abnormalities of *PRKD1* present	Also found in low-grade cribriform cystadenocarcinoma
Secretory carcinoma	*ETV6-NTRK3*	Defines the entity

tumours, more than one morphological type of carcinoma may be present. When the carcinoma component is still confined by the capsule of the pre-existing adenoma, the 'non-invasive' type, the tumour has an excellent prognosis, the same as for a pleomorphic adenoma. However, when there is infiltration of surrounding tissues, carcinoma arising in pleomorphic adenoma carries a poor prognosis. Five-year survival rates of about 55% falling to about 30% at 10 years have been reported.

Adenocarcinoma (not otherwise specified)

The diagnosis of adenocarcinoma not otherwise specified (NOS) is made by exclusion and is the term used for a tumour that does not fit into any of the other recognized types. Metastasis from a distant organ to the salivary gland should be considered before rendering a diagnosis of primary salivary adenocarcinoma NOS. Some examples may represent carcinoma arising in pleomorphic adenoma, where the adenoma remnant is not found. In the future, the use of molecular diagnostic tests may help to refine this diagnostic category.

Other types of salivary carcinoma

A variety of other histological types of salivary gland carcinomas are recognized in the WHO classification, but are rarely encountered. A pragmatic approach to risk stratification of salivary gland malignancy is outlined in Box 4.8.

Molecular pathology of salivary gland tumours

In recent years, a number of characteristic molecular alterations have been described in certain salivary gland neoplasms. Chromosomal translocations have been found, similar to those described in childhood sarcomas, and these may result in formation of abnormal fusion oncogenes (Table 4.4). The chromosomal translocations and 'signature' fusion products can be detected by fluorescence *in situ* hybridization (FISH), PCR, or next-generation sequencing techniques. Recently, a new type of salivary gland carcinoma, called secretory carcinoma, has been identified that has a microcystic architecture and cells with a fairly uniform nuclear appearance and granular or foamy eosinophilic cytoplasm (Fig. 4.36A). Morphologically, it most closely resembles acinic cell carcinoma, but secretory carcinoma is defined by a specific chromosomal translocation t(12;15)(p13;q25) leading

to formation of an *ETV6-NTRK3* fusion oncogene (Fig. 4.36B; Table 4.4). Advances in the understanding of the molecular pathogenesis of salivary gland tumours will facilitate accurate diagnosis and produce insights into the management of these rare cancers.

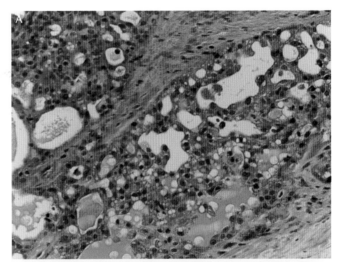

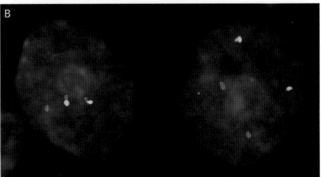

Fig. 4.36 Secretory carcinoma with a microcystic pattern composed of vacuolated cells. The FISH preparation shows that the malignant cells have the characteristic *ETV6-NTRK3* gene fusion demonstrated by close proximity of the red and green fluorescent probes (left). The normal cells have widely spaced fluorescent signals (right).
Courtesy of Professor Paul Speight.

5

Diseases of the teeth and supporting structures

Chapter contents

Developmental abnormalities of teeth

A wide variety of processes can affect the formation of teeth during development. The number, size, shape, and quality of dental hard tissue may be abnormal and teeth may erupt early or be prematurely shed or resorbed. When a child presents with a tooth abnormality, the clinical and radiographic features are often distinctive and management depends on diagnosis (Box 5.1). Broadly, developmental abnormalities of the teeth can be either genetically determined or acquired as a result of injurious processes affecting the developing teeth. It can be problematic to make a diagnosis, particularly when teeth initially erupt. Sometimes pathological examination of a shed or extracted tooth by ground sectioning (for enamel) or conventional sectioning of a decalcified tooth can provide a diagnosis. Research has provided insights into the genetic and structural basis of dental anomalies, and has resulted in a complex and extensive classification of subtypes. Minor abnormalities, such as failure of development of a few teeth or enamel erosion in adult life, may be dealt with in general dental practice, but it is advisable to refer younger patients with more complex or extensive dental abnormalities to a specialist in child dental health, with links to expert diagnostic facilities and input from orthodontic and restorative colleagues. The publically available Online Mendelian Inheritance in Man (OMIM) database provides an invaluable resource for genetic disorders, including dental abnormalities.

Disorders of number, size, and shape of teeth

Number

Supernumerary teeth are common and may be rudimentary in form or of normal morphology, when they are referred to as supplemental teeth. The most common supernumerary tooth occurs in the mid-line of the maxillary alveolus and is referred to as a mesiodens, which usually

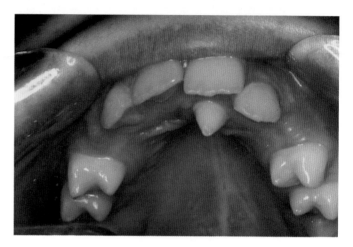

Fig. 5.1 Conical-shaped mesiodens in the palate.

has a conical shape (Fig. 5.1). Eruption of adjacent normal successor teeth may be impeded by a mesiodens, which is an indication for its removal. Most supernumerary teeth occur as a sporadic event in development, but multiple extra teeth can be found in certain developmental disorders (Table 5.1).

Failure of development of tooth germs results in teeth missing from the dental arch and is referred to as hypodontia (Fig. 5.2). Most often the missing teeth are third molars, second premolars, and upper lateral incisors. Hypodontia is more common in the permanent dentition than in the primary teeth. It is often symmetrical and severe forms can occur, with numerous missing teeth. Anodontia, where no teeth develop at all, is very rare. Hypodontia can be a feature of developmental disorders

---

Box 5.1 Establishing a history from a patient with a dental abnormality

- Primary dentition/secondary dentition/both affected
- Single tooth affected
- Multiple teeth affected—distribution (random/symmetrical)
- Location in the arch
- Crown—size, shape, colour (opaque white, yellow, brown, black), surface (smooth, ridged, pitted)
- Root—length, morphology, root canals (patent, obliterated), pulp stones
- Exfoliation—premature, delayed, root resorption
- Family history of tooth abnormalities
- Maternal medical problems and medications
- Childhood medical problems and medications
- Fluoride exposure
- Dental trauma/infection

Table 5.1 Hyperdontia associated with developmental disorders

Cleft lip/palate	Multiple teeth in anterior maxilla
Cleidocranial dysplasia OMIM 119600	Supernumerary teeth in all quadrants, retention of primary dentition, failure of eruption of secondary teeth, hypoplastic maxilla, high-vaulted narrow palate, flat cranial bones produce 'helmet-shaped' head, abnormal absent/hypoplastic clavicles.
Gardner's syndrome OMIM 175100	Supernumerary teeth, multiple odontomes, jaw osteomas, bowel polyps, and desmoid tumours.
Oculofaciocardiodental syndrome OMIM 300166	Double teeth, elongated dental roots, tall stature, microphthalmia.
Otodental syndrome OMIM 166750	Enlarged canine and molar teeth (globodontia), sensori-neural hearing loss, coloboma.

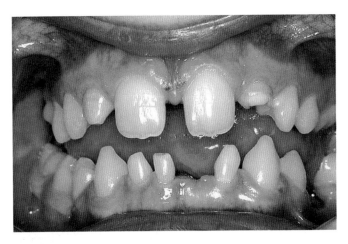

Fig. 5.2 Hypodontia with retention of deciduous teeth where successors are absent.

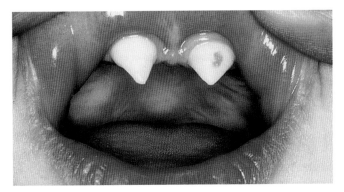

Fig. 5.3 Hypodontia and conical-shaped teeth associated with hypohidrotic ectodermal dysplasia.

maxillary lateral incisors. Abnormalities of tooth shape are outlined in Table 5.3 and illustrated in Figs 5.4 and 5.5.

Genetic disorders of dental hard tissues

Certain genetic disorders have systemic features that include dental abnormalities as part of the syndrome, whilst others affect teeth only.

Amelogenesis imperfecta

Amelogenesis imperfecta is a group of hereditary conditions affecting enamel formation. All the teeth, in both the primary and secondary dentitions, have abnormal enamel. The pattern of inheritance may be autosomal dominant, autosomal recessive, or X-linked. The molecular basis of amelogenesis imperfecta is complex and mutations have been described in a variety of genes; some encode enamel matrix proteins, such as enamelin, amelogenin, and matrix metalloproteinase 20 (Table 5.4).

Clinically it is possible to classify amelogenesis imperfecta into two main groups: hypoplastic types and hypomineralization (hypocalcified and hypomaturation) types.

Hypoplastic types

Secretion of enamel matrix is defective but mineralization is normal. The teeth may have enamel pits or grooves, but these are non-chronological in distribution. In some types of hypoplastic amelogenesis imperfecta,

(Table 5.2; Fig. 5.3). The genetic basis of hypodontia is complex; however, *MSX1* and *PAX9* genes are known key regulators of odontogenesis (Box 5.2).

Size and shape

Tooth size varies with both environmental and genetic factors, but precise definitions of normal size ranges have not been defined. An excessively large tooth is termed a macrodont and if the dentition is generally affected, it is known as macrodontia. Microdontia is associated with growth disorders, such as congenital heart disease and Down's syndrome. Some patients with Ehlers–Danlos syndrome, an inherited connective tissue disease, have microdontia, short roots, and pulp stones. The most common variations of the shape of crowns of teeth affect the

Table 5.2 Hypodontia associated with selected developmental disorders

Cleft lip/palate	Missing teeth anterior maxilla
Crouzon's syndrome OMIM 123500	Craniosynostosis, hypertelorism, exophthalmos, external strabismus, parrot-beaked nose, short upper lip, hypoplastic maxilla, mandibular prognathism.
Down's syndrome OMIM 190685	Intellectual disability, characteristic facies, trisomy 21.
Ellis–van Creveld syndrome OMIM 225500	Short limbs, short ribs, postaxial polydactyly, dysplastic nails, congenital cardiac defects.
Hypohidrotic ectodermal dysplasia OMIM 305100, other types known	Smooth dry skin, sparse fine hair, partial or complete absence of sweat glands (hyperthermia), nail abnormalities, severe hypodontia, conical teeth.
Oro-facialdigital syndrome OMIM 311200	Malformations of the face, oral cavity, and digits.

Box 5.2 Molecular basis of hypodontia

MSX1 and *PAX9* are part of a complex regulatory network of transcription factors and signalling molecules involved in odontogenesis.

In humans, heterozygous *MSX1* and *PAX9* gene mutations cause hypodontia.

Msx1 and *Pax9* are essential for tooth formation in mice. In the absence of either gene (gene knock out), tooth formation is arrested at the bud stage causing anodontia.

Pax9 hypomorphic mice (partial gene knock down) have hypodontia, indicating the importance of gene dosage for the development of individual teeth.

Table 5.3 Abnormalities of tooth shape

Peg-shaped maxillary lateral incisors	Maxillary lateral incisors are small and have a tapered or conical crown
	Common dental abnormality
Invaginated odontome (Dens in dente)	Ranges from deep cingulum pit to gross change with a dilated root (dilated or 'gestant' odontome)
	Usually maxillary lateral incisors
Evaginated odontome	Extra cusp-like tubercles, which usually arise from the palatal surfaces of maxillary incisors or occlusal surfaces of premolars
	'Talon cusps' on palatal surfaces of maxillary lateral incisors
Enamel pearl (Enameloma)	Small 'droplet' of enamel on root surface, usually near the furcation of the roots of maxillary permanent molar teeth
Conical teeth	Mesiodens
	Hypohidrotic ectodermal dysplasia (also have hypodontia)
Double teeth	Two teeth joined by fusion (joining of two separate tooth buds) or gemination (two teeth develop from one tooth bud)
	Sporadic or syndromic (e.g. oculofaciocardiodental syndrome)
Taurodontism	Elongated pulp chamber, greater occluso-apical height, no cervical constriction
	Sporadic or syndromic (e.g. Klinefelter's syndrome)
Dilaceration	Bent tooth, the crown of the tooth is displaced from its normal alignment with the root
	Association with trauma to the developing teeth, usually central incisors
Concrescence	Two tooth roots joined by cementum, acquired abnormality associated with hypercementosis
Congenital syphilis	Screw driver-shaped, notched incisors and 'mulberry' molars
	Historical interest, very rare

the enamel is very thin and translucent, giving the incisor teeth a chisel-like form (Fig. 5.6).

Hypomineralization (hypocalcified and hypomaturation) types

There is defective enamel mineralization producing a broad spectrum of clinical appearances. Generally, the enamel tends to be opaque, rather than translucent, producing discoloured teeth. In hypocalcified types, the enamel has a chalky texture and is often yellow or brown in colour. The hypocalcified enamel is prone to excessive wear and the underlying dentine becomes exposed, causing pain and hypersensitivity. In hypomaturation types, the enamel tends to be hard, yet brittle, and easily chips off the crown (Fig. 5.7).

Dentinogenesis imperfecta

Mutation of the *DSPP* gene that encodes dentine phosphoprotein and dentine sialoprotein causes dentinogenesis imperfecta (OMIM 125490). Dentinogenesis imperfecta affects only the teeth and must be distinguished from osteogenesis imperfecta with opalescent teeth, which is caused by mutation of the *COL1A1* and *COL1A2* genes (Chapter 7). In dentinogenesis imperfecta, the teeth are blue-grey or amber-brown and opalescent (Fig. 5.8). On radiographs, the teeth have bulbous crowns, slender roots, and have narrow or completely obliterated pulp chambers (Fig. 5.9). The enamel may split readily from the dentine when subjected to occlusal forces. Both primary and secondary dentitions are affected and, histologically, the dentine contains widely spaced and irregular dentinal tubules (Fig. 5.10).

Dentine dysplasia

Dentine dysplasia is a genetic disorder of teeth, commonly exhibiting an autosomal dominant inheritance. It is characterized by presence of normal enamel but atypical dentine with abnormal pulpal morphology. Two types of dentine dysplasia are described. Radicular dentine dysplasia (Type I, OMIM 125400) is characterized by microdontia and short roots. The teeth tend to exfoliate spontaneously because root formation is inadequate. On histological examination of exfoliated permanent teeth, the enamel and coronal dentine formation is normal but the root dentine shows a 'sand dune' or 'water flowing around boulders' appearance, fills the pulp chamber, and arrests, failing to form a functional root. Mutations in the *SMOC2* gene are reported. Coronal dentine dysplasia (Type II, OMIM 125420) is an allelic variant of dentinogenesis imperfecta and is caused by mutation in *DSPP*. The crowns may be normal but the pulps are enlarged and are described as having a 'thistle-shaped' appearance in the permanent dentition.

Cemental hypoplasia or aplasia

Mutations of the *ALPL* gene result in hypophosphatasia (OMIM 241510), in which there is defective alkaline phosphatase activity that results in abnormal bone mineralization. Tooth exfoliation results from lack of functional cemental attachment. Five clinical types of hypophosphatasia are described with very variable severity, ranging from infantile lethal to mild types that affect only the teeth.

Acquired disorders of dental hard tissues

Localized defects and chronological hypoplasia

Abnormalities of dental hard tissues may be acquired during development through injury to tooth germs or after teeth have erupted. Disturbance of ameloblast function during the formation of enamel can lead to the development of a groove or pit in the enamel surface. Shortly after eruption, the enamel defects are often colonized by bacteria and their products, together with dietary components, frequently stain the crown, resulting in an unsightly appearance.

Local factors, such as dental trauma and periapical infection of a primary tooth, are the most common causes of damage to successor tooth germs and developing teeth. Isolated idiopathic enamel opacities also occur. Teeth with such imperfections are called 'Turner teeth' (Fig. 5.11).

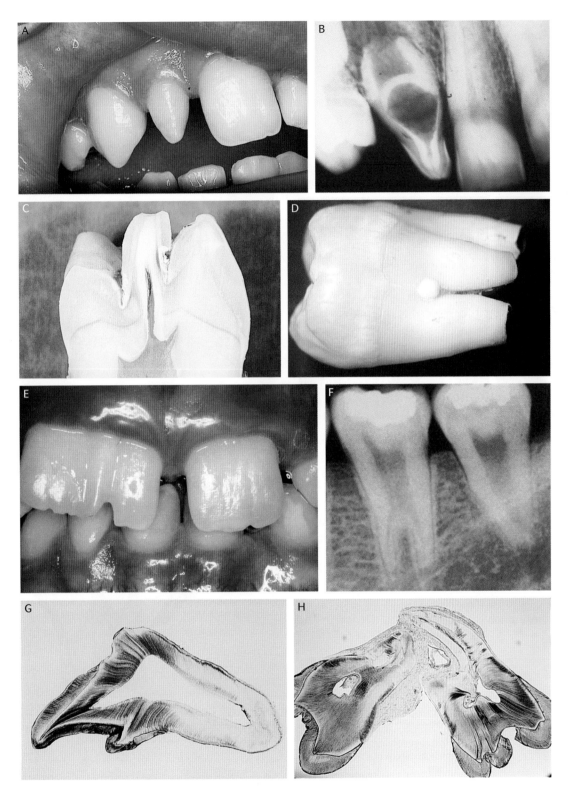

Fig. 5.4 (A) Peg-shaped maxillary lateral incisor. (B) Radiograph of an invaginated odontome (dens-in-dente). (C) Bisected evaginated odontome. (D) Enamel pearl. (E) Double teeth involving the maxillary incisors. (F) Taurodonts. (G) Ground section of a dilacerated central incisor. (H) Ground section of concrescence of maxillary molars.

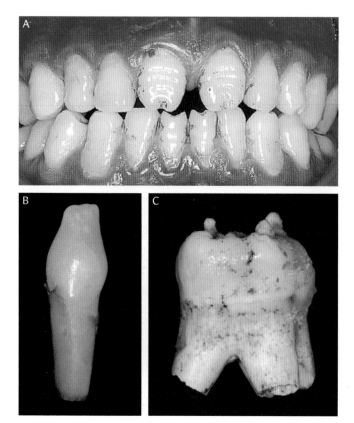

Fig. 5.5 Tooth abnormalities in congenital syphilis. Hutchinson's incisor and a mulberry molar.
Courtesy of Dr Pia Nystrom, University of Sheffield.

Systemic diseases acquired during the period of tooth development may affect multiple teeth at different stages of development, resulting in 'chronological' enamel hypoplasia. Systemic infection during the period of tooth formation is the most important cause, but metabolic disturbance and medications such as tetracycline can also cause enamel hypoplasia (Box 5.3). The temporal features of the disturbance will determine the pattern of enamel hypoplasia and the teeth that are affected. If the causative agent operates for a finite period, teeth will be

Table 5.4 Three genes mutated in amelogenesis imperfecta

Gene	Protein	Clinical features
ENAM	Enamelin	Most common, autosomal dominant and recessive forms known
AMELX	Amelogenin	X-linked, can produce alternating bands of normal and abnormal enamel
MMP20	Matrix metalloproteinase 20	Autosomal recessive, hypomineralized types as MMP20 required for removal of enamel matrix

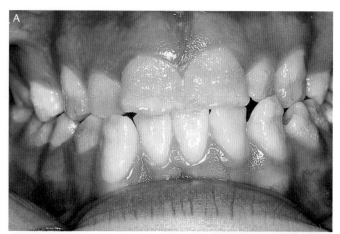

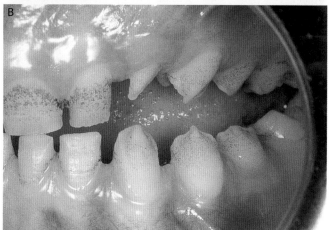

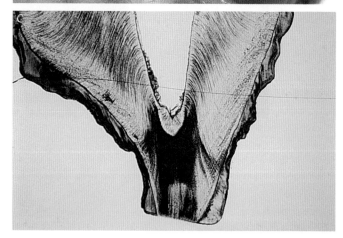

Fig. 5.6 Amelogenesis imperfecta, hypoplastic-types. Ground section showing pitting and roughness of the enamel.

affected according to the stage of development of the tooth germs, producing a band-like enamel defect (Figs 5.12 and 5.13).

Profound metabolic disturbances, e.g. rickets, hypophosphataemia (vitamin D resistant rickets), and hypophosphatasia, also affect the developing dentine. Typically, the predentine layer is expanded and there are increased amounts of interglobular dentine (Fig. 5.14). Enlarged pulp chambers, elongated pulp horns, and stunted roots are also a feature.

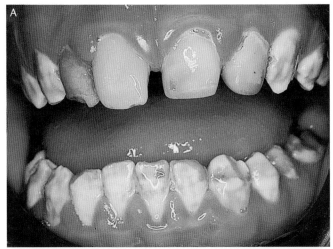

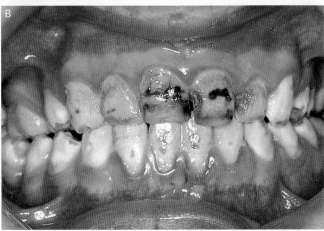

Fig. 5.7 Amelogenesis imperfecta, hypomineralization-types.

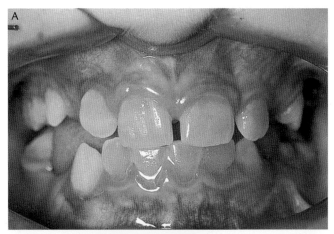

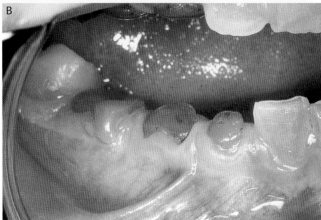

Fig. 5.8 Dentinogenesis imperfecta showing opalescent amber-like appearance of the teeth and marked attrition of the primary dentition.

Molar–incisor hypomineralization

Some patients present with a characteristic pattern of enamel hypomineralization affecting some or all of the first permanent molars and incisor teeth (often maxillary are more affected than mandibular incisors). The enamel has a yellow-brown appearance and may undergo rapid post-eruptive breakdown. It is suspected that a chronological defect in enamel maturation causes this condition and whilst many aetiological factors have been suggested, including childhood and maternal illness, medication, and toxins, the cause often remains elusive.

Regional odontodysplasia

Also known as 'ghost teeth', regional odontodysplasia typically involves one to three teeth in a quadrant of the jaw. The affected teeth typically show grossly abnormal development and usually fail to erupt. On radiographs, the affected teeth are distorted and misshapen, with abnormal enamel and dentine formation (Fig. 5.15). Often the pulp chamber is large and the root is curved or bent. The thin layer of poorly mineralized, circumpulpal dentine and abnormal enamel produces a ghostly outline of a tooth. Calcification of the follicle is typically found. The aetiology is unknown but vascular disturbance or viral infections have been suggested as possible causes. Segmental odontomaxillary dysplasia is a closely related condition, where missing or malformed teeth are found in an expanded area of abnormal fibrous alveolus in the posterior maxilla.

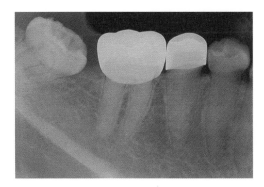

Fig. 5.9 Radiograph of teeth in dentinogenesis imperfecta showing obliteration of the root canals.

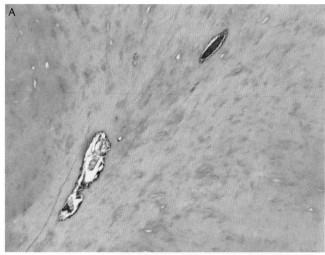

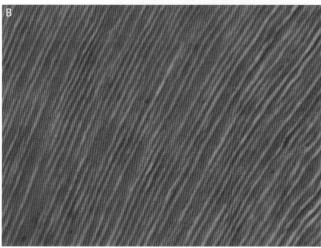

Fig. 5.10 Abnormal dentine in dentinogenesis imperfecta (A) and normal dentine tubules shown for comparison (B).

Box 5.3 Chronological enamel hypoplasia

Prenatal period

- Maternal infections (e.g. rubella, syphilis)
- Maternal systemic disease
- Excess fluoride

Neonatal period

- Premature birth
- Haemolytic disease of the newborn
- Hypocalcaemia
- Excess fluoride

Postnatal period

- Severe childhood infections (e.g. measles)
- Chronic diseases in childhood (e.g. congenital heart disease, gastrointestinal diseases, endocrine diseases)
- Nutritional deficiencies (e.g. vitamin D)
- Cancer chemotherapy
- Excess fluoride

Fluorosis

Enamel is mostly composed of the mineral hydroxyapatite and carbonated hydroxyapatite. When fluoride is taken up during tooth development, fluorapatite replaces part of the hydroxyapatite. Excessive fluoride can cause white spots and, in severe cases, brown stains, pitting, or mottling of the enamel (Fig. 5.16). Fluorapatite is beneficial because it is more resistant to dissolution by acids than other forms of apatite. Fluorosis usually affects permanent teeth but, occasionally, may involve the primary teeth. Clinically, concern in dental fluorosis is related only to the aesthetic changes to the permanent dentition.

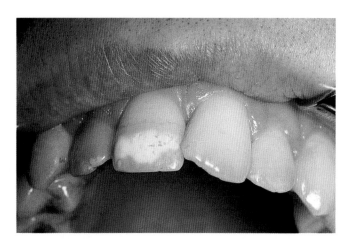

Fig. 5.11 Idiopathic enamel opacity.

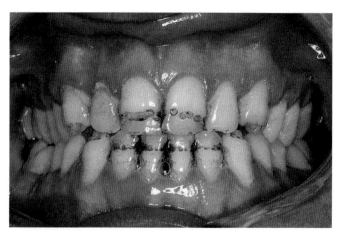

Fig. 5.12 Chronological hypoplasia of enamel associated with measles in early childhood.

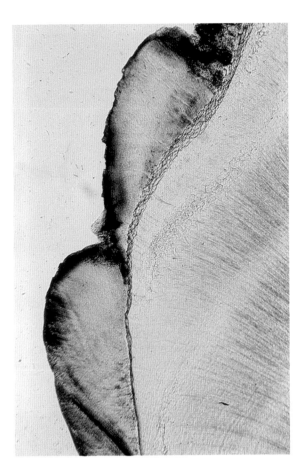

Fig. 5.13 Ground section of a tooth with pitting of enamel due to chronological hypoplasia.

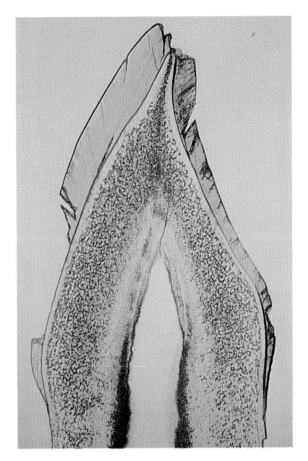

Fig. 5.14 Ground section of a tooth from a patient with hypophosphataemia showing prominent interglobular dentine.

Changes occur when excess fluoride exposure occurs between 1 and 4 years of age. The severity of dental fluorosis depends on the amount of fluoride exposure, the age of the child, individual response, weight, physical activity, nutrition, and bone growth. Over-exposure to fluoride may result from inappropriate use of fluoride supplements, diet, environmental pollution, and water supplies. Naturally high levels of fluoride in water occur in some rural areas. Fluoride at 1 ppm in water supplies is generally considered optimal for prevention of caries and avoidance of dental fluorosis.

Pigmentation of teeth

Tooth pigmentation may be classified as *intrinsic* or *extrinsic*. Generalized intrinsic tooth pigmentation is caused by the incorporation of pigment into dental hard tissue during development. Intrinsic pigmentation may be due to genetic factors such as porphyria, which results in red teeth or environmental factors such as tetracycline drugs taken before the age of 8 years, which results in grey-green tooth discoloration (Fig. 5.17). Intrinsic discoloration of individual teeth is usually caused by pulp necrosis and is due to leaching of haemoglobin-derived pigments into the dentinal tubules (Fig. 5.18). Extrinsic tooth pigmentation occurs when the teeth are normal after eruption but

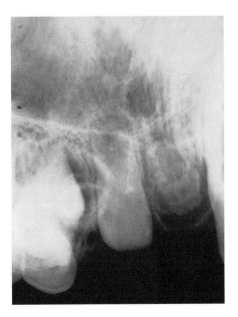

Fig. 5.15 Radiograph of anterior maxillary teeth in regional odontodysplasia.

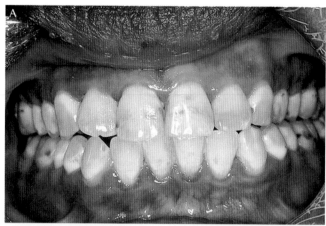

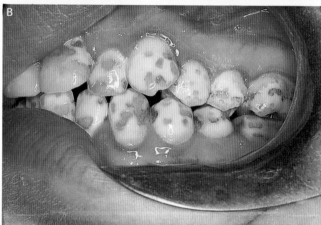

Fig. 5.16 Dental fluorosis.

pigment from bacteria, diet, habits such as paan chewing and smoking, or medicaments are deposited on the enamel surface (Fig. 5.19). Extrinsic pigment can usually be removed easily but if there is enamel pitting, it can be difficult.

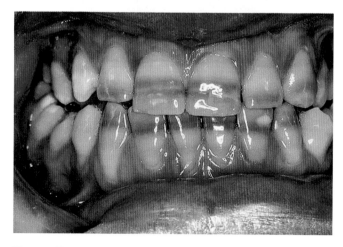

Fig. 5.17 Tetracycline staining. Note the chronological distribution.

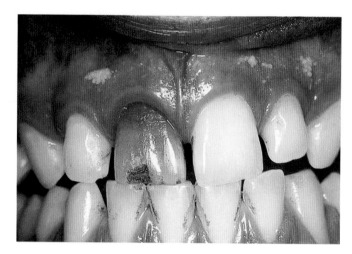

Fig. 5.18 Discoloration following pulpal necrosis.

Hypercementosis

The coronal third of the root is normally covered only by a thin layer of acellular (primary) cementum, whereas the apical two-thirds and furcation areas are covered by an additional thicker layer of cellular (secondary) cementum. Cellular cementum continues to be formed throughout the life of the tooth. The thickness of the cementum varies considerably between individuals but generally increases with age. Hypercementosis (Figs 5.20 and 5.21) may be idiopathic or the result of local or general disorders (Box 5.4). It may affect one or several teeth and it may be associated with root ankylosis, when cementum is directly continuous with the alveolar bone, or with concrescence (Fig. 5.4). Sometimes an ankylosed primary tooth may appear to 'submerge' back into the alveolus after eruption, as a result of jaw growth enveloping the crown (Fig 5.22).

Abnormal eruption

Natal and neonatal teeth are present at, or within a month of, birth. Commonly, such teeth are located in the anterior mandible or maxilla. Extraction may be necessary if the tooth interferes with feeding or is excessively mobile due to an incomplete or malformed root. Ectopic eruption may result in transposition of teeth. Local failure

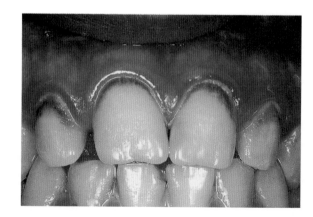

Fig. 5.19 Extrinsic staining associated with chromogenic bacteria.

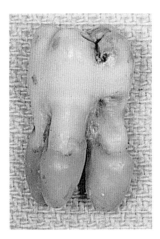

Fig. 5.20 Hypercementosis of a molar tooth.

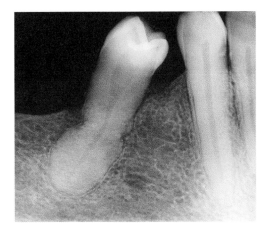

Fig. 5.21 Hypercementosis associated with excessive occlusal load.

Box 5.4 **Causes of hypercementosis**

Localized causes

- Periapical inflammation
- Excessive mechanical stimulation
- Functionless and unerupted teeth

Generalized causes

- Paget's disease of bone (Chapter 7).

of tooth eruption may result from a supernumerary tooth, an odontome, or ankylosis of a retained primary tooth. A dentigerous/eruption cyst may also impede the eruption of an affected successor tooth (Chapter 6). Generalized delayed eruption is a feature of cleidocranial dysplasia (Fig. 5.23), hypothyroidism (cretinism), and Down's syndrome.

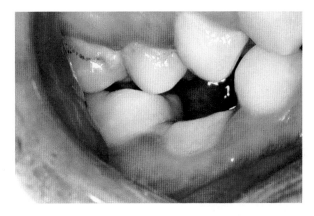

Fig. 5.22 Submerged mandibular primary second molar.

Tooth wear

Progressive loss of the tooth surface due to actions other than those that cause dental caries is commonly known as tooth wear. The prevalence and severity of tooth wear increases with age and it ranges from around 15% for 12-year-olds to 90% for over 65-year-olds. Tooth wear is caused

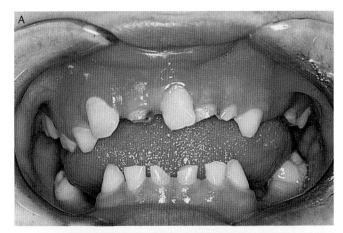

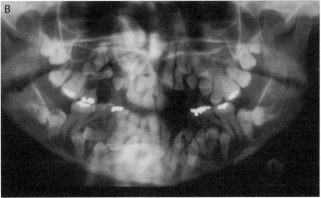

Fig. 5.23 Patients with cleidocranial dysplasia show retention of primary teeth, failure of eruption of secondary teeth, and multiple impactions.

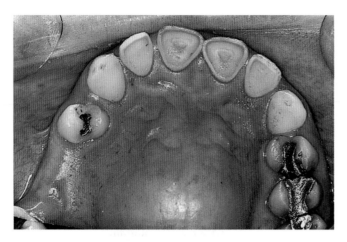

Fig. 5.24 Erosion of the palatal surfaces of the maxillary teeth in bulimia nervosa.

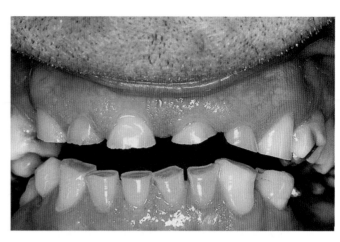

Fig. 5.25 Attrition.

by four phenomena: erosion, attrition, abrasion, and abfraction, though in many individuals tooth surface loss is multi-factorial and a combination of these processes.

Erosion is the progressive loss of tooth substance by chemical or acid dissolution, and no bacteria are involved. Erosion of tooth surfaces mostly results from excessive consumption of carbonated drinks (including sparkling water) and fruit juices with high levels of acidity. Severe enamel erosion of this type may be seen in teenagers and young adults. Typically, the labial enamel is smooth, shiny, and thin, sometimes with exposure of the underlying dentine. When erosion is due to gastro-oesophageal reflux disease or from bulimia, then the palatal enamel is more severely affected (Fig. 5.24). In addition, the risk of erosion is high in individuals with a low salivary flow rate.

Attrition is the progressive loss of dental hard tissue caused by mastication or grinding between opposing teeth. Mild attrition is normal in some populations where there is a coarse diet, but severe attrition from this may result in pulp exposure and overclosure. Habitual clenching or grinding of the teeth (bruxism) may also result in severe attrition (Fig. 5.25).

Abrasion is the progressive loss of tooth surface caused by mechanical actions other than tooth-to-tooth contacts. Abrasion is commonly associated with inappropriate toothbrushing technique, typically giving rise to cervical notching (Fig. 5.26). Abrasion may result from use of teeth as a tool to remove bottle tops or hold pins, clips, or nails. Oral piercing with the long-term use of intra-oral jewellery may also cause tooth abrasion and gingival injury.

Abfraction is the term used to describe the concentration of mechanical stresses around the amelo-cemental junction that may lead to tooth fracture.

Recognition of abnormal tooth wear is important. Patients should be advised on the best way to maintain dental health. This may include dietary and toothbrushing advice, as well as referral when an underlying

medical condition is present. Fluoride toothpaste is advocated as a surface coating of fluorapatite can form and is more resistant to wear than other forms of enamel apatites.

Resorption of teeth

External resorption

External resorption may be caused by inflammation or by mechanical stimulation. Inflammatory resorption typically involves the apical portion of the root, as a result of periapical inflammation (Fig. 5.27). Root resorption associated with mechanical stimulation may be seen in patients undergoing orthodontic treatment. External resorption at the cervical margin is usually idiopathic and has a burrowing pattern.

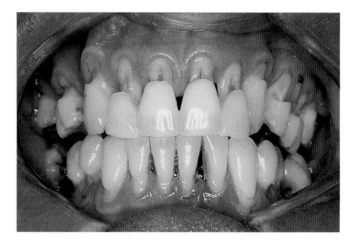

Fig. 5.26 Toothbrush abrasion.

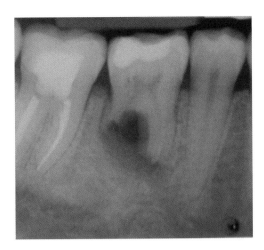

Fig. 5.27 Radiograph showing external root resorption associated with a periapical granuloma.

Internal resorption

Resorption starting from the pulpal surface (internal resorption) is usually associated with pulpitis (Fig. 5.28). When the coronal dentine is involved, the resorption may present clinically as a pink spot due to the vascular pulp tissue being visible through the overlying enamel.

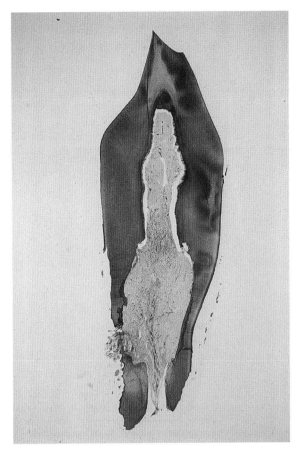

Fig. 5.28 Idiopathic internal root resorption.

Dental caries and its ramifications

Dental caries most often arises in fissures and in the regions of the crown that approximate adjacent teeth. Other distinct patterns occur, including cervical caries and root caries that often arises in older people with reduced salivary flow. If untreated, dental caries may progress to destroy dentine, ultimately leading to infection of the dental pulp, pulpal necrosis, and its consequences.

Pathology of dental caries

Enamel caries

The interactions between plaque biofilm, dietary carbohydrates, and oral environment on the enamel surface of the tooth can result in progressive loss of mineral from the enamel. Enamel caries arises in fissures and on approximal surfaces of teeth, and the first clinical sign is a 'white spot' lesion (Fig. 5.29), which gradually turns brown as the altered enamel surface becomes stained with extrinsic pigments in the oral environment. It is important to understand that enamel caries arises as a result of a dynamic process involving dissolution and re-precipitation of mineral within the lesion and on the surface of the tooth, which is bathed in saliva. Enamel caries is a reversible lesion that can be arrested by changing the oral environment, e.g. by dietary intervention, altering the biofilm, or introducing fluoride.

Ground sections of teeth have been used extensively to study enamel caries. The morphological descriptions are mainly based on examination of sections using transmitted and polarized light microscopy.

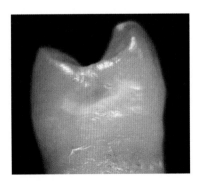

Fig. 5.29 White spot lesion of early enamel caries on the approximal surface of a premolar.

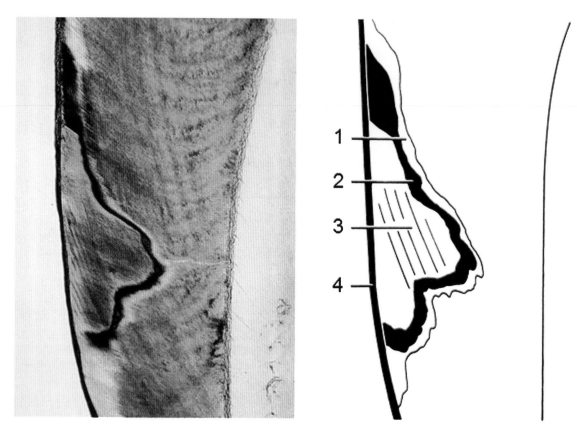

Fig. 5.30 Ground section through an early carious lesion in enamel showing zonation of the lesion. Diagramatic representation of the lesion: 1 translucent zone; 2 dark zone; 3 body of the lesion; 4 surface zone.

Biochemical analyses of carious enamel have also been carried out. Most investigations have focused on smooth surface caries to avoid the problems of interpretation of histological features imposed by the anatomy of pits and fissures. However, the pathological features are essentially similar at both sites. The established early lesion (white spot lesion) in smooth surface enamel caries is cone-shaped, with the base of the cone on the enamel surface and the apex pointing towards the amelo-dentinal junction. The shape is modified in pit and fissure caries. In ground sections, the enamel carious lesion consists of a series of zones, the optical properties of which reflect differing degrees of demineralization (Fig. 5.30).

Translucent zone

This is the first recognizable histological change at the advancing edge of the lesion. It is more porous than normal enamel and contains 1% by volume of spaces (pore volume), compared with the 0.1% pore volume in normal enamel. The pores are larger than the small pores in normal enamel, which approximate to the size of a water molecule. Chemical analysis shows that there is a fall in magnesium and carbonate when compared with normal enamel, which suggests that a magnesium- and carbonate-rich mineral is preferentially dissolved in this zone. Dissolution of mineral occurs mainly from the junctional areas between the prismatic and interprismatic enamel. The prism boundaries, which

are relatively rich in protein, allow ready ingress of hydrogen ions and the magnesium-rich and carbonate-rich mineral that is preferentially removed, may represent the surface layers of crystallites at the prism boundaries. The translucent zone is sometimes missing or present along only part of the lesion.

Dark zone

This zone has a pore volume of 2–4%. Some of the pores are large, but others are smaller than those in the translucent zone, suggesting that some remineralization has occurred due to reprecipitation of mineral lost from the translucent zone.

Body of the lesion

This zone has a pore volume of between 5% and 25%, and also contains apatite crystals larger than those found in normal enamel. It is suggested that these large crystals result from the re-precipitation of mineral dissolved from deeper zones. However, with continuing acid attack there is further dissolution of mineral both from the periphery of the apatite crystals and from their cores. The lost mineral is replaced by unbound water and, to a lesser extent, by organic matter, presumably derived from saliva and microorganisms. There is increased prominence of the striae of Retzius in the body of the lesion, the explanation for which is unknown.

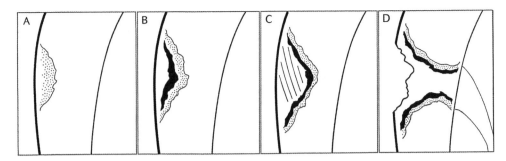

Fig. 5.31 Progress of approximal enamel caries: (A) subsurface translucent zone; (B) development of the dark zone; (C) typical zoned structure of the early carious lesion (white spot lesion); (D) cavitation of the surface, spread along amelo-dentinal junction, reactive changes in dentine.

Surface zone

This is about 40 µm thick and shows surprisingly little change in early lesions. The surface of normal enamel differs in composition from the deeper layers, being more highly mineralized and having, for example, a higher fluoride level and a lower magnesium level. The surface zone remains relatively normal despite subsurface loss of mineral, because it is an area of active re-precipitation of mineral derived both from the plaque and from that dissolved from deeper areas of the lesion as ions diffuse outwards.

Histopathogenesis of the early lesion

The development of enamel caries can be traced through the following stages when ground sections are examined by transmitted light (Fig. 5.31):

1. Development of a subsurface translucent zone, which is unrecognizable clinically and radiologically.

2. The subsurface translucent zone enlarges and a dark zone develops in its centre.

3. As the lesion enlarges, more mineral is lost and the centre of the dark zone becomes the body of the lesion. This is relatively translucent compared with sound enamel and shows enhancement of the striae of Retzius, interprismatic markings, and cross-striations of the prisms. The lesion is now clinically recognizable as a white spot.

4. The body of the lesion may become stained by extrinsic pigments from the oral environment. The lesion is now clinically recognizable as a brown spot.

5. When the caries reaches the amelo-dentinal junction it spreads laterally, undermining the adjacent enamel, giving the bluish-white appearance to the enamel, as seen clinically. Although lateral spread can occur before cavitation, it is more common and more extensive in lesions with cavity formation.

6. With progressive loss of mineral, a critical point is reached when the enamel is no longer able to withstand the loads placed upon it and the structure breaks down to form a cavity.

Caries in a fissure does not start at the base, but develops as a ring around the wall of the fissure, the histological features of the lesion being similar to those seen on smooth surfaces. As the caries progresses, it spreads outwards into the surrounding enamel and downwards towards the dentine, and eventually coalesces at the base of the fissure (Figs 5.32 and 5.33). This produces a cone-shaped lesion, but the base of the cone is directed towards the amelo-dentinal junction and is not on the enamel surface, as in smooth surface caries. The area of dentine ultimately involved is, therefore, larger than with smooth surface lesions.

Dentine caries

Dentine differs from enamel in that it is a living tissue and as such can respond to damage. It also has a relatively high organic content, approximately 20% by weight, which consists predominantly of collagen. In dentine caries it is, therefore, necessary to consider both the defence reaction of the pulpodentinal complex and the carious destruction of the tissue, which involves acid demineralization followed by proteolytic breakdown of the matrix. The defence reaction

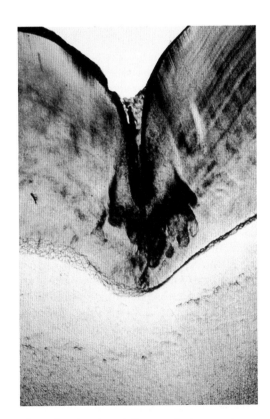

Fig. 5.32 Ground section through fissure caries in enamel.

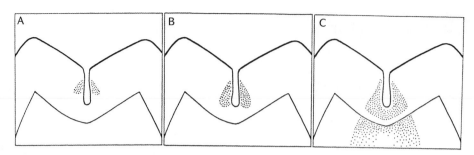

Fig. 5.33 Progress of enamel caries in a fissure.

may begin before the carious process reaches the dentine, presumably because of irritation to the odontoblasts transmitted through the weakened enamel, and is represented by the formation of reactionary (tertiary) dentine and dentinal sclerosis. However, in progressive lesions, the defence reaction is overtaken by the carious process as it advances towards the pulp.

Caries of the dentine develops from enamel caries: when the lesion reaches the amelo-dentinal junction, lateral extension results in the involvement of great numbers of tubules. The early lesion is cone-shaped, or convex, with the base at the amelo-dentinal junction. Larger lesions may show a broadening of the apex of the cone as it approaches the circumpulpal dentine. In caries of dentine, demineralization by acid is always in advance of the bacterial front, the subsequent bacterial invasion being followed by breakdown of the collagenous matrix. Because of the sequential nature of the changes, studies of ground and decalcified sections show a zoned lesion in which four zones are characteristically present (Fig. 5.34).

Zone of sclerosis

The sclerotic or translucent zone is located beneath and at the sides of the carious lesion. It is almost invariably present, being broader beneath the lesion than at the sides, and is regarded as a vital reaction of odontoblasts to irritation. Two patterns of mineralization have been described. The first is the result of acceleration of the normal physiological process of centripetal deposition of peritubular dentine, which eventually occludes the tubules. In the second, mineral first appears within the cytoplasmic process of the odontoblasts and the tubule is obliterated by calcification of the odontoblast process itself. Sclerosed dentine, therefore, has a higher mineral content.

Dead tracts may be seen running through the zone of sclerosis. They are the result of the death of odontoblasts at an earlier stage in the carious process. The empty dentinal tubules contain the remains of the dead odontoblast process and such tubules can obviously not undergo sclerosis. However, they provide ready access for bacteria to enter the pulp. To prevent this, the pulpal end of a dead tract is occluded by a thin layer of hyaline calcified material, sometimes called eburnoid, which is derived from pulpal cells. Beyond this, further, often very irregular, reactionary dentine may form following differentiation of odontoblasts or odontoblast-like cells from the pulp.

Zone of demineralization

In the demineralized zone, the intertubular matrix is mainly affected by a wave of acid produced by bacteria in the zone of bacterial invasion,

which diffuses ahead of the bacterial front. The softened dentine in the base of a cavity is, therefore, sterile but, in clinical practice, it cannot be distinguished reliably from softened, infected dentine. It may be stained yellowish-brown as a result of the diffusion of other bacterial products interacting with proteins in dentine.

Zone of bacterial invasion

In this zone, the bacteria extend down and multiply within the dentinal tubules (Fig. 5.35). The bacterial invasion probably occurs in two waves: the first wave consisting of acidogenic organisms, mainly lactobacilli, that produce acid that diffuses ahead into the demineralized zone. A second wave of mixed acidogenic and proteolytic organisms then attacks the demineralized matrix. The walls of the tubules are

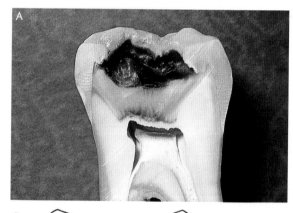

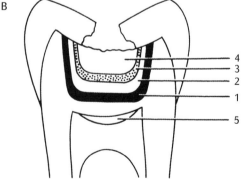

Fig. 5.34 Grossly carious molar. Spread of caries along the amelo-dentinal junction has resulted in undermining of the enamel. Diagramatic representation of the zones in established dentine caries: 1 sclerosis; 2 demineralization; 3 bacterial invasion; 4 destruction; 5 reactionary (tertiary) dentine beneath the lesion.

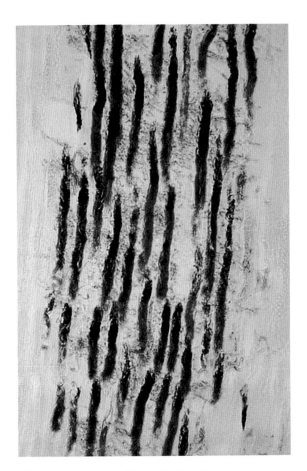

Fig. 5.35 Bacteria colonizing the dentinal tubules.

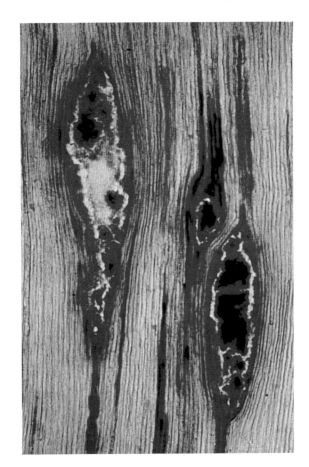

Fig. 5.36 Liquefaction foci in dentine caries.

softened by the proteolytic activity and some may then be distended by the increasing mass of multiplying bacteria. The peritubular dentine is first compressed, followed by the intertubular dentine, resulting in elliptical areas of proteolysis-liquefaction foci. Liquefaction foci run parallel to the direction of the tubules and may be multiple, giving the tubule a beaded appearance (Fig. 5.36).

Zone of destruction

In the zone of destruction, the liquefaction foci enlarge and increase in number. Cracks or clefts containing bacteria and necrotic tissue also appear at right angles to the course of the dentinal tubules forming transverse clefts (Fig. 5.37). Bacteria are no longer confined to the tubules and invade both the peritubular and intertubular dentine. Little of the normal dentine architecture now remains and cavitation commences from the amelo-dentinal junction. In acute, rapidly progressing caries, the necrotic dentine is soft and yellowish-white; in chronic caries it has a brownish-black colour and is of leathery consistency.

Reactionary (tertiary) dentine

A layer of reactionary (tertiary) dentine is often formed at the surface of the pulp chamber deep to the dentine caries, this dentine being localized to the irritated odontoblasts (Fig. 5.38). It varies in structure but the tubules are generally irregular, tortuous, and fewer in number than in primary dentine, or may even be absent. Its formation effectively increases the depth of tissue between the carious dentine and the pulp,

and in this way delays involvement of the pulp. Reactionary dentine is a non-specific response to odontoblast irritation, also being formed in reaction to tooth wear and restorative interventions.

In practice, the terms infected dentine (referring to the zones of bacterial invasion and destruction) and affected dentine (referring to the zone of demineralization) are used. Infected caries requires complete removal, but given the potential for remineralization, affected dentine may, in some cases, be left in order to protect the pulp. The criteria for

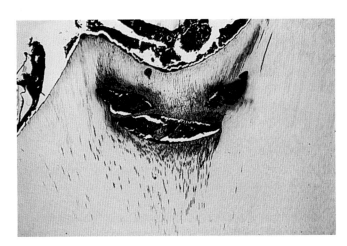

Fig. 5.37 Transverse cleft in dentine caries.

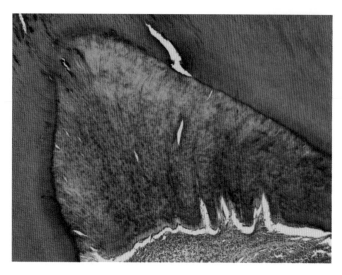

Fig. 5.38 Reactionary (tertiary) dentine in response to dentine caries.

Table 5.5 Typical symptoms of pulpitis

Site	Poorly localized
Severity	Severe pain
Onset	Spontaneous or associated with exacerbating factors
Nature	Stabbing pain with loss of sleep
Duration	Intermittent (10–15 min) or constant
Radiation	Jaws, face, ear, neck
Exacerbating factors	Hot, cold, sweet, lying down
Relieving factors	Analgesics minimal effect; dental treatment

doing so are beyond the scope of this book and the reader should refer to texts on operative dentistry for further detail.

Root caries

The primary tissue affected in root caries is cementum. The surface layer initially becomes hypermineralized due to reprecipitation and is analogous to the surface zone in enamel caries. Nevertheless, the subsurface cementum becomes progressively softer and bacteria invade along the exposed collagen fibres. The destruction of cementum occurs parallel to the root surface, spreading along the cemental lines, and eventually forming 'saucer-shaped' carious lesions that may encircle the root.

Pulpitis

The advance of cariogenic bacteria towards the vital pulp may cause acute and chronic inflammatory responses. Lymphocytes, plasma cells, and macrophages can appear in pulp in response to advancing dentine caries and this low-grade inflammatory process can spread through the root apex to involve the apical periodontal tissues without clinical symptoms. However, bacterial products may cause the pulp to develop hyperaemia and the patient may then experience acute pain (Table 5.5). It is generally recognized that early pulpitis is reversible but that when bacteria enter the pulp itself, then a pulp abscess can form or complete pulpal necrosis may occur (Fig. 5.39). There is a poor correlation between patient symptoms and the underlying histology of the pulp. Pulpitis and pulp necrosis may result from other causes, e.g. tooth wear, physical and chemical trauma (Table 5.6).

Pulp polyp

In primary or recently erupted permanent teeth with 'wide-open' carious cavities and a good apical blood supply, pulpitis may be associated with the production of exuberant granulation tissue. The hyperplastic pulpal granulation tissue protrudes from the cavity forming a dark red polyp that bleeds readily (Fig. 5.40). Over time, the polyp may become epithelialized, taking on a pinkish-white colour.

Pulp calcification

Pulp stones are calcified bodies with an organic matrix and occur most frequently in the coronal pulp. True pulp stones contain tubules (albeit few and irregular), and may have an outer layer of predentine and adjacent odontoblasts. False pulp stones are composed of concentric layers of calcified material with no tubular structure.

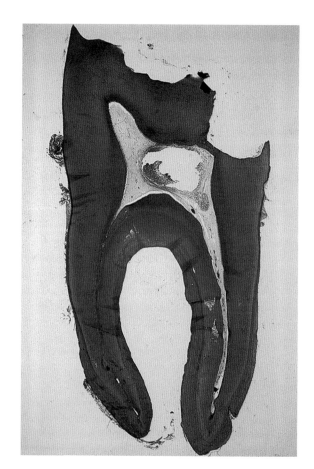

Fig. 5.39 Pulp abscess.

Table 5.6 Causes of pulpitis

Caries	Most common cause of pulpitis
Ingress of bacteria through exposed dentinal tubules	Invaginated odontome (dens in dente)
	Tooth wear (erosion, attrition, abrasion, abfraction)
	Fractured/cracked tooth
	Perio-endo lesion
Trauma	Mechanical injury to tooth e.g. sports injury, assault
	Thermal injury during cavity preparation
	Chemical injury from dental materials

According to their location in the pulp, stones may be described as free, adherent, or interstitial when they have become surrounded by reactionary dentine. When large they may be detected on radiographs. Dystrophic calcifications in the pulp consist of granules of amorphous calcific material that may be scattered along collagen fibres or aggregated into larger masses. They are most commonly found in the root canals. Dystrophic calcifications and pulp stones

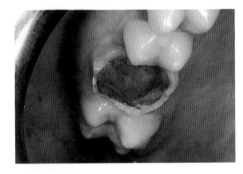

Fig. 5.40 Pulp polyp.

may obstruct endodontic therapy. Pulp obliteration may follow traumatic injury to the apical blood vessels, which is not sufficient to cause pulp necrosis. Large quantities of irregular dentine form in the pulp chamber and root canals, which become obliterated. Pulp obliteration is also seen in dentinogenesis imperfecta and dentine dysplasia.

Periapical disease

The consequences of pulp necrosis are outlined in Fig. 5.41. Spread of inflammation from the pulp chamber into periapical tissue causes a localized periodontitis, which usually presents as toothache (Table 5.7). Other causes of periapical periodontitis are listed in Table 5.8. The consequences of periapical periodontitis depend on the pathogens, host response, and the effectiveness of any dental treatment received.

Periapical granuloma

Persistent chronic inflammation results in the formation of an apical granuloma. Dental radiographs may show widening of the periodontal membrane space, loss of the apical lamina dura, and formation of a small, well-demarcated, rounded radiolucent area at the tip of the root apex (Fig. 5.42). The apical granuloma is composed of inflamed fibrous and granulation tissue (Fig. 5.43). There are numerous lymphocytes, plasma cells, and macrophages. It should be noted that the apical granuloma does not show granulomatous inflammation, which is a special type of inflammation associated with other diseases. The term apical granuloma is derived from granulation tissue formed after destruction of the periapical tissues by infection. In some patients, proliferation of the epithelial rests of Malassez within the apical granuloma may lead to the development of a radicular cyst (Chapter 6). The reasons why cysts develop in some granulomas but not others is unclear. Other changes in the apical region include focal sclerosing (condensing) osteitis (Chapter 7), root resorption (Fig 5.27), hypercementosis, and ankylosis.

Acute dentoalveolar abscess

If at any stage the diseased apical tissue undergoes suppuration, an acute dentoalveolar abscess (acute apical abscess) will form. Typically,

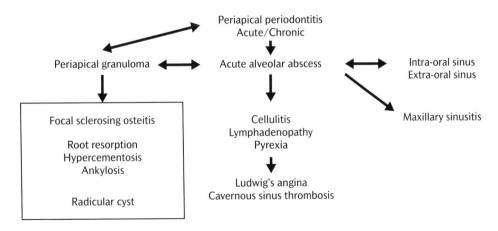

Fig. 5.41 Consequences of pulp necrosis.

Table 5.7 Typical symptoms of periapical periodontitis

Site	Localized
Severity	Severe pain or dull ache
Onset	Spontaneous or associated with exacerbating factors
Nature	Throbbing pain with loss of sleep
Duration	Constant (hours)
Radiation	Jaws, face, ear, neck
Exacerbating factors	Biting on affected tooth
Relieving factors	Analgesics minimal effect; dental treatment

Table 5.8 Causes of periapical periodontitis

Pulp necrosis	Most common cause of periapical periodontitis
Trauma	Mechanical injury to tooth, e.g. sports injury, assault, excessive orthodontic forces
	Excessive occlusal forces, e.g. 'high' restoration, attrition, bruxism
	Endodontic instrumentation and irrigation
	Root canal materials beyond the apical foramen

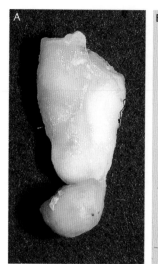
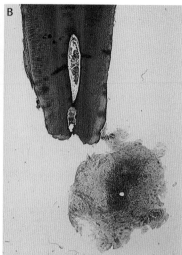
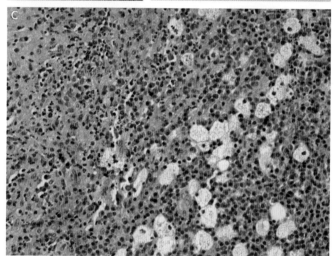

Fig. 5.43 Periapical granuloma attached to an extracted root. The root canal contains a necrotic pulp and the periapical granuloma contains a dense chronic inflammatory cell infiltrate.

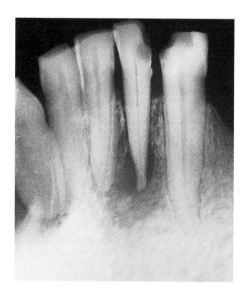

Fig. 5.42 Periapical radiolucency and apical resorption associated with a periapical granuloma.

the abscess will produce intra-oral pain and swelling (Fig. 5.44). Pus may drain into the oral cavity through the periodontal ligament or via a sinus tract, usually on the labial aspect of the alveolus (Fig. 5.45). Occasionally, the tract may open on to the facial skin, producing an extra-oral sinus (Fig 5.46). Spreading infection may produce a diffuse painful facial swelling (cellulitis), with lymphadenitis and pyrexia (Fig. 5.47). Life-threatening sequelae of spreading dental infection include Ludwig's angina and cavernous sinus thrombosis. Ludwig's angina is severe cellulitis involving the submandibular, sublingual, and submental spaces. The diffuse cellulitis produces a board-like swelling of the floor of the mouth, the tongue being elevated and displaced posteriorly. As a result, there is difficulty in eating, swallowing, and breathing. The latter is exacerbated as infection tracks backwards to involve the pharynx and larynx.

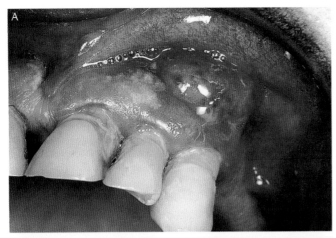

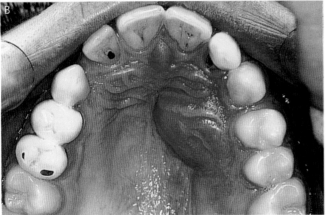

Fig. 5.44 Dentoalveolar abscess associated with a maxillary canine (A). A palatal abscess associated with a maxillary lateral incisor (B).

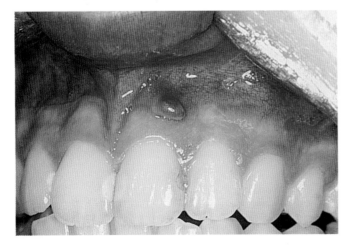

Fig. 5.45 Intra-oral sinus associated with a maxillary central incisor.

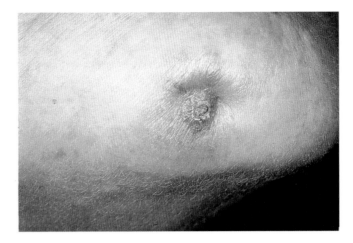

Fig. 5.46 Extra-oral sinus associated with a mandibular canine.

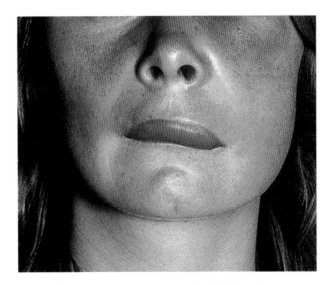

Fig. 5.47 Cellulitis associated with spread of infection from a dentoalveolar abscess associated with an anterior maxillary tooth.

Perio-endo lesions

Periapical inflammation may result from spread of infection originating in deep periodontal pockets. Conversely, inflammation originating from the pulp and periapical tissue may spread to involve periodontal tissue. The resulting lesions are known as perio-endo lesions and it is often impossible to know by which route the lesion developed. Generally, teeth associated with perio-endo lesions have a poor prognosis.

Gingivitis and periodontitis

Gingivitis and periodontitis are prevalent diseases; the UK Adult Dental Health Survey in 2009 indicated that 45% of adults have some degree of periodontitis and that the disease is a major cause of tooth loss. Gingivitis and periodontitis are typically caused by the accumulation of plaque, but non-plaque-induced gingivitis is occasionally encountered. Plaque-induced gingivitis and periodontitis are briefly described in this section and are covered in more detail in periodontology textbooks (see additional resources). Causes of non-plaque-induced gingivitis are described in more detail with cross-reference to Chapters 2 and 10, where necessary.

Necrotizing ulcerative gingivitis and pericoronitis

Necrotizing ulcerative gingivitis (NUG) typically presents with sudden onset of painful gingival erythema and swelling with characteristic halitosis and punched out ulceration of the gingival papillae (Fig. 5.48). There is a mixed bacterial infection (Box 5.5). The clinical features are distinctive and biopsy is not usually required. The condition may be related to local causes, such as poor oral hygiene and tobacco smoking, but can also be the presenting sign of an immunosuppressive disorder. NUG usually responds to antibiotic therapy but management should also be directed towards elimination of any underlying predisposing factors. The more aggressive necrotizing ulcerative periodontitis (NUP), where underlying periodontal tissues and alveolar bone are lost, is a disease strongly associated with HIV infection (Chapter 10).

Noma (cancrum oris) is a severe, rapidly developing gangrene of the oro-facial tissues and jaws that occurs almost exclusively in sub-Saharan Africa (Fig. 5.49). The majority of cases are preceded by NUG and tend to occur in malnourished, immunocompromised children.

Gingival inflammation around an erupting tooth is known as pericoronitis and is most often seen around partially erupted third molars. When ulceration occurs in the operculum overlying the crown, there may be pain and trismus. The microbiology is similar to that seen in NUG. Repeated episodes of pericoronitis can be one of the indications for surgical extraction of partly erupted third molar teeth.

Chronic gingivitis

In health, the marginal gingiva is pink and 'knife edged' to facilitate food shedding during mastication. The gingival crevice is a highly specialized structure with a biology that preserves the breach in mucosal

> ### Box 5.5 **Microorganisms implicated in necrotizing ulcerative gingivitis**
> - *Treponema vincentii*
> - *Prevotella intermedia*
> - *Porphyromonas gingivalis*
> - *Selenomonas sputigena*
> - *Fusobacterium fusiformis*

integrity that results from tooth eruption. A delicate balance between the microflora of the oral cavity and the gingival tissue is maintained and this relies principally on neutrophil activity. Patients with certain rare genetic disorders of neutrophil function typically develop severe gingivitis. In healthy patients, accumulation of dental plaque biofilm on the cervical and approximal surfaces of teeth can lead to a chronic inflammatory reaction in the gingival tissue. Studies conducted on human volunteers showed that after withdrawal of oral hygiene, there is first an acute inflammatory response in the marginal gingival tissue. The response is characterized by hyperaemia, fluid exudation resulting in oedema, and accumulation of neutrophils. Clinically, the gingiva lose their stippled appearance and become swollen and erythematous (Fig. 5.50). Neutrophils transmigrate through the crevicular epithelium in large numbers. With time, lymphocytes and macrophages accumulate in the gingival tissue and as the inflammatory reaction develops, plasma cells secreting local antibodies are found. False pocketing, where the inflamed gingival tissue swells above the cervical region to cover part of the crown, may result in trapping of plaque biofilm. When oral hygiene measures were re-introduced, the inflammatory process was found to be reversible, clinically. In patients with poor oral hygiene, the dental plaque biofilm may mineralize, forming calculus. Chronic gingivitis may progress into chronic periodontitis but can remain stable for years. Individual patient susceptibility and risk factors such as smoking, xerostomia, and diabetes mellitus are important determinants of progression to destructive periodontal disease.

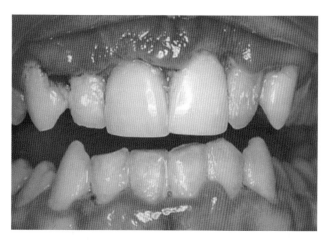

Fig. 5.48 Necrotizing ulcerative gingivitis.

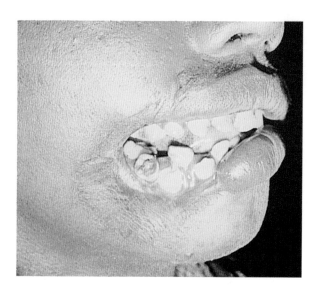

Fig. 5.49 Cancrum oris (Noma).

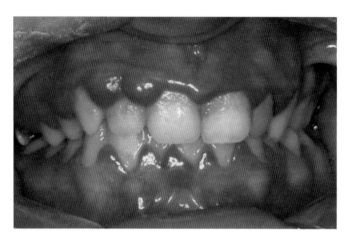

Fig. 5.50 Acute gingivitis.

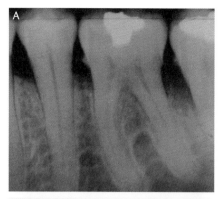

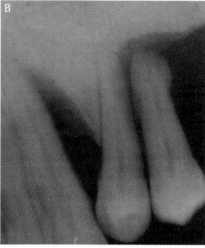

Fig. 5.51 Radiograph showing a mandibular molar with calculus deposits and horizontal bone loss (A). Radiograph showing calculus on the apical portion of the root of a maxillary second premolar and extensive vertical bone loss (B).

Chronic periodontitis

Chronic periodontitis results from spread of inflammation from the gingiva into the cervical periodontal ligament and alveolus. As in chronic gingivitis, there is marked variation in susceptibility and some patients with very poor oral hygiene never develop significant periodontitis. Slow progressive loss of periodontal tissue occurs and the cervical part of the tooth root may become exposed. The crevicular epithelium migrates apically and periodontal pockets develop. Biofilm accumulates and may mineralize forming subgingival calculus that is often hard and darkly coloured. Ultimately, the teeth may become mobile, if sufficient alveolar bone loss occurs. The rate of destruction may be so slow as to not cause a clinical problem during the patient's lifetime. Periodontal therapy aims to arrest or slow the rate of periodontal destruction. Histologically, the periodontal tissue contains an infiltrate of neutrophils, lymphocytes, macrophages, and plasma cells, typically located in the gingival connective tissue just below the crevicular epithelium. Multiple antigenic stimulation from plaque biofilm results in plasma cell accumulation. Plasma cell cytoplasmic fragments are frequently seen in the inflammatory infiltrate in the connective tissue. Proliferation and migration of the crevicular epithelium down the root face may result in formation of complex rete processes forming arcades and loops. Transmigrating neutrophils are typically present within the pocket epithelium. Resorption of the alveolar crest is mediated by osteoclasts. Bone destruction in chronic periodontitis typically manifests on radiographs as loss of definition of the lamina dura of the alveolar crests and progressive resorption creating horizontal and angular (vertical) alveolar bone defects (Figs. 5.51).

Aggressive periodontitis

In some individuals, periodontal destruction progresses relatively rapidly, even in the absence of known risk factors. A variety of terms have been used in the past to describe this disorder, including periodontosis, early onset periodontitis, and juvenile periodontitis, but these conditions overlap and have now been grouped together under the heading of aggressive periodontitis. Various clinical patterns are described, including localized and generalized forms, but all forms of aggressive periodontitis share the features of onset in childhood or young adult life, deep infra-bony pockets (Fig 5.51B), marked gingival inflammation, and, occasionally, relentless progression despite treatment. In milder clinical forms of aggressive periodontitis, the aim of treatment is to arrest or slow the disease with periodontal interventions and by improving oral hygiene. A number of distinctive syndromes are known where there is destruction of the alveolus with exfoliation of teeth in both the primary and secondary dentitions. Most of these are autosomal recessive genetic disorders that affect neutrophil function (Table 5.9). The best known of these is Papillon–Lefevre syndrome, where progression of periodontitis and rapid tooth exfoliation is accompanied by palmar plantar keratosis (OMIM 245000; Fig 5.52). Mutation of the gene that codes for cathepsin C (*CTSC*) is found; the enzyme is an important trigger of neutrophil elastase. Interestingly, patients with Papillon–Lefevre syndrome appear otherwise unaffected by their genetic defect.

Lateral periodontal abscess

The lateral periodontal abscess is a localized area of suppurative inflammation arising within the periodontal tissues alongside a tooth. The affected tooth is vital, which distinguishes it from the more common acute dentoalveolar abscess caused by a non-vital

Table 5.9 Genetic disorders of neutrophil function associated with periodontal disease

Neutrophil defect	Functional defect	Gene & OMIM	Clinical features
Agranulocytosis	Absence of neutrophils or all polymorphonuclear leukocytes	*HAX1* OMIM 610738	Necrotizing mucosal ulceration and rapid periodontal breakdown
Chediak–Higashi syndrome	Defects in chemotaxis, degranulation and bacterial killing	*LYST* OMIM 214500	Severe gingivitis and periodontal breakdown, ulceration
Cyclical neutropenia	Periodic fall in neutrophil numbers that resolves and recurs	*ELANE* OMIM 162800	Recurring oral ulcers, gingivitis, and mild periodontitis
Leukocyte adherence deficiency	Defective chemotaxis and phagocytosis	*LAD1* most common OMIM 116920 *ITGB2* *LAD 2, LAD3* rare	Frequent infections and severe periodontal breakdown
Papillon–Lefevre syndrome	Defects in chemotaxis and lack of NETosis (type of cell death)	*CTSC* OMIM 602365	Exfoliation of primary and secondary teeth; palmar plantar keratosis
Specific granule deficiency	Lactoferrin and defensin deficiency, defective in multiple functions	*CEBPE* OMIM 245480	Severe periodontal breakdown
Others	Several neutrophils defects are not characterised	Unknown	Mucosal ulceration, infections and periodontal inflammation

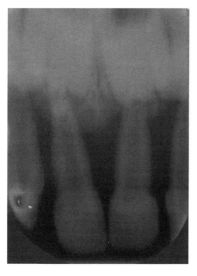

Fig. 5.52 Radiograph of a child with Papillon–Lefevre syndrome showing extensive bone loss.

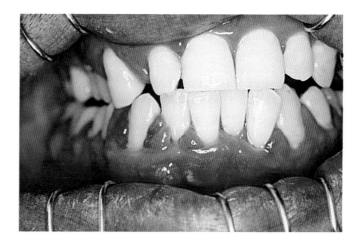

Fig. 5.53 Lateral periodontal abscess.

tooth. Clinically, periodontal abscesses may be acute or chronic. An acute abscess develops rapidly and is accompanied by pain and swelling of the overlying mucosa. The abscess may discharge spontaneously through the periodontal pocket, but in deep-seated lesions or where drainage is obstructed, it may track and present with a sinus opening on the mucosa somewhere along the length of the root (Fig. 5.53). Discharge of pus relieves the acute symptoms and the lesion may heal or become chronic with intermittent discharge. Radiographic appearances are very variable and depend on the extent of previously existing bone destruction, the stage of the abscess, and its location.

Non-plaque-induced gingivitis

Gingivitis caused by dental plaque is common, however, gingival inflammation caused by other diseases is important to recognize as it may lead to the diagnosis of an underlying systemic disease with broader implications for the patient's general health (Box 5.6).

Acute herpetic gingivo-stomatitis

Herpes simplex infection is common in children and young adults and may present as gingival erythema (Fig. 2.28). Small grey or yellow vesicles that quickly break down to form small ulcers can be present in the gingival tissue. The other features of herpetic gingivo-stomatitis and the recurrent herpes labialis that may follow are described in Chapter 2.

Desquamative gingivitis

A number of disorders can present on the gingiva with erythematous (often fiery red) atrophic lesions and these are often described clinically as desquamative gingivitis (Box 5.7). The term is a useful descriptor—desquamation relates to loss of the protective gingival epithelium—but is not a diagnosis. Differing pathological processes may underlie desquamative gingivitis and it is important to distinguish between these because the management differs depending on the nature of the underlying disorder.

Gingival lichen planus

Lichenoid inflammation is common in the oral cavity and is covered in detail in Chapter 2. Although lichen planus typically manifests as white hyperkeratotic striae in a lacy pattern with intervening erythematous areas in mobile oral mucosa, it may present as a purely erythematous lesion in the gingival tissue (Fig. 2.64A, Fig. 2.65B). The gingiva may be sore and assume a bright red shiny appearance due to epithelial atrophy. The presence of a few white striae or lichenoid lesions elsewhere in the oral cavity may provide a valuable clinical

clue to diagnosis. Incisional biopsy is necessary to obtain a diagnosis. The gingival margin should be avoided as a biopsy site because the gingival contour may be damaged and the histological features may be obscured by chronic inflammatory processes related to plaque. Sections of a representative site will show a sub-epithelial band containing lymphocytes and histiocytes. Basal cell degeneration, and the other features of lichenoid inflammation described in Chapter 2, may be observed. Once the diagnosis is established, symptomatic lesions can be treated with topical steroid therapy and non-symptomatic lesions may be observed.

Vesiculobullous disorders

Gingival erythema can be caused by autoimmune diseases, in which antibodies directed against mucosal components are produced. Small blisters (vesicles) or larger blisters (bullae) may form by accumulation of fluid in the damaged mucosa. The vesiculobullous disorders must be distinguished from other causes of gingival erythema, such as gingival lichen planus. Biopsy is used to make the diagnosis. When a vesiculobullous disorder is suspected, additional biopsy tissue must be submitted fresh to the cellular pathology laboratory, so that autoantibodies can be detected in frozen sections by direct immunofluorescence.

Mucous membrane pemphigoid

In pemphigoid, autoantibodies bind to the basement membrane. This results in activation of complement and separation of the epithelium from the lamina propria producing a sub-epithelial blister. Various types of pemphigoid are known. Bullous pemphigoid occurs in skin, typically in elderly patients. Mucosal involvement in bullous pemphigoid is rare. Mucous membrane pemphigoid, also known as cicatricial pemphigoid, does not affect skin, and lesions may occur in the oral mucosa, conjunctiva, and genital mucosa. When the gingivae are involved, the tissue shows bright erythema and blisters form that often contain blood (Fig 2.49). The blisters are typically flaccid and often break down to form shallow ulcers. Biopsy shows sub-epithelial splitting, and eosinophils are often present in the blister fluid that accumulates in the space between the lamina propria and epithelial basal layer. In frozen sections of intact mucosa, there is linear binding of IgG and C3 to the basement membrane. Mucous membrane pemphigoid is described in more detail in Chapter 2.

Pemphigus

Pemphigus vulgaris is caused by autoantibodies that react with desmoglein, which is an important component of the desmosome. Binding of autoantibodies causes separation of keratinocytes, known as acantholysis, that results in formation of an intra-epithelial bulla. The damaged squamous cells become rounded in form and if blister fluid is sampled by cytology, they have a characteristic appearance and are known as Tzank cells. Histologically, intra-epithelial separation occurs above the basal and suprabasal layer, leaving an intact layer of cells that line the bulla floor known as the 'tombstone' layer. Early in pemphigus, the autoantibodies are directed against desmoglein 3, which is abundant in oral epithelium, and consequently many cases of pemphigus present first with oral lesions. With time, there is antigenic drift and other desmogleins are affected, particularly desmoglein 1 in skin, and then cutaneous blisters appear. Direct immunofluorescence shows binding of IgG to desmosomes resulting in a net-like pattern. Pemphigus is a serious disease that is treated by immunosuppressive drugs and is described more fully in Chapter 2.

Granulomatous gingivitis

Erythematous and hyperplastic gingivitis is a feature of oro-facial granulomatosis and an oral manifestation of Crohn's disease and sarcoidosis (Chapter 10). Biopsy of the gingiva demonstrates small, non-caseating granulomas. Clinico-pathological correlation is required to establish the definitive diagnosis.

Plasma cell gingivitis

Plasma cell gingivitis or gingival plasmacytosis is a rare disorder that is characterized by erythema and papillary hyperplasia of the gingiva (Fig 5.54). Occasionally, the oral mucosa and other parts of the upper aerodigestive tract are also affected, termed plasma cell mucositis. Biopsy shows accumulation of mature plasma cells that expand the connective tissue papillae. The plasma cells are polyclonal, expressing a mixture of kappa and lambda immunoglobulin light chains. The cause is not always known but in some cases an allergen can be identified. The condition is

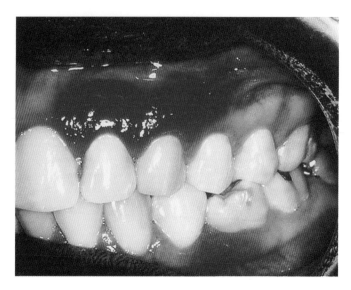

Fig. 5.54 Plasma cell gingivitis.

sometimes associated with a change the brand of toothpaste used. Plant products such as herbal extracts and khat (Qat) have been associated with plasma cell mucositis and cessation brings about resolution.

Generalized gingival overgrowth

This section describes generalized gingival overgrowth (Box 5.8). Localized gingival overgrowths, the epulides, are covered in Chapter 2.

Hereditary gingival fibromatosis

Genetic forms of generalized gingival overgrowth are known and the most common type is associated with gene *SOS1* (OMIM 135300).

Typically, the gingiva are enlarged but minimally inflamed and expand to partly cover the tooth crowns (Fig. 5.55). Multiple gingivectomy procedures may be needed to re-contour the gingival tissues to maintain oral health. Other genetic loci have been identified, and both autosomal dominant and recessive forms have been described. Symmetrical fibrous enlargement of the gingiva in the maxillary tuberosity region (Fig. 5.56) is not uncommon, but its relationship to hereditary gingival fibromatosis is uncertain.

Box 5.8 Generalized gingival enlargement

- Hereditary gingival fibromatosis
- Chronic hyperplastic gingivitis
  - puberty
  - oral contraceptives
  - pregnancy
- Drug-induced gingival overgrowth (DIGO)
  - phenytoin
  - calcium channel blockers
  - ciclosporin
- Granulomatous gingivitis
  - oro-facial granulomatosis/Crohn's disease
  - sarcoidosis
  - granulomatosis with polyangitis
- Ligneous gingivitis
- Acute leukaemias

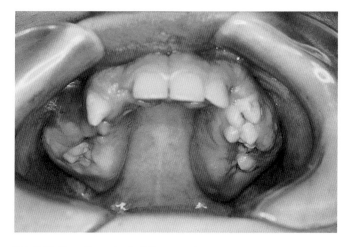

Fig. 5.55 Hereditary gingival fibromatosis.

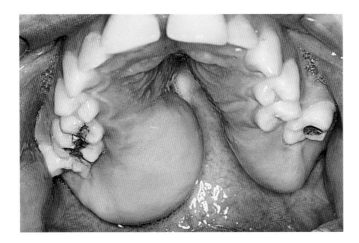

Fig. 5.56 Fibrous enlargement of the maxillary tuberosities.

Chronic hyperplastic gingivitis

Florid chronic gingivitis may result in chronic generalized gingival enlargement due to oedema and fibrosis. Local factors such as mouth breathing and systemic factors such as the hormonal changes associated with puberty and pregnancy may predispose to such gingival overgrowth. Maintaining good oral hygiene helps to eliminate the problem.

Drug-induced gingival overgrowth

Generalized gingival enlargement can be caused by a variety of drugs (Fig 5.57). The first class of drug described was anticonvulsants, principally phenytoin that was once widely prescribed for epilepsy. In recent years, the use of phenytoin has declined due to the availability of alternative therapy. Calcium channel blocking drugs, such as nifedipine, amlodipine, and verapamil, are widely prescribed for control of hypertension and may cause drug-induced gingival overgrowth (DIGO). The immunosuppressive drug, ciclosporin, also causes gingival overgrowth and in some patients florid overgrowth necessitates repeated gingivectomy. Ciclosporin was once widely used for transplant patients, but the introduction of tacrolimus, with other immunosuppressant drugs in a cocktail, has largely replaced ciclosporin in that role. However, ciclosporin is still used for dermatological inflammatory disorders.

If alternative drugs to those causing DIGO are not appropriate, it may be necessary to perform repeated gingivectomy to control the overgrowth. The gingival tissue in ciclosporin-related DIGO can be richly vascular and excessive postoperative bleeding has been described after gingivectomy. Rigorous oral hygiene measures can minimize DIGO and may be sufficient to control the gingival condition clinically, whilst allowing the drug regime to be maintained. As with any drug-related oral disease, it is important not to discontinue the drug therapy without prior consultation with the clinician responsible for prescribing the drug.

Granulomatosis with polyangitis

Enlargement of multiple gingival papillae with erythema, known as 'strawberry gingivitis' is a classic oral manifestation of granulomatosis with polyangitis (GPA) (Fig 5.58). Diagnosis is made by biopsy of a gingival papilla and this will reveal vasculitis, often with accumulations of neutrophils. GPA is a multisystem vasculitis that usually presents clinically with lesions in the kidney, lung, or nasal septum, often with a skin rash, conjunctivitis, or hearing loss. Histologically, the walls of small vessels are destroyed and there may be focal necrosis of tissue due to vascular obstruction. Granulomas (accumulations of macrophages) are typically found and these are non-caseating. Often, fused macrophages with multiple nuclei arranged in a horseshoe-shaped ring are present. The diagnosis can be confirmed by serological testing for c-ANCA and PR3. Additional testing for p-ANCA and MPO may be performed to exclude other types of vasculitis. Therapy can involve cytotoxic drugs or the newer monoclonal antibody therapies such as rituximab. In strawberry gingivitis, the full spectrum of histological changes is not always seen and there may be just small-vessel involvement (called leukocytoclastic capillitis).

Ligneous gingivitis

Ligneous gingivitis is rare and caused by a plasminogen deficiency. Fibrin deposits accumulate in the lamina propria, producing generalized nodular gingival enlargement; progression to aggressive periodontitis has been documented.

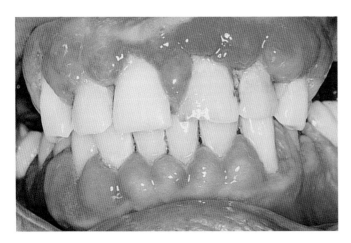

Fig. 5.57 Nifedipine-induced gingival overgrowth.

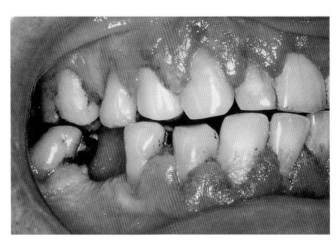

Fig. 5.58 Strawberry gingivitis in granulomatosis with polyangiitis.

Oral malignancy mimicking periodontal disease

Malignant neoplasms can invade and destroy the periodontal tissues mimicking plaque-induced periodontal destruction (Chapter 3). An important radiographic sign of a jaw malignancy is irregular periodontal destruction with displacement of teeth. This is particularly significant if the periodontal destruction is focal and there is little evidence of dental plaque. Squamous cell carcinoma, the most common oral malignancy, occasionally presents clinically with periodontal destruction and the rare histological variant carcinoma cuniculatum can arise in the gingiva, from where it may invade the alveolus in a burrowing, destructive pattern. Leukaemic infiltration of the periodontal tissues, typically in acute lymphoblastic leukaemia, can cause gingival enlargement and bleeding, periodontal destruction and tooth loosening, and may be the first signs of a potentially fatal haematological malignancy. Multiple myeloma, a malignant neoplasm of plasma cells in the marrow, may destroy the supporting alveolus causing tooth mobility. In Langerhans cell histiocytosis (LCH), infiltration of the periodontal tissues by abnormal Langerhans cells can lead to tooth exfoliation, with the classic radiological description of 'teeth floating in air'. In children under 2 years of the age, LCH is typically a disseminated disease with skin rash, periodontal destruction, pulmonary and bone lesions, requiring systemic therapy. In adult patients, periodontal destruction may be focal or multi-focal, with destructive bone lesions elsewhere in the skeleton. Osteosarcoma and chondrosarcoma of the jaw can mimic periodontitis and sometimes osteosarcoma presents with widening of the periodontal ligament on dental radiography. Kaposi sarcoma can occur on the gingiva as a red raised patch or an epulis, and is classified as a lesion strongly associated with HIV infection (Chapter 10). Metastatic malignancy from a distant site to the jaws may erode the alveolus causing tooth mobility and occasionally mimics an epulis.

6

Jaw cysts and odontogenic tumours

Introduction

Odontogenic cysts and tumours arise from inclusion of tooth-forming epithelium and mesenchyme in the jaw bones during development. Cysts also arise from non-odontogenic epithelium trapped during fusions or from vestigial structures. In addition, bone cysts that can arise at other skeletal sites may also occur in the jaws.

Odontogenic cysts and tumours may be classified according to their putative developmental origins and biology. The classification of jaw cysts is shown in Fig. 6.1. Odontomes are hamartomatous developmental lesions of the tooth-forming tissues. Odontogenic tumours are uncommon and are usually benign. Ameloblastoma is the most common odontogenic tumour and is described in detail. The other odontogenic tumours are rare and only the principal features are presented. Very rare congenital lesions of possible odontogenic origin are mentioned in the final section.

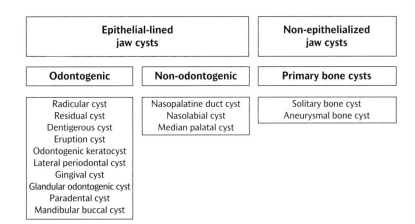

Fig 6.1 Classification of jaw cysts.

Jaw cysts

A cyst may be defined as pathological cavity lined by epithelium with fluid or semi-fluid contents. However, clinically, the term encompasses a broader range of benign fluid-filled lesions, some of which do not possess an epithelial lining. The preferred definition is, therefore, 'a pathological cavity having fluid or semi-fluid contents that has not been created by the accumulation of pus'. Cysts are commonly encountered in clinical dentistry and are generally detected on radiographs or as expansions of the jaws. Most cysts have a radiolucent appearance and are well circumscribed, often with a corticated outline. At least 90% of jaw cysts are of odontogenic origin. The clinico-pathological features of jaw cysts are summarized in Table 6.1. The incidence of the four most common jaw cysts are provided in Table 6.2.

Odontogenic cysts

The epithelial lining of odontogenic cysts originates from residues of the tooth-forming organ.

- *Epithelial rests of Serres* are remnants of the dental lamina and are thought to give rise to the odontogenic keratocyst, lateral periodontal, and gingival cysts.
- *Reduced enamel epithelium* is derived from the enamel organ and covers the fully formed crown of the unerupted tooth. The dentigerous (follicular) and eruption cysts originate from this tissue, as do the mandibular buccal and paradental cysts.
- *Epithelial rests of Malassez* form by fragmentation of Hertwig's epithelial root sheath that maps out the developing tooth root. Radicular cysts originate from these residues.

Radicular cyst

Clinical and radiographic features

Radicular cysts are the most common type of jaw cyst. They are frequently referred to as dental cysts or periapical cysts, but the term 'radicular cyst' is preferred because the cyst arises in relation to a tooth root. Radicular cysts are subdivided into apical, lateral, and residual types, depending on the anatomical relationship to the root of the tooth. Apical radicular cysts are the most common cystic lesions in the jaws and are always associated with the apices of non-vital teeth. They account for about 75% of all radicular cysts. When small, they are frequently symptomless and are usually discovered during routine radiological examination. As they enlarge they expand the alveolar bone and, ultimately, may discharge through a sinus. Most radicular cysts do not grow to large dimensions. The expansion of the alveolar bone is accompanied by deposition of successive layers of new bone by the overlying periosteum. This results in a bony-hard expansion. However, the rate of expansion tends to outstrip the rate of sub-periosteal deposition, leading to progressive thinning of the cortex, which can be deformed on palpation, producing the clinical signs of 'oil-can bottoming' and 'egg-shell crackling' (Fig. 6.2). Eventually, radicular cysts may perforate the cortex and present as a bluish, fluctuant, submucosal swelling. The rate of expansion of radicular cysts has been estimated at approximately 5 mm in diameter per year. Pain is seldom a feature, unless there is acute infection, which may progress to abscess formation. Radicular cysts can arise at any age after tooth eruption but are rare in the deciduous dentition. They are most common between 20 and 60 years of age and can occur in relation to any tooth in the arch.

Table 6.1 Summary of the clinico-pathological features of jaw cysts

Type of cyst	Location	Clinical features	Histopathology
Radicular cyst	Always associated with a non-vital tooth Periapical region, especially anterior maxilla	Most common jaw cyst, often symptomless, incidental finding on radiographs, slowly expansile Peak 30–50 years	Thick, inflamed fibrous capsule; non-keratinizing squamous epithelial lining; mural cholesterol nodules; Rushton's bodies
Residual cyst	At the site of a previously extracted non-vital tooth Most common in mandibular premolar area	Slowing enlarging swelling, frequently symptomless Peak 40–60 years	Thick fibrous capsule; variable non-keratinizing squamous epithelial lining; mural cholesterol nodules; minimal inflammation unless infected
Dentigerous cyst	Always associated with an unerupted tooth Mandibular third molar, maxillary canine, maxillary third molar, premolars	Develop around crowns of unerupted teeth; may displace the tooth and become lateralized Peak 30–50 years	Capsule resembles dental follicle, myxoid areas and odontogenic rests; lined by reduced enamel epithelium, squamous metaplasia common
Eruption cyst	Always associated with a partially erupted tooth Primary and permanent teeth, usually anterior to first molar	Bluish fluctuant swelling over an erupting tooth, may spontaneously burst Peak 10–30 years	Capsule resembles dental follicle, myxoid areas and odontogenic rests; lined by reduced enamel epithelium
Odontogenic keratocyst	Majority, angle of mandible, posterior maxilla	Typically multilocular radiolucency; expands through medullary bone; minimal, cortical expansion; can recur after enucleation Peak 20–40 years	Thin, fibrous capsule, lined by parakeratotic squamous epithelium 7–10 cell layers thickness, basal cell palisade; satellite cysts; occurs in basal cell nevus syndrome (Gorlin–Goltz syndrome)
Lateral periodontal cyst	Mandibular premolar and canine regions	Lateral periodontal cysts often symptomless; incidental finding on radiographs; botryoid cysts are larger and expand jaw Peak 50–80 years	Related to roots of vital teeth; thin, fibrous capsule; non-keratinizing squamous lining with focal thickenings
Gingival cyst	Inter-premolar region	Perinatal period: Bohn's nodules, multiple 2-mm nodules on alveolar ridge Adult type: 50–70 years, 5 mm bluish nodule on gingiva	Childhood-type often multiple; keratin-filled nodules on alveolar ridge Adult-type is the extra-osseous, soft-tissue counterpart of lateral periodontal cyst
Glandular odontogenic cyst	Majority in anterior mandible	Unilocular or multilocular, may be locally destructive, tend to recur after enucleation Peak 50–70 years	Non-keratinizing squamous epithelial lining; intracapsular islands of cells forming mucinous ducts
Paradental cyst	Mandibular third molar	Buccal to impacted third molars; enamel spur often present; may discharge contents Peak 20–40 years	Pouch arising from pericoronal tissue; thick capsule of inflamed fibrous tissue; lined by hyperplastic non-keratinizing squamous epithelium
Mandibular buccal cyst	Mandibular first molar	Expansion of buccal soft-tissue around erupting first molars Peak 5–10 years	Similar to paradental cyst
Nasopalatine duct cyst	Floor of nose to incisive papilla	Swelling, palatine papilla to floor of nose; displace central incisors; salty taste, radiolucency >6 mm, vital adjacent teeth Any age, peak 40-70 years	Fibrous capsule, may contain neurovascular bundles; lined by respiratory or simple squamous epithelium or both
Nasolabial cyst	Nasolabial fold	Fluctuant swelling of skin or labial vestibule close to nasal alar Peak 40–60 years	Fibrous capsule; lined by cuboidal, columnar or simple squamous epithelium (or mixed)

(*continued*)

Table 6.1 *Continued*

Type of cyst	Location	Clinical features	Histopathology
Median palatal cyst	Mid-line palate	Mid-line fluctuant swelling posterior to nasopalatine duct area; remnants of palatal shelf fusion Perinatal period: Epstein's pearls	Fibrous capsule with included epithelial remnants; lined by respiratory epithelium; often shows squamous metaplasia and may form keratin
Solitary bone cyst	Mandible	Non expansile, radiolucent lesion with scalloping between roots of teeth; clear fluid or air on aspiration Peak 10–20 years	Delicate granulation tissue lining with osteoclast-like giant cells and blood clot; clear fluid contents or air
Aneurysmal bone cyst	Mandible and maxilla	Rapidly expanding destructive lesion in jaws; bleeds copiously at biopsy; may be associated with other bone lesions Peak 10–20 years	Dense granulation tissue, fibrin, osteoclast-like giant cells, blood clot, bone fragments

Radiographically, the apical radicular cyst presents as a round or ovoid radiolucency at the root apex (Fig. 6.3). The lesion is often well circumscribed and may be demarcated by a peripheral radiopaque (corticated) margin continuous with the lamina dura of the involved tooth. Radicular cyst develops within an apical granuloma and whether or not an apical radiolucency represents a granuloma or a cyst cannot reliably be determined from the radiographic features. Only around 15% of apical radiolucencies are found to be cysts.

The other varieties of radicular cyst are less common. The residual cyst is a radicular cyst that has remained in the jaw and failed to resolve following extraction of the involved tooth (Fig. 6.4). About 20% of radicular cysts are residual in type. However, it should be noted that most periapical inflammation resolves after elimination of the non-vital pulp, either by endodontic therapy or tooth extraction. The lateral type is very uncommon and arises as a result of extension of inflammation from the pulp into the lateral periodontium along a lateral root canal.

Pathogenesis

Radicular cysts arise from proliferation of the epithelial rests of Malassez within chronic periapical granulomas (Fig. 5.43), but not all granulomas progress to cysts. The factors that determine why cystic transformation occurs in some, and the mechanisms involved in the formation of the cyst, are uncertain. Persistence of chronic inflammatory stimuli derived from the necrotic pulp, particularly bacterial endotoxin, appears essential since most periapical inflammation will resolve spontaneously once the causative agent has been removed. It is assumed that the environment within the chronically inflamed granuloma, which is likely to be rich in cytokines, including growth factors, stimulates the epithelial rests of Malassez to proliferate. Strands and sheets of squamous epithelium derived from proliferation of the rests are common findings in periapical granulomas.

Table 6.2 Incidence of the most common jaw cysts

Radicular cyst	60–75%
Dentigerous cyst	10–15%
Odontogenic keratocyst	5–10%
Nasopalatine duct cyst	5–10%

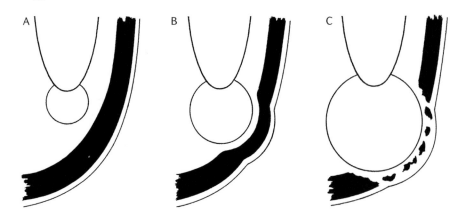

Fig. 6.2 Enlargement of a radicular cyst (A), causing cortical expansion (B), and then cortical thinning (C).

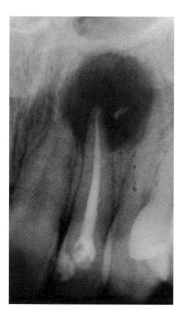

Fig. 6.3 Radiograph of a radicular cyst.

Two main mechanisms of formation have been proposed:

- Degeneration of central cells within a proliferating mass of epithelium. It is thought that a microcyst may form then continue to expand. Neutrophils frequently accumulate within the proliferating rests and may also contribute to cavitation.

- Necrosis and cavitation of granulation tissue. It is suggested that stromal areas within the granuloma may cavitate after enclavement by proliferating strands of epithelium or as a result of release of toxic products from the dead pulp or infecting organisms. Epithelial proliferation around the cavity results in the formation of a cyst.

Histopathology

Radicular cysts are lined wholly or in part by non-keratinized stratified squamous epithelium supported by a chronically inflamed fibrous tissue capsule (Fig. 6.5). In some cases the cyst may surround the root apex and such lesions have been referred to as 'pocket cysts' or 'strap cysts'. It has also been suggested that this type is more likely to heal

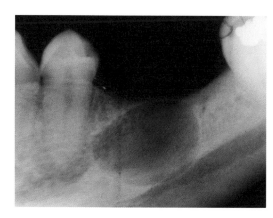

Fig. 6.4 Radiograph of a residual cyst.

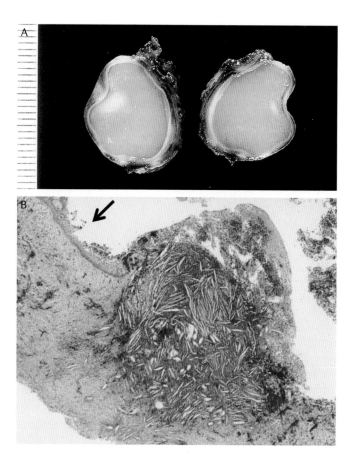

Fig. 6.5 Radicular cyst bisected to show the contents. Histology shows the epithelial lining (arrow) and a cholesterol nodule.

after endodontic treatment. However, some radicular cyst cavities are separated from the apex by the chronically inflamed capsule. In newly formed cysts, the epithelial lining is irregular and may vary considerably in thickness (Fig. 6.6A). Hyperplasia of the epithelium is a prominent feature resulting in long, anastomosing cords forming complex arcades extending into the surrounding capsule. The fibrous capsule is richly vascular and diffusely infiltrated by inflammatory cells. In established cysts, the epithelial lining is more regular in appearance and of fairly even thickness. Epithelial discontinuities are common and mural cholesterol nodules may be present. Metaplasia of the epithelial lining may give rise to respiratory-type epithelium and is found in about 40% of radicular cyst linings. In approximately 10% of cases the lining contains hyaline eosinophilic bodies—Rushton bodies—of varying size and shape (Fig. 6.6B). They have no diagnostic significance and are likely to be a product of the odontogenic epithelium. With time, the connective tissue capsule tends to become more fibrous, less vascular, and less inflamed. Deposits of cholesterol crystals are common within the capsules of many radicular cysts (Fig. 6.7A). In histological sections, cholesterol clefts may be few in number or form large mural nodules, in which case they are often associated with epithelial discontinuities and project into the cyst lumen (Fig. 6.5B). They are the probable origin of cholesterol crystals found in the cyst fluid. Mural cholesterol clefts are associated with foreign-body giant cells. As in periapical granulomas, the cholesterol is probably derived from the breakdown of red blood cells as a result of haemorrhage into the cyst

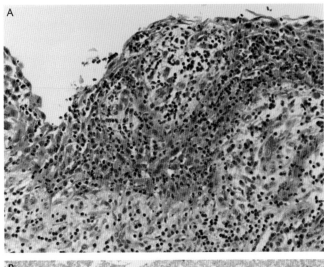

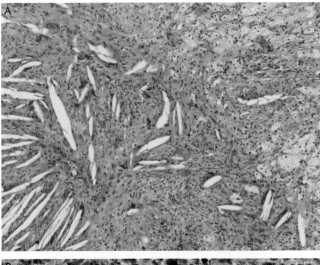

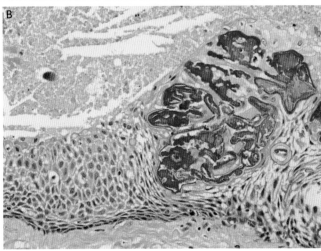

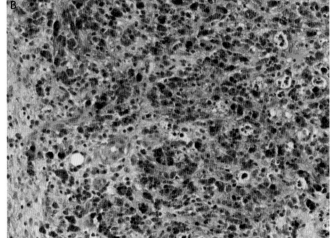

Fig. 6.6 Acutely inflamed non-keratinized squamous epithelium lining a radicular cyst (A). Eosinophilic hyaline material (Rushton bodies) within the cyst lining (B).

Fig. 6.7 The wall of a radicular cyst showing cholesterol clefts (needle-like spaces) and foamy macrophages (A). There is abundant haemosiderin deposition (brown deposits) (B).

capsule, and deposits of haemosiderin are commonly associated with the clefts (Fig. 6.7B).

Cyst contents

On aspiration, radicular cyst content typically varies from a watery, straw-coloured fluid through to semi-solid, brownish material of paste-like consistency (Fig. 6.5). Cholesterol crystals impart a shimmering appearance.

The composition of cyst fluid is complex and variable. It is hypertonic compared with serum and contains:

- Breakdown products of degenerating epithelial and inflammatory cells, and connective tissue components.
- Serum proteins; the soluble protein level is 50–110 g/l. Cyst fluid contains higher levels of immunoglobulin compared to plasma, probably due to local production by plasma cells in the capsule.
- Water and electrolytes.
- Cholesterol crystals.

Cyst expansion

Once formed, radicular cysts tend to progressively expand equally in all directions. The rate of expansion is governed by the rate of local bone resorption and, as bone is resorbed, the hydrostatic pressure of the contents causes the cyst to enlarge. Bone resorption is associated with activation of osteoclasts by factors released by inflammatory and other cells within the capsule. The hydrostatic pressure of the cyst fluid is increased because the contents are hypertonic compared with plasma, and water is drawn into the cyst cavity along this osmotic gradient. This movement of fluid increases the hydrostatic pressure within the cyst causing it to expand in a unicentric 'ballooning' pattern.

Dentigerous and eruption cysts

A dentigerous cyst encloses part or the whole of the crown of an unerupted tooth. It is attached to the amelo-cemental junction and arises in the follicular tissues covering the fully formed crown of an unerupted tooth. Radiographically, other cysts may present in apparent

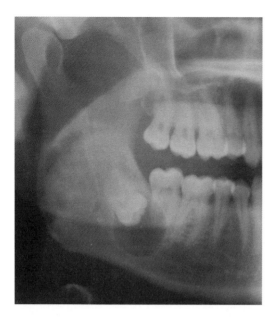

Fig. 6.8 Dentigerous cyst associated with a mandibular third molar.

(false) dentigerous relationship due to superimposition. An eruption cyst is a dentigerous cyst that arises outside the alveolar bone over an erupting tooth.

Clinical and radiographic features

Dentigerous cysts occur over a wide age-range and, although many are detected in adolescents and young adults, there is an increasing prevalence up to the fifth decade. They are about twice as common in males as in females and twice as common in the mandible than in the maxilla. The cysts most frequently involve teeth that are commonly impacted or erupt late. Most are associated with the mandibular third molar and then, in order of decreasing frequency: the maxillary permanent canines, maxillary third molars, and mandibular premolars. Uncommonly, they are associated with supernumerary teeth or with odontomes. Although a tooth of the permanent series will be missing from the arch (with possible exceptions where a supernumerary or cystic odontome is responsible), a dentigerous cyst may go undetected until it has enlarged sufficiently to produce expansion of the jaw. Alternatively,

a cyst may be detected on routine radiographic examination or on seeking a cause for a retained deciduous tooth. Pain is not a feature unless there is secondary inflammation.

Radiographically, the dentigerous cyst typically presents as a well-defined, unilocular radiolucency associated with the crown of an unerupted tooth (Figs 6.8–6.10). The tooth may be displaced for a considerable distance.

Eruption cysts involve both the primary and secondary dentitions. Because they arise in an extra-alveolar location, they present as fluctuant swellings on the alveolar mucosa and are often bluish in colour (Fig. 6.11). Haemorrhage into the cyst cavity is common as a result of trauma.

Pathogenesis and cyst expansion

Dentigerous cysts develop from the follicular tissues investing the crown of an unerupted tooth. Less than 1% of unerupted teeth develop cysts. The cyst cavity develops between the crown of the unerupted tooth and the reduced enamel epithelium, but the mechanisms of cyst formation are unknown. One hypothesis suggests that compression of the follicle by a potentially erupting but impacted tooth increases the venous pressure in the follicle, leading to increased transudation of fluid. Pooling of this transudate separates the follicle from the crown, resulting in cyst formation. Another hypothesis suggests that the cysts arise as a result of proliferation of the outer layers of the reduced enamel epithelium, as would normally occur in tooth eruption, followed by apoptosis of cells within the epithelial islands, leading to cyst formation. In a few cases, a dentigerous cyst may arise as a result of spread of periapical inflammation from a deciduous predecessor to involve the follicle of the permanent successor, accumulation of inflammatory exudate leading to cyst formation. Such inflammatory dentigerous cysts most often involve premolar teeth and are much more common in the mandible than in the maxilla. The mechanism of expansion of dentigerous cysts is probably similar to that of radicular cysts. The rate of cyst expansion in children may be rapid but enlargement is much slower in adults.

Histopathology

Macroscopically, dentigerous cysts are attached to the amelo-cemental junction (Fig. 6.12A). In most cases, the cyst completely surrounds the crown of the associated tooth (central type). Less frequently, the cyst projects laterally from the side of the tooth and does not completely

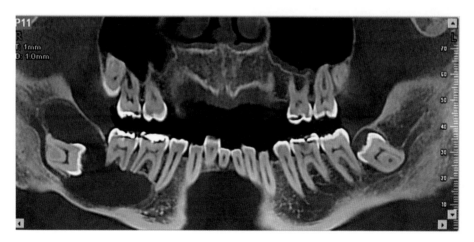

Fig. 6.9 Dentigerous cyst associated with a right mandibular third molar (Cone beam CT).

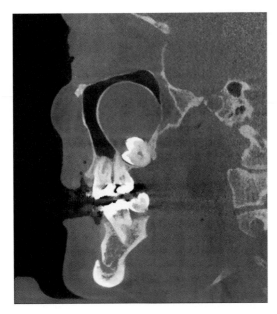

Fig. 6.10 Dentigerous cyst associated with a maxillary third molar (Cone beam CT).

enclose the crown (lateral type). The lining of dentigerous cysts is typically a thin, regular layer, some two to five cells thick, of non-keratinized, stratified squamous or flattened/low cuboidal epithelium (Fig. 6.12B). It resembles the reduced enamel epithelium from which it is derived. Mucous cell metaplasia is common and epithelial discontinuities are frequently observed. The capsule is fibrous and often contains loose myxoid areas resembling the dental follicle, from which it is derived. Islands and small strands of odontogenic epithelium are also occasionally observed. Inflammation is only present if there is secondary infection. Rarely the lining of a dentigerous cyst undergoes squamous metaplasia and shows orthokeratosis. Dentigerous cysts contain a proteinaceous, yellowish fluid, and cholesterol crystals are common. The soluble protein content is around 50–70 g/l. The lining of eruption cysts may be similar to a dentigerous cyst but is usually modified by chronic inflammation and haemorrhage, possibly as a result of trauma.

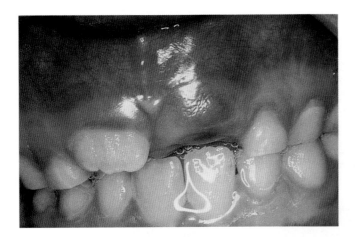

Fig. 6.11 Eruption cyst.

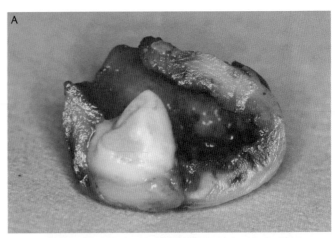

A

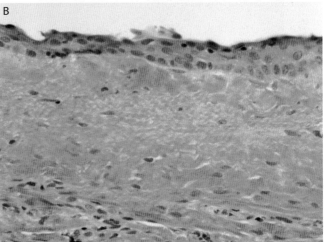

B

Fig. 6.12 Dentigerous cyst showing the relationship of the cyst to the crown of the tooth. The cyst lining is attenuated and resembles reduced enamel epithelium.

Odontogenic keratocyst

Although only accounting for 5–10% of jaw cysts, the odontogenic keratocyst is noteworthy because of its unusual growth pattern, tendency to recur and its association with an inherited syndrome.

Clinical and radiographic features

Odontogenic keratocysts occur over a wide age-range, but there is a pronounced peak incidence in the second and third decades, with a second smaller peak in the fifth decade. The cysts are more common in males than females, and 70–80% occur in the mandible. The most common site, accounting for at least 50% of all cases, is the third molar region and ascending ramus of the mandible. In both the mandible and maxilla, the majority of cysts occur in the region posterior to the first premolar.

Odontogenic keratocysts give rise to remarkably few symptoms, unless they become secondarily inflamed, and this probably accounts for why some do not present until the fifth decade. Unlike radicular and dentigerous cysts that tend to expand in a unicentric 'ballooning' pattern, odontogenic keratocysts enlarge predominantly in an antero-posterior direction and can reach large sizes without causing gross bone

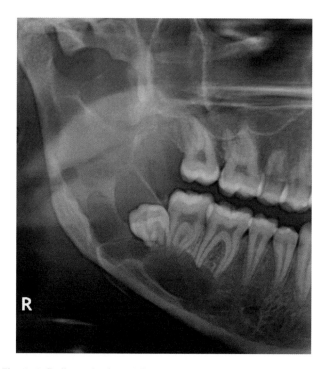

Fig. 6.13 Radiograph of a multilocular odontogenic keratocyst.

expansion (Fig. 6.13). In the mandible, odontogenic keratocyst often extends into the horizontal and vertical ramus resulting in a dumb-bell-shaped profile. Odontogenic keratocysts may be unilocular but frequently appear multilocular on radiographs (Fig. 6.13). They are often discovered, incidentally, on routine radiographic examination. Many odontogenic keratocysts are found in apparent dentigerous relationship with unerupted third molars, but the crowns of such teeth are usually separated from the cyst cavity, the pericoronal tissues being continuous with the cyst capsule. Odontogenic keratocysts may also present with the radiographic features of a lateral periodontal cyst, underscoring the need to submit every cyst that is removed surgically for histopathological examination.

The majority of odontogenic keratocysts arise sporadically and present as solitary lesions, although in a few patients two or more cysts may develop (Fig. 6.14). Multiple cysts are associated with the the basal cell naevus syndrome (BCNS; Gorlin–Goltz syndrome; OMIM 109400), inherited as an autosomal dominant trait with variable expressivity (Table 6.3). BCNS can be caused by mutations in the *PTCH1* gene on chromosome 9q22, the *PTCH2* gene on 1p32, or the *SUFU* gene on 10q24-q25. All of these mutations affect the Sonic Hedgehog signalling pathway. Mutations in *PTCH* have also been found in sporadic odontogenic keratocysts.

An important clinical feature of odontogenic keratocysts is their tendency to recur after surgical treatment. Recurrence rates vary in different reported series from 3 to 60%. The lining of odontogenic keratocyst is thin and tears easily on removal. Carnoy's solution, a tissue fixative, may be applied to eliminate cyst remnants and surgical marsupialization can also be employed to reduce the chances of recurrence.

Histopathology

The cyst wall is usually thin and often folded. Typically, it is lined by a regular continuous layer of stratified squamous epithelium between five and ten cells thick (Fig. 6.15A). The interface between the epithelial lining and the capsule is typically smooth. The basal cell layer is well defined and consists of palisaded columnar or occasionally cuboidal cells. The suprabasal cells resemble those of the stratum spinosum of oral epithelium and there is an abrupt transition between these and the surface layers that differentiate towards parakeratin production (Fig. 6.15A). The cells desquamate into the cyst lumen where they accumulate. Mitotic activity is higher than in other types of odontogenic cysts and sparse mitotic figures are found in basal and suprabasal cells. The fibrous capsule wall of the cyst is usually thin and generally free from inflammatory cell infiltration. If the cyst becomes secondarily inflamed, the epithelial lining loses its characteristic histology and proliferates to resemble that of a radicular cyst. Small groups of epithelial cells resembling dental lamina rests are often found in the cyst wall and these can give rise to independent satellite cysts around the main lesion (Fig. 6.15B). Satellite cysts are more common in cysts associated with the BCNS. Odontogenic keratocysts contain thick, creamy-white, cheesy material consisting of keratinous debris. There is little free fluid and the contents have a low soluble protein level, less than 40 g/l, composed predominantly of albumin.

The term odontogenic keratocyst should not be used to describe any odontogenic cyst producing keratin; it refers to a specific

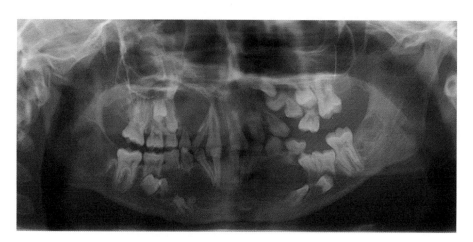

Fig. 6.14 Multiple odontogenic keratocysts in basal cell naevus syndrome (13, 33, 43, 48 regions).

Table 6.3 Basal cell naevus syndrome

Cutaneous	Multiple naevoid basal cell carcinomas are not restricted to sun-exposed skin and commonly appear from puberty onwards
Oral	Multiple odontogenic keratocysts may arise at varying intervals throughout the lifetime of the patient but tend to appear earlier than single sporadic cases
Skeletal	Rib abnormalities, vertebral deformities, polydactyly, cleft lip/palate
CNS	Calcified falx cerebri, brain tumours (medulloblastoma)

clinico-pathological entity. Other jaw cysts, such as radicular and dentigerous cysts, may produce keratin by metaplasia, but the epithelial linings of such cysts are usually orthokeratinized and lack the distinctive histopathological features of odontogenic keratocyst. There is an uncommon entity called orthokeratinized odontogenic cyst, which is lined entirely by orthokeratinized epithelium, but this should not be confused with odontogenic keratocyst, as it is effectively treated by enucleation and rarely recurs.

Growth of the odontogenic keratocyst

The odontogenic keratocyst has a destructive pattern of growth, burrowing through cancellous bone in a predominantly antero-posterior direction, this distinguishes it from the other odontogenic cysts that tend to expand in a unicentric ballooning pattern. The unique pattern of growth of the odontogenic keratocyst, in comparison to the other cysts, suggests that different mechanisms of enlargement are involved. The major factors thought to cause this are:

- Active epithelial growth. The epithelial lining of keratocysts shows a higher rate of mitotic activity than other odontogenic cysts. The proliferation is not uniform but tends to occur in clusters, which may account for foldings in the cyst lining and projections of the cyst into cancellous spaces.
- Cellular activity in the connective tissue capsule. Active growth of the capsule occurs in association with the proliferating areas of the epithelium. Osteoclasts tend to be located around the tips of the projections of the lining that are growing into the cancellous spaces.

Gingival cyst

Gingival cysts are of little clinical significance. They are common in neonates when they are often referred to as Bohn's nodules. Most disappear spontaneously by 3 months of age. They arise from remnants of the dental lamina that proliferate to form small keratinizing cysts. Gingival cysts in adults are rare. They occur most frequently in females and in the inter-premolar region of the mandible (Fig. 6.16).

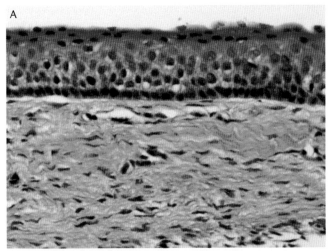

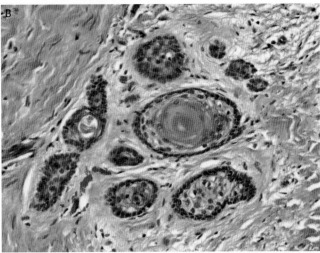

Fig. 6.15 Odontogenic keratocyst showing the typical thin parakeratinized squamous epithelial lining and odontogenic epithelial rests and satellite cysts in the wall.

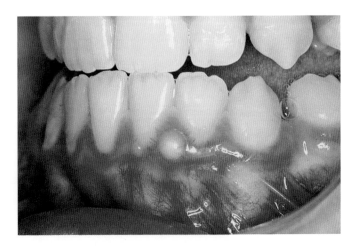

Fig. 6.16 Gingival cyst.

Lateral periodontal cyst

The lateral periodontal cyst is an uncommon lesion that must be distinguished from a lateral radicular cyst associated with a non-vital tooth and from an odontogenic keratocyst arising alongside the root of a tooth. Clinically, the lateral periodontal cyst occurs mainly in the canine and premolar region of the mandible in middle-aged patients. It may present with expansion or be discovered on routine radiographic examination as a well-defined radiolucent area with corticated margins (Fig. 6.17A). Histologically, the cyst is lined by thin non-keratinized squamous or cuboidal epithelium resembling reduced enamel epithelium, with focal thickenings (Fig. 6.17B). Its pathogenesis is uncertain but it is probably derived from either the reduced enamel epithelium or Serres' rests. Occasionally, lateral periodontal cysts are multilocular and may be described as 'botryoid' because of their resemblance to a bunch of grapes (botryoid odontogenic cyst).

Paradental cyst

This type of cyst arises alongside a partly erupted third molar involved by pericoronitis. Almost all occur in the mandible and most are located on the buccal or distobuccal aspect of the tooth (Fig. 6.18). The teeth associated with these cysts may show an enamel spur extending from the buccal cervical margin to the root furcation. Radiographically, the paradental cyst appears as a well-defined radiolucency related to the neck of the tooth and the coronal third of the root. The cysts are of inflammatory origin and probably arise as a result of extension of inflammation stimulating proliferation and cystic change in the reduced enamel epithelium covering the unerupted part of the crown. Histologically, paradental cysts resemble inflammatory radicular cysts.

Mandibular buccal cyst

Some authors consider the mandibular buccal cyst as a variant of the paradental cyst. Clinically, the cyst typically occurs in children aged 6–9 years and in the buccal aspect of mandibular first and second molars, often in the bifurcation. The cyst can be enucleated without necessarily extracting the adjacent tooth, depending on the clinical circumstances.

Glandular odontogenic cyst

The glandular odontogenic cyst (also known as sialo-odontogenic cyst) is a rare developmental odontogenic cyst. Most reported cases have occurred in the anterior part of the mandible where they presented as a slow-growing, painless unilocular or multilocular radiolucency. Histologically, the cyst is lined by epithelium of varying thickness with a superficial layer of columnar or cuboidal cells and occasional mucous cells. Crypts or small cyst-like spaces are present within the thickness of the epithelium and the lining has a distinctly glandular structure, with mucin formation. The cyst has a potentially destructive, locally invasive nature and a tendency to recur.

Key points Odontogenic cysts
- Arise from remnants of odontogenic epithelium
- Often symptomless and discovered on radiographs
- May expand the jaws and perforate the bone cortex

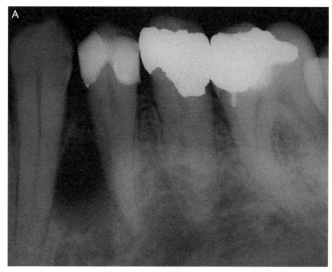
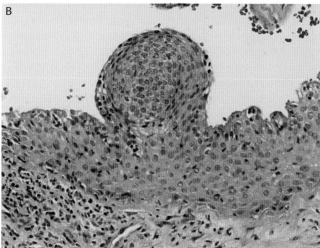

Fig. 6.17 Radiograph of lateral periodontal cyst. Cyst lining showing a characteristic focal thickening of the epithelium.

- Radicular cyst is the most common
- Typically radiolucent with corticated outline
- Clinico-pathological correlation essential for diagnosis
- Recurrence rare in radicular and dentigerous cysts
- Odontogenic keratocyst and glandular odontogenic cyst may recur after enucleation

Non-odontogenic cysts

Nasopalatine duct (incisive canal) cyst

The nasopalatine duct cyst is a distinct clinico-pathological entity and is the commonest of the non-odontogenic cysts. It is a developmental lesion thought to arise from epithelial remnants of the nasopalatine duct that connects the oral and nasal cavities in the embryo. The stimulus for cystic change is unknown.

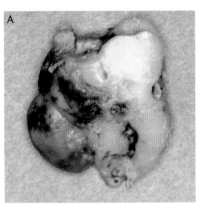
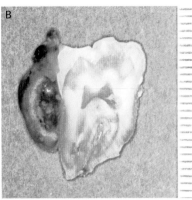

Fig. 6.18 Paradental cyst associated with a mandibular third molar.

Clinical and radiographic features

Nasopalatine duct cyst presents most commonly in the fifth and sixth decades and occurs more frequently in males than in females. It may be asymptomatic and discovered on routine radiographic examination, or present as a slowly enlarging swelling in the anterior region of the mid-line of the palate. Occasionally, it discharges into the mouth when the patient may complain of a salty taste. Pain may occur if the cyst becomes secondarily inflamed. Although cysts can arise at any point along the nasopalatine canal, most originate in the lower part and some arise entirely within the soft tissue of the incisive papilla. Such lesions are often designated cysts of the palatine papilla (Fig. 6.19A).

Radiographically, nasopalatine duct cysts present as well-defined, round, ovoid, or heart-shaped radiolucencies, often with a corticated rim (Fig. 6.19B). They are usually symmetrical about the mid-line, but some are displaced to one side. The cyst must be distinguished from the normal incisive fossa and it is generally accepted that a radiolucency not greater than 6 mm wide may be considered within normal limits. Where there are standing teeth, the lesion must also be differentiated from a radicular cyst and pulp vitality testing should be undertaken.

Histopathology

Nasopalatine duct cysts may be lined by a variety of different types of epithelium. Stratified squamous epithelium, pseudostratified ciliated columnar (respiratory) epithelium, often containing mucous cells, cuboidal epithelium, or columnar epithelium may be seen alone or in any combination. The epithelial lining is supported by a connective tissue capsule that usually includes prominent neurovascular bundles from the terminal branches of the long sphenopalatine nerve and vessels. Collections of mucous glands and a scattered chronic inflammatory cell infiltrate are frequently present.

Nasolabial cyst

The nasolabial cyst is a rare lesion that arises in the soft tissue of the upper lip just below the alar of the nose. Clinically, it presents as a slowly enlarging soft-tissue swelling obliterating the nasolabial fold and distorting the nostril. The cyst may arise bilaterally. The majority of cases present in the fourth decade and over 75% occur in women. The cysts are usually lined by pseudostratified columnar epithelium but stratified squamous epithelium, mucous cells, and ciliated cells may also be present. Nasolabial cyst is thought to originate from remnants of the lower part of the embryonic nasolacrimal duct.

Median palatal cyst

The median palatal cyst is very rare and is thought to originate from epithelium remnants included at the time of fusion of the palatal

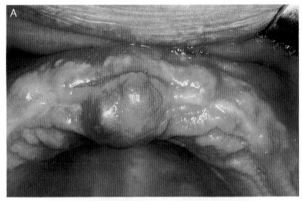

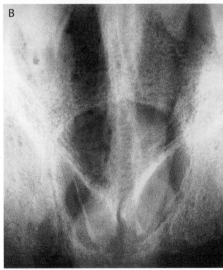

Fig. 6.19 Nasopalatine duct cyst presenting as an enlarged incisive papilla and a well-demarcated radiolucency on an upper occlusal radiograph.

shelves. Most cases have occurred in very young patients and are called Epstein's pearls. The cyst always arises in the mid-line of the palate, posterior to the incisive canal. The histological features are similar to nasopalatine duct cyst and some published cases may represent displaced nasopalatine duct cysts.

Key points Non-odontogenic epithelialized jaw cysts

- Arise from vestigal entrapped epithelium
- Nasopalatine duct cyst is the most common
- Recurrence is unlikely after enucleation
- Clinico-pathological correlation essential for diagnosis

Primary bone cysts

Primary bone cysts occur most often in long bones but are occasionally seen in the jaws, almost exclusively in the mandible.

Solitary bone cyst

A variety of terms have been used to designate this lesion, including simple bone cyst, traumatic bone cyst, haemorrhagic bone cyst, and unicameral bone cyst.

Clinical and radiographic features

The solitary bone cyst occurs predominantly in children and adolescents, with a peak incidence in the second decade. The cyst arises most frequently in the premolar and molar regions of the mandible. Maxillary lesions are rare. The majority of solitary bone cysts are asymptomatic and are chance radiographic findings; some degree of bony expansion occurs in about 25% of cases.

Radiographically, the lesion presents as a radiolucency of variable size and irregular outline. Scalloping is a prominent feature, particularly around and between the roots of standing teeth (Fig. 6.20). The margins of the lesion are usually well defined. In some circumstances, if the radiographic diagnosis can be made with confidence, then observation may be all that is required.

Histopathology

Surgical exploration typically reveals an empty cavity with a little clear or blood-stained fluid. Rapid healing follows surgical exploration but, even without surgical intervention, the cyst may resolve spontaneously over time. Microscopic examination of curettings from the lesion shows that the bony walls are covered by a delicate layer of loose, vascular fibrous tissue containing extravasated red blood cells and deposits of haemosiderin. There is no epithelial lining. The pathogenesis of the solitary bone cyst is unknown. It is commonly believed that there is a relationship to trauma, but the evidence is not convincing. A history of trauma can be elicited in only around a half of cases.

Aneurysmal bone cyst

The aneurysmal bone cyst is rare in the jaws. It arises either as a primary lesion or as a secondary change in some other pre-existing disorder of bone. Most of the reported cases of primary aneurysmal bone cysts have arisen in the mandible, usually the posterior part of the body or angle, and have occurred in children or young adults. Aneurysmal bone cyst presents as a firm and often rapidly growing expansile swelling causing facial deformity, and may be associated with pain. Radiographs show a uni- or multilocular radiolucency that may have a ballooned-out appearance due to gross cortical expansion. Secondary aneurysmal bone cysts in the jaws have been reported, mainly in association with fibro-osseous lesions and central giant cell granuloma (Chapter 7). Microscopically, aneurysmal bone cyst consists of numerous, non-endothelial-lined, blood-filled spaces of varying size, separated by cellular fibrous tissue. Multinucleated osteoclast-like giant cells, and evidence of old and recent haemorrhage, are common in the fibrous septa. The pathogenesis of aneurysmal bone cyst is unknown, but some have a USP6 fusion gene.

Key points Primary bone cysts

- No epithelial lining present
- May occur in other parts of the skeleton
- Solitary bone cyst not usually expansile or symptomatic
- Aneurysmal bone cyst typically rapidly expands the jaw

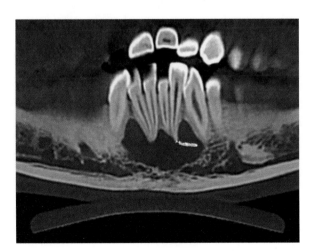

Fig. 6.20 Solitary bone cyst (Cone beam CT).

Lesions that may simulate cysts on radiographs

Stafne's idiopathic bone cavity is a developmental anomaly of the mandible. It typically appears as a round or oval, well-demarcated radiolucency between the premolar region and angle of the jaw, and is usually located beneath the inferior alveolar canal (Fig. 4.1). Occasionally, the anomaly is bilateral. The radiographic appearance is due to a saucer-shaped depression on the lingual aspect of the mandible that contains ectopic salivary tissue in continuity with the submandibular salivary gland. It is important to be aware of Stafne's cavity in order to avoid unnecessary investigations for a bone cyst.

Primary bone lesions, such as central giant cell granuloma, myeloma, Langerhans cell histiocytosis, Ewing's sarcoma, and even metastatic deposits of carcinoma in bone, may also simulate cysts clinically and radiographically (Chapter 7). Odontogenic tumours are more commonly mistaken for cysts, initially. Discovery of a significant solid component during surgical removal points to cystic degeneration of a neoplasm rather than a simple cyst. When enucleating a cyst, the material should be submitted for histopathological examination to derive a definitive diagnosis.

Management of cysts

Small, radicular cysts may be treated by orthograde endodontic treatment or apicectomy; larger cysts are generally treated by enucleation, which aims to remove the entire cyst by separating the cyst wall from the adjacent bone. Dentigerous cysts are usually enucleated and the associated unerupted tooth is removed, whilst eruption cysts may be observed or 'de-roofed' to encourage eruption of the associated tooth. Odontogenic keratocyst has a high potential rate of recurrence and may require adjunctive treatment such as application of Carnoy's solution after enucleation. All other types of cyst are treated by enucleation, with the exception of glandular odontogenic cyst, which may require local conservative excision.

Odontomes

Complex odontome

The complex odontome is a developmental tumour-like mass consisting of disorderly arranged dental tissues. It has a limited growth potential and can be considered as a dental hamartoma. The complex odontome occurs predominantly in the second and third decades of life and the majority arise in the molar region of the mandible. They are often associated with the crowns of unerupted teeth (Fig. 6.21A) and, occasionally, may take the place of a tooth. For these reasons they may be discovered, when small, as incidental findings when investigating a patient with a tooth missing from the dental arch. As the lesion enlarges, it usually presents as a painless, slow-growing expansion of the jaw, but may become infected and present with pain and swelling, particularly if it communicates with the oral cavity. Multiple odontomes are rare and may be part of Gardner's syndrome (OMIM 175100; Chapter 7).

Radiographically, a fully formed complex odontome appears as a radiopaque lesion, sometimes with a radiating structure (Fig. 6.21A), but in the developing stages it shows as a well-defined radiolucent lesion in which there is progressive deposition of radiopaque material as mineralization of the dental tissues proceeds. The mature lesion is surrounded by a narrow radiolucent zone analogous to the pericoronal space around unerupted teeth.

Histologically, the fully developed complex odontome consists of a mass of disorderly arranged, but well-formed enamel, dentine, and cementum (Fig. 6.21B). Dentine forms the bulk of the lesion and, on surfaces not covered by enamel or cementum, is in contact with tissue resembling the normal pulp. In decalcified sections, the areas occupied by enamel appear as empty spaces, except where enamel maturation is incomplete, when the spaces contain remnants of enamel matrix with a 'fishscale' appearance. The developing complex odontome contains ameloblasts, odontoblasts, and cementoblasts, with associated hard tissues at all stages in odontogenesis

Compound odontome

The compound odontome is a developmental tumour-like mass that, unlike the complex odontome, consists of numerous, small, discrete, tooth-like structures called denticles. They do not resemble the teeth of the normal dentition but each one consists of normal enamel, dentine,

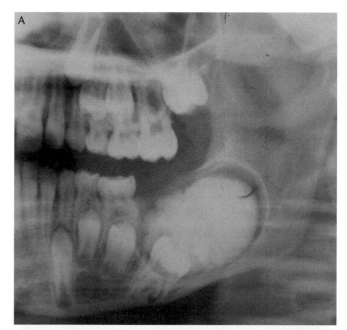

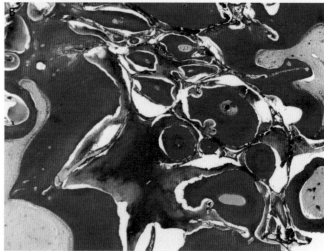

Fig. 6.21 Complex odontome showing a well-demarcated radiodense lesion. Histology shows a haphazard mixture of hypomineralized enamel, dentine, and pulpal tissue.

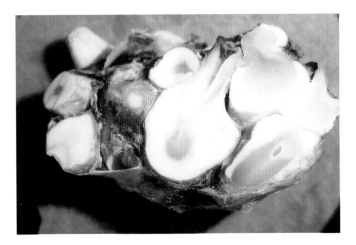

Fig. 6.22 Macroscopic appearance of the cut surface of a compound odontome showing separate denticles.

cementum, and pulp arranged as in a normal tooth (Fig. 6.22). The compound odontome occurs predominantly in the first two decades of life

and the majority arise in the anterior maxilla. In many cases, the lesion overlies the crown of an unerupted tooth and is discovered incidentally when investigating the cause of a missing tooth from the dental arch. It appears to have a more limited growth potential than the complex odontome and so expansion of bone is less prominent. The compound odontome may also, occasionally, be associated with an odontogenic tumour.

Radiographically, the developing compound odontome may appear as a radiolucent or mixed radiopaque and radiolucent lesion but, by the time most are detected, they contain recognizable distinct denticles.

> **Key points Odontomes**
> - Hamartomatous developmental lesions
> - May cause delay in eruption of a permanent tooth
> - Can become infected if covering mucosa breaks down
> - Complex odontome is a fused mass of dental hard-tissues
> - Compound odontome is comprised of multiple denticles
> - Multiple odontomes present in Gardner's syndrome

Odontogenic tumours

Odontogenic tumours originate from remnants of the tooth-forming tissues. They are broadly classified as epithelial, mixed, and mesenchymal, depending on the predominate constituent elements. Only when both odontogenic epithelial and specialized dental mesenchyme are present can dental hard-tissue form, though hard tissue is not always present in such tumours. It is also important to understand that the tooth-forming tissue is intimately related to bone during development. The majority of odontogenic tumours are benign and do not metastasize; however, some are characterized by local invasion and bone destruction. This unusual biological property may be due to the normal requirement for the odontogenic apparatus, including the cells of the dental lamina, to migrate and 'invade' into the jaw during development. The classification outlined in Box 6.1 is modified from the WHO classification published in 2005. Malignant odontogenic tumours, capable of local destruction and metastasis, are recognized but are rare.

Benign odontogenic tumours

Ameloblastoma

Ameloblastoma is the most frequent odontogenic tumour. There are several variants and the most common type is known as 'conventional' or 'solid/multicystic' ameloblastoma. It is a slowly growing, locally invasive epithelial neoplasm with a high rate of recurrence if not removed adequately. There is no gender predilection and ameloblastoma occurs over a wide age-range. Most cases present between 30 and 60 years of age, and the tumour is rare below the age of 20 years. Geographic and racial differences are well recognized.

Clinical and radiographic features

Ameloblastoma occurs mainly in the jaws but, rarely, also can arise in the sinonasal cavities. Approximately 80% occur in the mandible, with a marked predilection for the posterior region, except in African Black people where the anterior mandible is more frequently involved. Most maxillary ameloblastomas occur in the posterior region. Ameloblastoma may be asymptomatic or cause swelling of the jaw (Fig. 6.23). Radiographs show a unilocular or multilocular radiolucency resembling a cyst (Fig. 6.24). Scalloped borders are sometimes seen and an unerupted tooth may be present. Resorption of the roots of adjacent teeth is common. Ameloblastoma is locally invasive and infiltrates through the medullary spaces. The neoplasm expands cortical bone and eventually may erode the cortical plate and extend into adjacent tissues (Fig. 6.25). In the posterior maxilla, ameloblastoma obliterates the maxillary sinus and may invade the skull base.

Histopathology

Macroscopically, conventional ameloblastoma may show extensive cystic change. Thickened, mural areas must be sampled by biopsy to establish the diagnosis. Two basic histopathological patterns, follicular and plexiform, are recognized (Fig. 6.26). The follicular pattern consists of islands of odontogenic epithelium within a fibrous stroma. The basal cells of these islands are columnar, hyperchromatic, and lined up in a palisaded arrangement. They resemble pre-ameloblasts morphologically. Typically, their nuclei are displaced away from the basement membrane, called reverse nuclear polarity, the basal cytoplasm

---

Box 6.1 Odontogenic tumours

| **Benign odontogenic tumours** | **Malignant odontogenic tumours** |

Epithelial lesions

Without odontogenic mesenchyme

- Ameloblastoma
- Squamous odontogenic tumour
- Calcifying epithelial odontogenic tumour
- Adenomatoid odontogenic tumour
- Keratocystic odontogenic tumour (odontogenic keratocyst)

With odontogenic mesenchyme (mixed lesions)

- Ameloblastic fibroma
- Ameloblastic fibrodentinoma
- Ameloblastic fibro-odontoma
- Calcifying odontogenic cyst
- Dentinogenic ghost cell tumour

Mesenchymal lesions

- Odontogenic fibroma
- Odontogenic myxoma
- Cementoblastoma

Malignant odontogenic tumours

Odontogenic carcinomas

- Ameloblastic carcinoma
- Primary intra-osseous squamous cell carcinoma
- Clear cell odontogenic carcinoma
- Ghost cell odontogenic carcinoma
- Malignant change in odontogenic cyst

Odontogenic sarcomas

- Ameloblastic fibrosarcoma
- Ameloblastic fibro-odontosarcoma

Congenital tumours of possible odontogenic origin

- Congenital epulis
- Melanotic neuroectodermal tumour of infancy
- Congenital odontogenic myxoma

Source data from Chapter 6 Odontogenic Tumours, in *Pathology and Genetics of Head and Neck Tumours*, Fifth edition, Barnes L, Eveson L W, Reichart P, and Sidransky D. (eds), 2005.

---

is abundant, and sometimes vacuolated, lacking Tomes' processes. The central cells may be loosely arranged, resembling stellate reticulum. Squamous differentiation may be seen and granular cells may be present. The plexiform pattern contains basal cells arranged in anastomosing strands with an inconspicuous stellate reticulum. The fibrous stroma is variable and can be delicate or densely fibrotic. No dental hard-tissue formation is observed in ameloblastoma. Cyst-like degeneration may be seen in both the stromal and epithelial components. The two patterns, follicular and plexiform, have no clinical significance and both may occur in areas of an individual neoplasm. Mitotic activity and cellular pleomorphism are rarely found.

Management

Biopsies of ameloblastoma may show mainly cystic areas of the tumour and, in these cases, it is often necessary to correlate the biopsy and imaging appearances to reach a definitive diagnosis. Current treatment aims at achieving complete excision with a small margin of uninvolved tissue. In some cases a more conservative approach may be adopted for

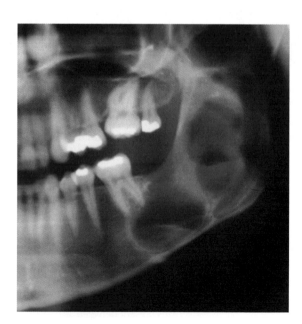

Fig. 6.23 Facial deformity associated with ameloblastoma.

Fig. 6.24 Ameloblastoma presenting as a multilocular radiolucency at the angle of the mandible.

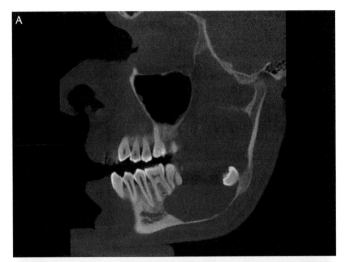

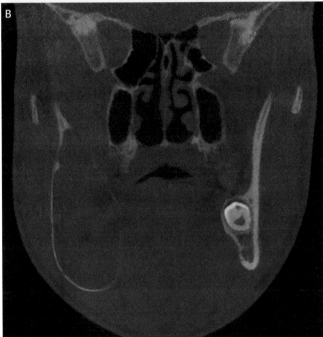

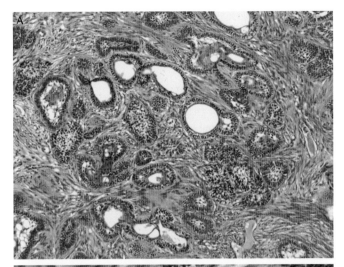

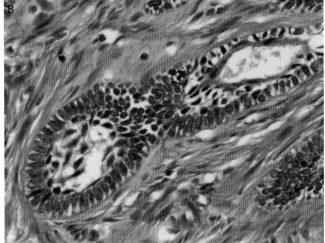

Fig. 6.26 Ameloblastoma (solid/multicystic-type) showing the follicular pattern of the epithelial component embedded in a mature fibrous stroma.

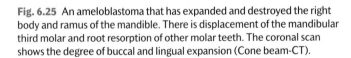

Fig. 6.25 An ameloblastoma that has expanded and destroyed the right body and ramus of the mandible. There is displacement of the mandibular third molar and root resorption of other molar teeth. The coronal scan shows the degree of buccal and lingual expansion (Cone beam-CT).

clinical reasons. Radiotherapy and chemotherapy are not advocated. Long-term follow-up is mandatory because recurrence has been found after more than 10 years.

Variants of ameloblastoma

Peripheral ameloblastoma

This distinctive variant presents as a red, sometimes papillary, mucosal patch often involving the gingiva. The lesion may be raised and, although there may be 'saucerization' of the underlying bone, the

tumour is entirely extra-osseous. Histologically, there are sheets and islands of cells resembling conventional ameloblastoma and, in many cases, the neoplasm appears to originate from the surface epithelium. Some authors regard peripheral ameloblastoma as the oral counterpart of basal cell carcinoma of skin (Chapter 8). The tumour is treated by local excision, often involving a rim resection or block of underlying alveolar bone to ensure clearance. In rare cases, peripheral ameloblastoma can de-differentiate and give rise to ameloblastic carcinoma that invades the underlying jaw.

Desmoplastic ameloblastoma

This variant occurs most frequently in the anterior mandible and maxilla. It occurs over a similar age-range to conventional ameloblastoma. Radiographs show a distinctive appearance consisting of a mottled, diffuse, mixed radiodense and radiolucent lesion, often associated with tooth displacement and/or resorption. A diagnosis of destructive fibro-osseous lesion may be suggested. Microscopically, desmoplastic ameloblastoma has an abundant stromal component with compressed islands of odontogenic epithelium. These resemble ameloblastoma but often lack the peripheral palisade and are jagged in outline. Metaplastic bone trabeculae, microcytic change, and myxoid areas may be present. Treatment is similar to that of conventional ameloblastoma—complete excision.

Unicystic ameloblastoma

This type of ameloblastoma presents as a unilocular cyst. Over 90% occur in the posterior mandible. The age-range is younger than in conventional ameloblastoma. In many cases an unerupted third molar tooth is present, sometimes in a dentigerous relationship. On radiographs, the cyst is unilocular and has a well-corticated, smooth outline (Fig. 6.27). Histological diagnosis on a small amount of cyst lining is challenging because the typical morphological features of ameloblastoma are inconspicuous and may lead to the erroneous diagnosis of a developmental odontogenic cyst. Three histological variants of unicystic ameloblastoma are recognized:

Luminal-type—the cyst is lined by attenuated 'ameloblastomatous' epithelium.

Intra-luminal-type—the cyst has projections of plexiform ameloblastoma into the central cystic cavity.

Mural-type—the ameloblastomatous cyst lining shows complex budding and invasion of the cyst wall.

The luminal and intra-luminal types show no invasion of the cyst wall and the majority are eradicated by enucleation. The mural-type has a risk of recurrence and treatment is the same as for conventional ameloblastoma—complete excision.

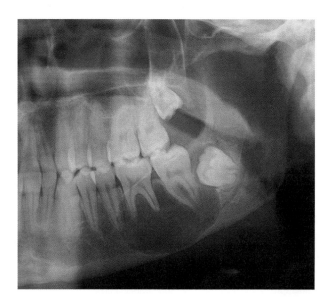

Fig. 6.27 Unicystic ameloblastoma with features similar to a large dentigerous cyst.

Odontoameloblastoma

This rare tumour has histological features of developing odontome admixed with conventional solid/multicystic ameloblastoma. Clinically it is treated as conventional ameloblastoma.

Key points Ameloblastoma

- Most common odontogenic tumour
- Predilection for the mandible
- Typically expands both cortical plates
- Often multilocular radiolucent lesion
- Follicular and plexiform histological patterns
- Pre-ameloblast-like cells show reversed nuclear polarity
- Treatment is by excision with a small margin
- Unicystic ameloblastoma and other variants occur

Squamous odontogenic tumour

This is a rare neoplasm that typically occurs between the roots of teeth. It most often produces a triangular or unilocular radiolucent area but larger examples may be multilocular. Histologically, there are islands of squamous cells, sometimes with a peripheral layer of cuboidal cells. Treatment is by local excision and recurrence is rare.

Calcifying epithelial odontogenic tumour

The calcifying epithelial odontogenic tumour (CEOT) is a locally invasive neoplasm, characterized by the presence of amyloid material that may become calcified. The CEOT is also widely known as Pindborg tumour. CEOT is rare and accounts for only 1% of all odontogenic tumours occurring in patients between 20 and 60 years of age, with a mean around 40 years. Most cases are intra-osseous but a peripheral variant is recognized. The premolar area of the mandible is most commonly affected, but CEOT may arise in any part of the alveolus.

Clinical and radiographic features

CEOT typically presents as an asymptomatic, slow-growing mass expanding the jaw. Peripheral gingival lesions are firm, painless masses. In radiographs, the CEOT shows a mixed radiolucent and radiopaque appearance and the lesion may be unilocular or multilocular (Fig. 6.28). An unerupted tooth, most often a mandibular third molar, is often associated with CEOT.

Histopathology

On gross section, CEOT has a solid, pale white appearance with variable foci of calcification. Cystic change is not a common feature. Microscopically, CEOT consists of islands and sheets of polyhedral epithelial cells with abundant eosinophilic cytoplasm, sharply defined cell borders, and well-developed inter-cellular bridges (Fig. 6.29A). The nuclei are frequently pleomorphic and enlarged nuclei are common.

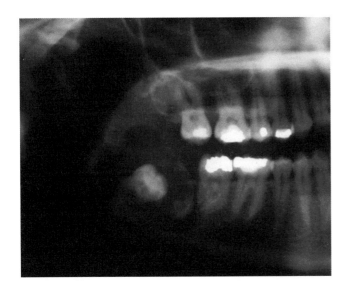

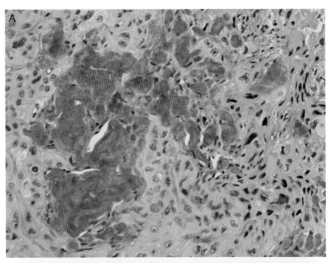

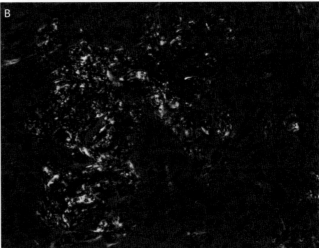

Fig. 6.28 Radiograph of a calcifying epithelial odontogenic tumour in the mandibular third molar region.

Mitotic figures are sparse. The sheets of tumour cells are supported by a fibrous stroma. Amyloid, appearing as an eosinophilic, homogeneous hyaline material that is often calcified in the form of concentric rings, is present within or around the sheets of neoplastic cells. The amyloid can be demonstrated by the histochemical stain Congo Red; the pink-staining material has a characteristic 'apple green' birefringence when viewed under cross-polarized light (Fig. 6.29B). It is likely that the amyloid is derived from secreted enamel proteins. Clear cells may be present and in some cases make up a significant proportion of the tumour.

Management

Local excision is recommended with a margin of normal tissue. Recurrence is noted in around 20% of cases and is more frequent when a clear cell component is present. Rare malignant variants of CEOT have been described.

Adenomatoid odontogenic tumour

The adenomatoid odontogenic tumour (AOT) usually presents during the second and third decades of life. It is classified as a benign neoplasm; however, the age-profile, slow growth, and innocuous clinical behaviour suggest that it may be a dental hamartoma. AOT is usually intra-osseous and is more frequent in the maxilla than in the mandible. The rare peripheral type occurs almost exclusively in the anterior maxillary gingiva.

Clinical and radiographic features

AOT is typically found in association with unerupted permanent teeth, particularly maxillary canines. Most AOTs are asymptomatic but may cause jaw expansion or displacement of neighbouring teeth. Radiographically, AOT appears as a well-defined, radiolucent lesion with a corticated outline, often resembling a dentigerous cyst (Fig. 6.30A).

Fig. 6.29 Calcifying epithelial odontogenic tumour stained with Congo red showing pleomorphic epithelial cells with dark nuclei and pink-staining amyloid. The amyloid has a characteristic apple-green colour when viewed with cross-polarized light.

Histopathology

Most AOTs are treated by enucleation, with removal of the unerupted tooth, if present. On gross section, the cut surface is solid with focal microcystic changes. Microscopically, AOT shows variably sized, solid nodules of cuboidal or columnar cells of odontogenic epithelium forming nests or rosette-like structures with minimal stromal connective tissue (Fig. 6.30B). Eosinophilic amorphous material, as droplets or short bars, is often present and can be demonstrated with the histochemical stain DPAS. Tubular duct-like spaces lined by a single row of columnar epithelial cells, with the nuclei polarized away from the luminal surface, are characteristic. Nodules consisting of polyhedral, eosinophilic epithelial cells of squamous appearance are also seen. Globules of amorphous amyloid-like material and calcified osteodentine may be found in the AOT.

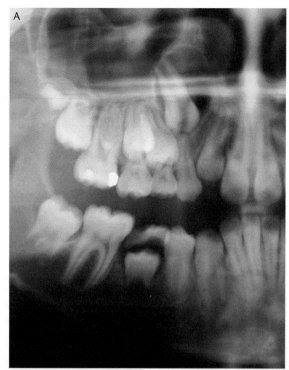

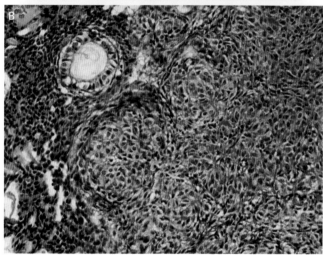

Fig. 6.30 Radiograph showing an adenomatoid odontogenic tumour associated with the maxillary canine. Histology showing epithelial rosettes and a 'duct-like' structure.

Management

Enucleation or conservative local excision is curative.

Keratocystic odontogenic tumour (odontogenic keratocyst)

This lesion is more widely known as odontogenic keratocyst and has been described earlier in this chapter. The WHO introduced the term 'keratocystic odontogenic tumour' into the 2005 classification of odontogenic tumours, to reflect the aggressive behaviour by comparison to other odontogenic cysts, but the terminology is controversial.

Ameloblastic fibroma

Ameloblastic fibroma is a rare odontogenic tumour that occurs mostly in the posterior mandible of children and young adults. The tumour consists of odontogenic mesenchyme resembling the dental papilla. Epithelial strands and nests are present but dental hard-tissue formation is not seen. If dentine forms, then the tumour is referred to as ameloblastic fibrodentinoma. The term ameloblastic fibro-odontoma is used if all the dental hard tissues are present; however, it is thought that these calcifying lesions simply represent developing odontomes.

Clinical and radiographic features

Ameloblastic fibroma typically presents as a painless swelling or failure of a permanent tooth to erupt. Radiographically, the tumour presents as a well-demarcated radiolucency, often in connection with a displaced tooth.

Histopathology

On gross section, ameloblastic fibroma has a uniform, creamy-white, slightly mucoid appearance. Microscopically, the major component is an immature cell-rich myxoid tissue with stellate-shaped fibroblasts possessing elongated slender cytoplasmic extensions resembling embryonic tooth pulp. Strands and islands of epithelial cells are distributed throughout the myxoid component. These show features of pre-ameloblasts and stellate reticulum, and they resemble ameloblastoma.

Management

The approach to treatment is enucleation and curettage. Recurrence may occur but is readily curable. Rarely, ameloblastic fibroma may undergo progressive malignant change to become an ameloblastic fibrosarcoma.

Calcifying odontogenic cyst

Calcifying odontogenic cyst (COC) is a simple cyst lined by ameloblastoma-like epithelium with ghost cells that may calcify.

Clinical and radiographic features

Intra-osseous COC typically presents as a painless swelling resembling a cyst. Peripheral (extra-osseous) COC forms an elevated red mass on the gingiva or alveolus. Radiographs of peripheral COC may show saucerization and sometimes displacement of adjacent teeth. Intra-osseous COC is typically seen as a unilocular radiolucency with a well-circumscribed outline (Fig. 6.31A). A variable amount of radiopaque flecking may be seen. Root resorption is common and an associated unerupted tooth may be present.

Histopathology

Macroscopically, COC consists of pale grey-brown tissue with cream flecks. In both the peripheral and intra-osseous variants, the cyst wall is lined by a thin ameloblastomatous epithelium with the formation of 'ghost' cells (Fig. 6.31B). These show a distinctive form of keratinization in which eosinophilic material accumulates in the cytoplasm that obscures the nuclear detail. The ghost cells often undergo calcification. Dysplastic dentine resembling bone may form in the capsule in COC.

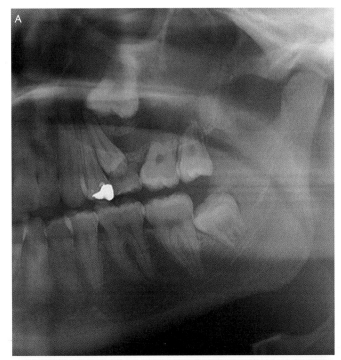

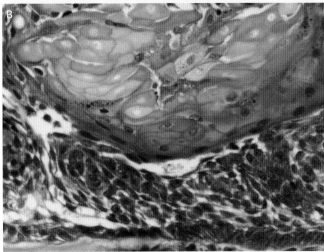

Fig. 6.31 Radiograph of a calcifying odontogenic cyst in the left maxilla. The maxillary first molar has been displaced. Histopathology of the cyst lining shows odontogenic epithelium and keratinized 'ghost' cells.

Management

Enucleation or conservative excision is considered appropriate for COC and recurrence is rare.

Dentinogenic ghost cell tumour

Dentinogenic ghost cell tumour (DGCT) is a locally invasive neoplasm related to COC and characterized by ameloblastoma-like islands of epithelial cells in a mature connective tissue stroma. Ghost cells are characteristic and there may be dysplastic dentine formation. Most examples are intra-osseous but a peripheral variant is recognized to occur.

Clinical and radiographic features

Intra-osseous DGCT is usually asymptomatic. There may be bony expansion and cortical bone destruction with extension into soft tissues. Adjacent teeth may be displaced and mobile. Radiographs show a mixed radiolucent and radiopaque appearance due to calcification. Most are unilocular and show well-defined borders. Resorption of adjacent teeth is a common finding.

Histopathology

DGCT is comprised of tumour islands that resemble ameloblastoma. The distinguishing feature is the presence of ghost cells. Individual ghost cell keratinization, as well as large islands of ghost cells, may be seen. Some ghost cells undergo calcification and dysplastic dentin may be formed. Invasion of the medullary spaces is seen and the biological behaviour is similar to ameloblastoma.

Management

Local resection is normally performed, particularly if the tumour margins are poorly defined. Enucleation or conservative excision may be appropriate for peripheral DGCT. Rare malignant transformation to dentinogenic ghost cell carcinoma has been reported.

Odontogenic fibroma

Odontogenic fibroma is a rare neoplasm characterized by varying amounts of inactive-looking odontogenic epithelium embedded in a mature, fibrous stroma.

Clinical and radiographic features

Odontogenic fibroma presents as a slowly enlarging, painless, jaw swelling, often with cortical expansion. Most often the tumour appears as a unilocular radiolucent area with a well-defined corticated outline. Calcified material may produce a mixed radiolucent and radiopaque appearance. Scalloped margins may be present and adjacent teeth may be displaced.

Histopathology

Odontogenic fibroma is composed of cellular, fibroblastic, and collagenous connective tissue interwoven with less cellular and often vascular areas. Small islands or short strands of inactive-appearing odontogenic epithelium are present and may be sparse or abundant. Some authors recognize epithelial-rich and poor-types as distinct variants.

Management

Odontogenic fibroma is generally treated by local enucleation and curettage. Recurrence is thought to be rare and is attributed to incomplete removal. Rarely, odontogenic fibroma can reach a large size causing facial deformity, particularly in those lacking access to healthcare.

Odontogenic myxoma

Odontogenic myxoma (fibromyxoma) is an intra-osseous neoplasm characterized by stellate and spindle-shaped cells embedded in an abundant myxoid extracellular matrix. The tumour is the second most frequent odontogenic tumour after ameloblastoma. Most occur in children and young adults. Two-thirds of odontogenic myxomas are located in the mandible, most frequently in the molar region.

Clinical and radiographic features

Odontogenic myxoma expands the jaw and, when present in the maxilla, tends to obliterate the maxillary sinus. On radiographs there is typically a unilocular or multilocular radiolucency. A fine 'soap bubble' or 'honeycomb' appearance may be present and fine bony trabeculations are often seen on CT (Fig. 6.32A). The borders of the neoplasm are frequently well defined and corticated but can be poorly demarcated or diffuse. Tooth displacement and root resorption may occur.

Histopathology

On sectioning after excision, the tumour appears as a grey-white mass with a translucent mucinous appearance. Fine, white collagenous

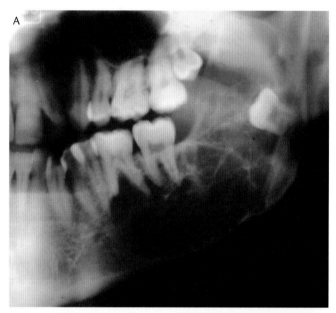

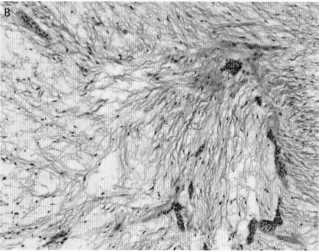

Fig. 6.32 An odontogenic myxoma presenting as a multilocular radiolucency. Histology showing loose myxoid fibrous tissue containing a few nests of odontogenic epithelium.

bands may traverse the tumour. Microscopically, randomly oriented oval, stellate, and spindle-shaped cells with long, slender, anastomosing cytoplasmic processes extending from the centrally placed nucleus are seen. Rests of odontogenic epithelium may be present but are not always seen. Some odontogenic myxomas contain a collagenous fibrous component (Fig. 6.32B). The neoplasm often permeates into the marrow spaces in an infiltrative pattern.

Management

Small odontogenic myxomas have been successfully treated by currettage but larger lesions require complete excision with free margins. Recurrence rates average about 25% but metastasis does not occur and the prognosis is good. Maxillary lesions may extend into the cranial base.

Cementoblastoma

Cementoblastoma is a benign neoplasm and is characterized by the formation of cementum-like tissue around the root of a tooth. The age range is from 8 up to 44 years, the mean being approximately 20 years. The majority of cementoblastomas are located in the mandible, particularly related to the permanent first molar; association with a primary tooth is exceptional.

Clinical and radiographic features

Cementoblastoma typically presents as a painful swelling of the buccal and lingual aspects of the alveolus. The involved tooth remains vital. Radiographically, cementoblastoma is well defined and is comprised of a central radiopaque nidus surrounded by a thin radiolucent zone (Fig. 6.33A). Root resorption, loss of root outline, and obliteration of the periodontal ligament space are common findings.

Histopathology

On removal, a hard nodular mass firmly attached to one or more tooth roots surrounded by thin fibrous tissue is typically found (Fig. 6.33B). Microscopically, cementoblastoma consists of dense masses of acellular cementum-like material in a fibrous stroma that may contain multinucleated cells. The tumour merges with the root of the tooth. At the periphery, sheets of unmineralized tissue with plump cementoblasts may be seen, often arranged in radiating columns (Fig. 6.34).

Management

Conservative surgical removal is indicated. Recurrence is common and is usually a consequence of incomplete removal.

Key points Benign odontogenic tumours

- Can be locally invasive but lack metastatic potential
- Ameloblastoma is the most common
- Some resemble cysts on imaging
- Histopathology must be correlated with imaging
- May show destructive features and displace teeth
- Malignant odontogenic tumours are very rare

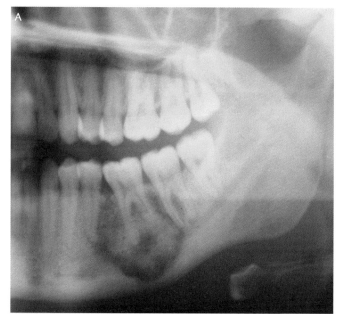

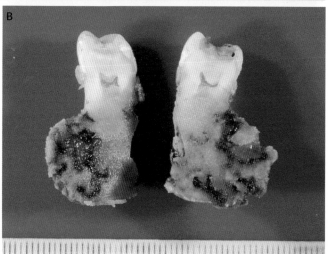

Fig. 6.33 Radiograph of a cementoblastoma and the surgical specimen bisected.

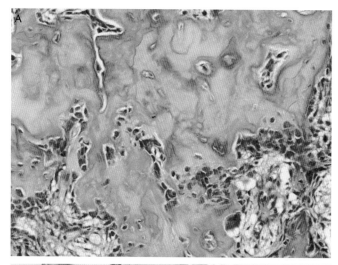

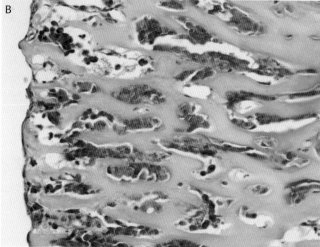

Fig. 6.34 Cementoblastoma composed of basophilic cementum and plump cementoblasts. At the periphery there are radiating seams of cementum.

Malignant odontogenic tumours

Odontogenic carcinomas are very rare and odontogenic sarcomas are extremely rare. It is increasingly recognized that malignant variants, or transformation of benign odontogenic tumours such as calcifying epithelial odontogenic tumour, exist. Sometimes squamous cell carcinoma arises from a pre-existing benign odontogenic tumour or cyst. The clinical presentation is variable, but 'red flag' signs and symptoms include extensive bone destruction, mobile teeth, a non-healing tooth socket, mucosal ulceration, paraesthesia or anaesthesia of the trigeminal nerve, and lymphadenopathy.

Ameloblastic carcinoma

This rare malignant neoplasm is highly invasive and can metastasize to regional lymph nodes and distant sites. Some ameloblastic carcinomas appear malignant from the outset. Others appear to arise by de-differentiation from conventional ameloblastoma. Malignant peripheral ameloblastic carcinoma is also recognized. Microscopically, there are sheets and islands of basaloid cells with peripheral palisading. Mitotic figures, nuclear and cellular pleomorphism, and necrosis may be present. Neural and vascular invasion are often found. Treatment is similar to that for oral squamous cell carcinoma and involves surgical excision with clear margins. Depending on the clinical stage of disease, a neck dissection may be required to remove the regional lymph nodes.

Primary intra-osseous squamous carcinoma

Although the majority of oral squamous cell carcinomas arise from surface mucosa, a small number arise from odontogenic epithelium included in the jaws. Some arise *de novo* and others in a pre-existing odontogenic cyst. These neoplasms expand the jaws, show rapid growth, and may cause pathological fracture. Microscopically, they resemble conventional squamous cell carcinoma and treatment is along similar lines.

Clear cell odontogenic carcinoma

The clear cell odontogenic tumour is rare and behaves in a malignant fashion with potential to spread to regional lymph nodes and distant sites, including lungs and bone. Microscopically, a biphasic pattern is often present with islands of epithelial cells possessing clear to faintly eosinophilic cytoplasm along with cords of dark-staining basaloid cells. Treatment is along the lines of that given for oral squamous cell carcinoma.

Ghost cell odontogenic carcinoma

This very rare malignant neoplasm is the counterpart of the DGCT and only a small number of cases have been reported. The biological behaviour is uncertain but some reported cases have metastasized. Treatment is decided on a case by case basis but if worrying features are present, then treatment is planned as for oral squamous cell carcinoma.

Odontogenic sarcomas

These are extremely rare lesions and two variants are recognized. These are the ameloblastic fibrosarcoma, the malignant counterpart of amleoblastic fibroma, and the ameloblastic fibrodentinoma (ameloblastic fibroodontosarcoma), in which dental hard tissue formation may additionally be seen. Both are treated by surgery with wide margins to ensure clearance.

Congenital tumours of possible odontogenic origin

Congenital epulis

This rare lesion presents in neonates most often in the anterior maxillary ridge. The swelling is rounded and often pedunculated (Fig. 6.35). Histologically, there are closely packed granular cells covered by oral mucosa. The lesion is also known as congenital gingival granular cell tumour, but it is unlikely to be neoplastic and does not recur after local excision.

Melanotic neuroectodermal tumour of infancy

This unusual lesion affects infants under 1 year of age. The most common site is the anterior maxilla but the lesion can occur in the mandible and also at extragnathic sites around the cranium. Also known as melanotic progonoma, the lesion behaves aggressively and tends to recur, requiring multiple attempts at excision to gain control.

Congenital odontogenic myxoma

Rarely, odontogenic myxoma is present at birth. The lesion expands the jaw and treatment is often delayed to allow some facial growth, with removal in early childhood.

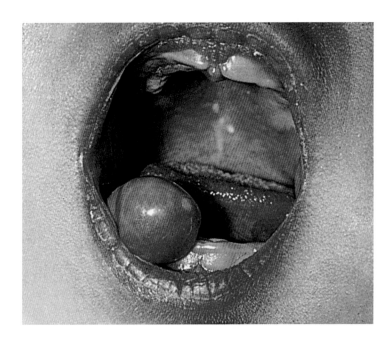

Fig. 6.35 Congenital epulis.

Summary of the radiological features of odontogenic lesions

The radiological features of the most important odontogenic lesions are summarized in Table 6.4. The differential diagnosis of a multilocular radiolucency at the angle of the mandible is presented in Box 6.2.

Table 6.4 Radiological features of important odontogenic lesions

	Radicular cyst	**Dentigerous cyst**	**Odontogenic keratocyst**	**Ameloblastoma**
Site	Apex of non-vital tooth	Crown of an unerupted tooth	Body and angle of mandible	Body and angle of mandible
Size	Variable	Variable	Variable	Variable
Shape	Round, unilocular	Round, unilocular	Unilocular, multilocular	Unilocular, multilocular
Outline	Well defined, corticated	Well defined, corticated	Well defined, corticated	Well defined, corticated
Radiodensity	Radiolucent	Radiolucent	Radiolucent	Radiolucent
Effects on adjacent stuctures	Buccal expansion Tooth displacement Root resorption (20%)	Bucco-lingual expansion Tooth displacement Root resorption (50%)	Minimal effects on adjacent structures Expands through medullary bone	Cortical expansion Tooth displacement Root resorption

---

Box 6.2 Differential diagnosis of a multilocular radiolucency at the angle of the mandible

Most common lesions

- Odontogenic keratocyst
- Ameloblastoma

Rare odontogenic tumours

- Ameloblastic fibroma
- Calcifying epithelial odontogenic tumour
- Odontogenic myxoma

Giant cell lesions

- Central giant cell granuloma
- Hyperparathyroidism
- Cherubism
- Aneurysmal bone cyst

Malignancy

- Metastases

7

Disorders of bone

Chapter contents

Introduction

Most invasive dental procedures involving removal of teeth or bone are followed by uneventful healing. However, dentists should be aware that generalized abnormalities of bone, such as osteoporosis and Paget's disease of bone, may complicate these procedures and, rarely, can lead to ongoing clinical problems. The effects of radiotherapy to the jaws and bisphosphonate treatment are well-described causes of osteonecrosis and delayed healing. Diagnosis of bone disorders often depends on integrating the results of clinical, imaging, pathological, genetic, and biochemical investigations.

Normal bone architecture

Although the bony skeleton is often thought of as forming just a rigid framework, it should be remembered that bone is a living, responsive tissue that plays an important role in metabolism. During development, some bones develop from a cartilaginous template and others, such as most of the craniofacial bones, form in fibrous membranes. Bone matrix is laid down by osteoblasts that are derived from the extensive meshwork of bone-lining cells that cover the bone surfaces. The bone matrix contains osteocytes that are responsive to mechanical stresses. Bone matrix is removed by osteoclasts that move over the bone surface, resulting in scalloped pits termed Howship's lacunae. Bone matrix can be woven or lamellar in pattern (Figs 7.1 and 7.2). Pathologists often examine sections of bony lesions in polarized light to determine

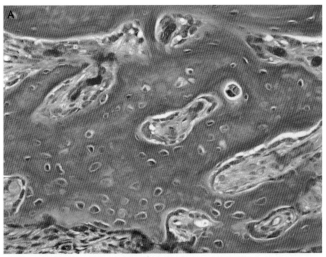

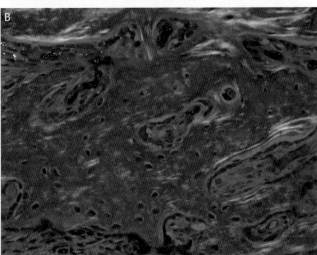

Fig. 7.1 Recently formed woven bone. Plump osteoblasts line the bone surface. In polarized light the woven texture of the bone matrix can be seen.

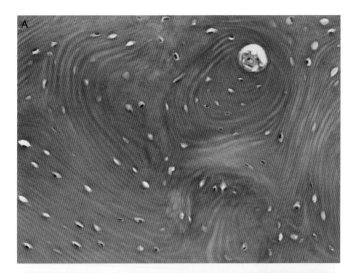

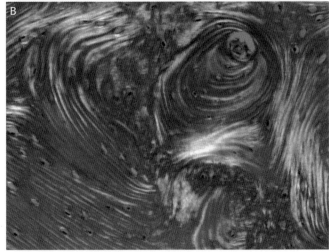

Fig. 7.2 Lamellar bone from the mandibular cortex. In polarized light the organized layers of bone matrix are evident.

Table 7.1 Woven and lamellar bone

Woven bone	• Immature bone with course collagen bundles arranged in an interwoven fashion • Remodelled to lamellar bone over time	Laid down during: • Intra-membranous ossification (skull and clavicles) • Healing of tooth sockets • Healing of fractures • Bone disease
Lamellar bone	• Mature bone with collagen bundles laid down in organized parallel sheets or lamellae • Compact cortical bone • Cancellous medullary bone	Laid down during: • Endochondral ossification • Replacement of woven bone • Circumferential bone growth

whether the pattern of the collagenous matrix is woven or lamellar, because it can be pivotal for diagnosis (Table 7.1).

It is also important for clinicians to be aware that, in order to produce a histological section of bone, the tissue must first be fixed and then demineralized to soften the matrix. When a bone biopsy is performed, the patient should be made aware that additional time will be needed to process the biopsy.

Bone healing

Normal extraction socket healing

Following extraction of a tooth, the socket rapidly fills with blood, which then clots. Granulation tissue, which consists of proliferating endothelial cells and fibroblasts derived from remnants of the periodontal ligament and surrounding alveolar bone, grows into the clot and organization commences. Osteoclasts begin to remodel the crestal bone and remove any small spicules of bone detached during the extraction. Squamous epithelium from the gingiva migrates across the defect, between the blood clot and the proliferating granulation tissue (Fig. 7.3A). Epithelial continuity is normally restored 10–14 days after the extraction. The regenerating squamous epithelium is thin initially, and then gradually thickens and develops keratinization. Osteoblasts appear in the granulation tissue towards the base of the socket and the granulation tissue is gradually replaced by woven bone (Fig. 7.3B). After approximately 6 weeks the regenerated epithelium over the socket appears normal, the supra-alveolar connective tissues have healed by repair, and the socket is filled by woven bone. However, the outline of the socket can still be discerned both radiologically and histologically (Fig. 7.4). Subsequently, the lamina dura and newly formed woven bone is remodelled with the formation of cortical and cancellous bone to form a smooth, rounded alveolar ridge. The height of the alveolar ridge in the area of the extraction reduces with time and 'knife-edged' ridges result if one alveolar plate is fractured away during the extraction. The socket outline remains detectable on radiographs for up to 30 weeks after the extraction.

Osseointegration of implants

Osseointegration is the term used to describe the healing of bone around an endosseous implant that results in a close interface between the bone and the implant. The healing process is essentially similar to that seen in a healing socket. Blood clots form at the interface between the bone and the implant. There is organization by granulation tissue, removal of dead bone by osteoclasts, deposition of woven bone, and then remodelling occurs. Vital bone is apposed to the implant surface and a very thin interface, similar to a reversal line in normal bone matrix, can be seen. The gingival epithelium becomes arranged as a collar around the implant post and attaches to the implant surface by formation of a basal lamina and hemidesmosomes, in a similar arrangement to that seen linking normal junctional epithelium to enamel and cementum.

Plaque accumulation can lead both to inflammatory changes around the implant and to alveolar bone loss, similar to that seen in chronic periodontal disease, and is referred to as 'peri-implantitis'. There are few contraindications to implants and, even though, very rarely, malignancy may develop around an implant, they can be used in the rehabilitation of the jaws after treatment for oral cancer.

Fracture healing

Healing of jaw fractures is similar to that in other bones. The fracture line fills with a blood clot, which is gradually replaced by granulation tissue. Maturation of the granulation tissue is accompanied by the deposition of woven bone. Callus may be produced by the

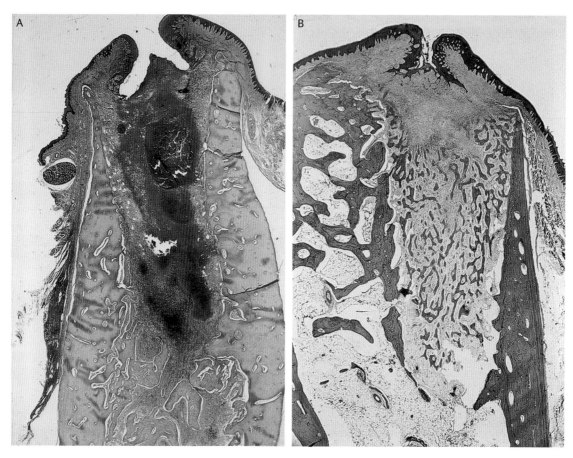

Fig. 7.3 Healing tooth socket seven days after extraction showing early organization of blood clot (A). Four weeks after extraction the socket is filled by fibrous tissue containing trabeculae of woven bone and the mucosal surface is covered by squamous epithelium (B).

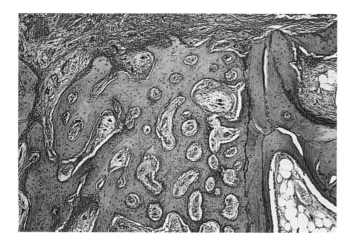

Fig. 7.4 Healing tooth socket 6 weeks after extraction. The socket is filled by interconnected trabeculae of woven bone. The socket wall is shown on the right and the alveolar crest has remodelled to form a smooth surface.

periosteum, which may be separated from the cortex by oedema, to aid temporary union. The bone in the fracture site remodels over time, and the normal cortical and trabecular architecture is restored. Consideration of the treatment of fractures is outside the scope of this text but it is important to understand that management should aim to ensure that the fractured bone ends are immobile relative to each other. Fibrous healing or non-union may occur if the bone ends can move freely.

Bone atrophy

Following extraction of the teeth and subsequent wearing of dentures for many years, the alveolar bone may undergo atrophy. This is thought to result from loss of mechanical stresses from the teeth that are necessary to maintain the bone mass. The mandibular ridge may become flattened and flabby ridges may occur in the maxillary alveolus. Edentulous patients with osteoporosis often show excessive bone loss, reducing the mandible to a thin fragile strip of bone.

Inflammatory disorders of bone

The term 'osteitis' is generally used to describe a localized inflammation of bone with no progression through the medullary cavity, particularly that associated with dry socket (alveolar osteitis). Osteomyelitis is a more extensive inflammation of the interior of the

Table 7.2 Inflammation and necrosis of bone

Osteitis	Localized inflammation of the bone with no progression through medullary cavity
Osteomyelitis	Inflammation of the interior of the bone usually involving the medullary cavity; may progress to erode or even perforate the cortex
Periostitis	Inflammation of the periosteal surface of the bone; may cause superficial erosion of the cortex
Osteonecrosis	Death of bone tissue; areas of non-vital bone are separated by osteoclasts and form sequestra; occurs in osteomyelitis, after radiotherapy, bone infarction, and in relation to drugs (bisphosphonates and denosumab) and chemicals (phosphorus exposure)

bone involving, and typically spreading through, the marrow spaces. Periostitis refers to inflammation of the periosteal surface of the bone and may or may not be associated with osteomyelitis. Oedema can separate the periosteum from the cortical bone surface and successive 'onion skin' layers of reactive woven bone can be deposited (Table 7.2).

Dry socket (alveolar osteitis)

This unpredictable complication in the healing of extraction wounds occurs in 1–3% of all extractions. Known risk factors are molar extraction, particularly a lower molar, difficult extractions, and smoking. The condition most commonly follows extraction of impacted lower third molars. Dry socket is a localized inflammation of the alveolar bone following either a failure of blood clot formation in the socket, or the premature loss or disintegration of the clot. Failure of a clot to form may be due to a relatively poor blood supply to the bone, such as that found in osteopetrosis, Paget's disease of bone, or following radiotherapy, or it might result from the excessive use of vasoconstrictors in local anaesthetics. Where an adequate blood clot forms, it may be washed away by excessive mouth rinsing or it may disintegrate prematurely due to fibrinolysis of the clot, often as a result of infection by proteolytic bacteria. No specific bacteria have been implicated, the infection being of mixed type. Food debris, saliva, and bacteria collect in the empty socket, and the adjacent bone becomes infected and necrotic. The inflammatory reaction in the adjacent marrow localizes the infection to the walls of the socket, as otherwise spread of infection through the medullary cavity would ensue. Any non-vital bone is gradually separated by osteoclasts and sequestra may be formed. Healing is extremely slow and follows the ingrowth of granulation tissue from the surrounding vital bone.

Dry socket is typically associated with severe pain developing 2–3 days after an extraction. The pain often radiates and ear pain may be experienced. The socket often contains foul-tasting and smelling decomposing food debris that can be washed away to reveal the denuded bone lining the cavity. The denuded bone is exquisitely tender to probing and halitosis is usually present.

Identification of risk factors by taking an apposite history and undertaking a thorough clinical examination is important. Preventive actions should be taken where possible. These include treating infection, improving oral hygiene, providing smoking-cessation advice, minimizing trauma during extractions, and advising the patient to avoid excessive rinsing in the post-extraction period. Written advice sheets can be a useful aid.

When dry socket has been diagnosed, it may be appropriate to first radiograph the socket to exclude the possibility of retained fragments of tooth or foreign material. The affected socket should be gently irrigated with warmed saline. Any debris should be gently dislodged and aspirated. Local anaesthesia may be required and regional nerve blocks should be used whenever possible. Once cleansed, the socket should be lightly packed with a dressing that contains an obtundant for pain relief and a non-irritant antiseptic to inhibit bacterial and fungal growth. The aim is to prevent accumulation of food debris and to protect the exposed bone from local irritation. Appropriate analgesics should be prescribed and the patient kept under review until they are pain-free and socket healing is ensured. Dry socket may persist for 40 days and irrigation with application of a dressing may need to be repeated.

Key points Alveolar osteitis

- Occurs mainly in the mandible
- Incidence after surgical removal of third molars in 20–30%
- Failure of formation, dislodgement, or breakdown of clot
- Post-extraction written instructions for prevention
- Treat by gentle irrigation, obtundant dressing, and analgesics

Focal sclerosing (condensing) osteitis

Osteosclerosis commonly follows chronic periapical inflammation. It is typically found in relation to the apex of a tooth, most commonly the first permanent molar (Fig. 7.5), and often remains as a sclerotic area of bone after extraction. It is usually asymptomatic. Histologically, a localized increase in the number and thickness of the bone trabeculae

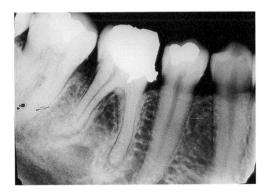

Fig. 7.5 Focal sclerosing osteitis around the roots of a non-vital mandibular first molar tooth.

is seen, and there may be scattered lymphocytes and plasma cells in the surrounding scanty fibrosed marrow. Small areas of sclerotic bone, known as a dense bone islands, are well recognized in the jaws and these enter the differential diagnosis. Focal infection (chronic pulpitis) requires treatment by endodontics or extraction, but focal sclerosing osteitis itself does not require any other intervention.

Osteomyelitis

Although osteomyelitis of the jaws was a common complication of dental sepsis before the advent of antibiotics, it is now a rare disease. Various clinical subtypes may be recognized, but the pathological features of osteomyelitis are best considered as comprising a spectrum of inflammatory and reactive changes in bone and periosteum. Osteomyelitis reflects a balance between the nature and severity of the irritant, the host defences, and local and systemic predisposing factors. The latter relate mainly to local factors that compromise the vascularity and vitality of bone, and to systemic conditions that compromise the host defence systems.

Suppurative osteomyelitis is usually divided clinically into acute and chronic types, depending on the severity of symptoms and time course of the disease. Disease persisting for longer than a month is usually referred to as chronic suppurative osteomyelitis. The source of the infection is usually a dental abscess or local trauma, such as a fracture, penetrating wound, or extraction. A mixed infection including anaerobic organisms is typical. The mandible is more frequently involved than the maxilla because the vascular supply is more readily compromised. Thrombosis of the mandibular artery or of its branching loops can lead to extensive necrosis of bone. By contrast, there is a rich collateral circulation in the mid-face area and osteomyelitis of the maxilla is rare.

Following entry into the bone, bacteria proliferate in the marrow spaces giving rising to an acute inflammatory reaction. Tissue necrosis and suppuration rapidly ensue and the necrosis may be widespread because of thrombosis of neighbouring vessels. Inflammation, suppuration, and necrosis continue, and the marrow spaces become filled with pus. The suppurative inflammation tends to spread through the adjacent marrow spaces and may extend through the cortical bone to involve the periosteum. Stripping of the periosteum compromises the blood supply to the cortical plate and predisposes to further bone necrosis. Eventually, a mass of necrotic bone (a sequestrum), covered by pus, becomes separated from the surrounding vital bone by the action of osteoclasts (Fig. 7.6). The sequestrum may spontaneously exfoliate through a sinus tract. Radiographic examination may be normal in the early stages of the disease, but after 10–14 days, sufficient bone resorption may have occurred to produce irregular, moth-eaten areas of radiolucency (Fig. 7.7). Clinically, acute suppurative osteomyelitis presents with pain, swelling, pyrexia, and malaise. Trismus is frequent and there may be paraesthesia of the lip and mobility of teeth if they are involved. Disease of more chronic nature also presents with pain and swelling associated with chronic suppuration and discharge of pus through one or more intra-oral or extra-oral sinuses.

Chronic sclerosing osteomyelitis is a less clearly defined condition. Localized lesions are identical to focal sclerosing osteitis. However, diffuse sclerosing lesions of the mandible have been reported as a

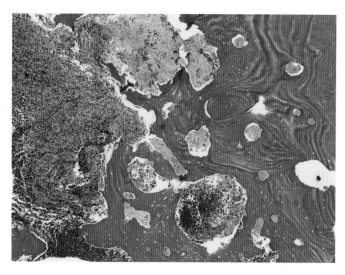

Fig. 7.6 Bone sequestrum in acute osteomyelitis. The osteocyte lacunae are empty and the bone surface is scalloped due to the action of osteoclasts. The bone surfaces are coated in biofilm.

complication of spread from a contiguous focus of low-grade infection, such as a periapical granuloma.

Garré's osteomyelitis is a distinct clinico-pathological entity characterized by a proliferative sub-periosteal reaction, rather than inflammation of the interior of the bone. It is essentially a periostitis, rather than a deep-seated osteomyelitis. The condition is a type of sclerosing osteomyelitis found almost exclusively in the mandible in children and young adults. Garré's osteomyelitis presents clinically as a bony, hard swelling on the outer surface of the mandible. The periosteal reaction is thought to result from the spread of a low-grade, chronic inflammation through the cortical bone, stimulating a proliferative reaction of the periosteum. Occlusal radiographs show a

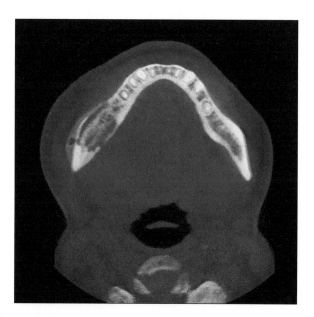

Fig. 7.7 Osteomyelitis showing medullary bone destruction (Cone beam CT).

focal sub-periosteal overgrowth of bone with a smooth surface on the outer cortical plate, and often showing a multi-layered appearance. The sub-periosteal mass consists of irregular trabeculae of actively forming woven bone with scattered chronic inflammatory cells in the fibrous marrow. Resolution follows successful treatment of the inflammatory focus.

Vegetable pulse granuloma

An unusual form of chronic periostitis in the jaws is associated histologically with hyaline ring-shaped bodies accompanied by a foreign body type, giant cell reaction (Fig. 7.8). The hyaline rings are formed by deposition of collagen on the cellulose rims of vegetable pulse material that has been implanted in the tissues. Fibrous thickening of the periosteum occurs with chronic inflammation and there may be chronic suppuration. Local bone resorption can produce an underlying cortical defect. Vegetable pulse material may enter the tissue through ulceration or a periodontal pocket. Biopsy often removes sufficient foreign material to facilitate resolution.

Osteoradionecrosis

Radiation, as part of the therapy for oral malignancy, reduces the vascularity of the bone by causing a proliferation of the intima of the blood vessels (endarteritis obliterans). This can have serious consequences in the mandible with its end-artery supply, and the inferior alveolar artery or its branches may be obstructed by organization or thrombosis. The non-vital bone that results from the reduction in blood supply is sterile and asymptomatic, but is very susceptible to trauma and supervening infection (Fig. 7.9). If the mucosa is breeched, infection may spread rapidly, resulting in extensive osteomyelitis and painful necrosis of the irradiated bone, referred to as osteoradionecrosis. When radiotherapy is planned, the clinical team, which should include a dentist, aims to render the patient dentally fit beforehand, and teeth with sepsis or of poor prognosis in risk areas are extracted. Modern methods of

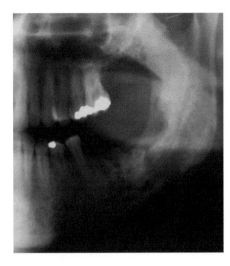

Fig. 7.9 Osteoradionecrosis of the mandible.

delivering radiotherapy have greatly reduced the incidence of osteoradionecrosis, but good dental care is an important part of the patient's overall management for oral cancer.

Medication-related osteonecrosis of the jaw

Bisphosphonate-related osteonecrosis of the jaw (BRONJ), now termed medication-related osteonecrosis of the jaw (MRONJ), is a well-recognized side-effect of bisphosphonate therapy. It is usually identified by the appearance of exposed bone in the oral cavity in persons taking bisphosphonates for more than 8 weeks. In addition to exposed bone, there may be localized pain, loosening of teeth, and swelling of the gingival or adjacent mucosa, with infection and inflammation. Bisphosphonates are widely prescribed to prevent loss of bone mass in cancer patients, particularly those with breast, prostate, and haematological malignancy, and are also used to treat Paget's disease, osteoporosis, and other conditions associated with bone fragility and fractures. The drug inhibits osteoclast action and thus interferes with normal bone turnover. In the jaws, this appears to render the bone more susceptible to infection and loss of vitality, particularly when the integrity of the mucosa is compromised.

Bisphosphonates bring enormous clinical benefits and only a small proportion of patients taking the drugs develop MRONJ. The risk of developing MRONJ correlates with the dose, the duration of therapy, and the number of intravenous administrations given. The majority of patients on bisphosphonates take a low dose orally for osteoporosis prevention. Their risk of developing MRONJ is significantly less than those patients on a high dosage taken intravenously for malignancy affecting the bones. Around two-thirds of MRONJ cases are associated with a previous dental procedure, such as extraction or implant placement. Oral lesions of MRONJ are progressive and are thought to commence with just exposed bone (Stage 1), followed by the development of areas of mucosal or bone inflammation with pain (Stage 2). Ultimately, there may be extensive bone exposure (Fig. 7.10), pathological fracture, and severe pain with florid necrosis, infection, and inflammation in both mucosa and bone (Stage 3). Preventive measures for those on bisphosphonates include good oral hygiene, regular

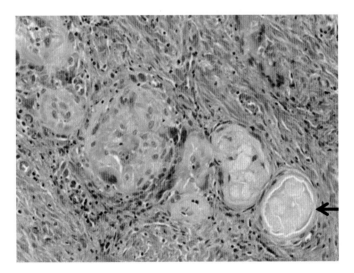

Fig. 7.8 Vegetable pulse granuloma showing a foreign-body giant response to plant material (arrow).

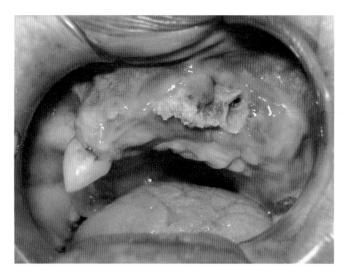

Fig. 7.10 Medication-related osteonecrosis of jaws (MRONJ). Necrotic infected bone is seen through a dehiscence in the alveolar mucosa.

dental check-ups, and self-examination. Treatment of MRONJ can be challenging and measures may include daily irrigation, antibiotic therapy, surgical removal of necrotic bone, and covering of affected areas to prevent trauma.

Denosumab, a monoclonal antibody drug that inhibits osteoclast action through the RANKL pathway, also causes MRONJ. The drug is licensed for a number of applications and is increasingly used in place of bisphosphonates as part of cancer therapy. Monoclonal antibodies used in cancer treatments may also be a risk factor for the development of MRONJ. Bevacizumab, a monoclonal antibody that inhibits vascular endothelial growth factor, used in the treatment of metastatic colorectal cancer, and sunitinib, a tyrosine kinase inhibitor, used in the treatment of renal cell carcinoma, have both been implicated.

Key points Bone necrosis

- Radiotherapy to bone reduces blood supply, causes osteoradionecrosis
- Bisphosphonates and denosumab predispose to jaw osteonecrosis
- Infection of necrotic bone may progress to osteomyelitis
- Avoid trauma and extractions when predisposition to osteonecrosis known
- Treat dehiscence of mucosa conservatively
- Major surgery may be required to remove dead bone

Swellings of bone

Torus palatinus, torus mandibularis, and other exostoses

The term 'exostosis' is used clinically to describe a bony outgrowth. A torus is an exostosis that occurs at a characteristic site, either in the mid-line of the palate (torus palatinus; Fig. 7.11) or on the lingual surface of the mandible, usually in the premolar region above the mylohyoid line (torus mandibularis; Fig. 7.12). Mandibular tori are frequently bilateral and may be multiple. It is important to recognize these common lesions because patients may become concerned about the swelling and need reassurance that tori are harmless developmental lesions that do not require intervention. Tori are rarely seen in childhood and have a slow growth. They may vary considerably in size and shape, ranging from flat and small elevations to large, nodular growths. They may be

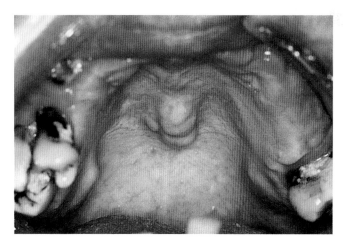

Fig. 7.11 Torus palatinus.

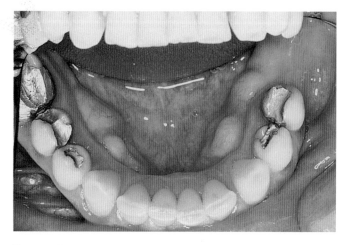

Fig. 7.12 Torus mandibularis.

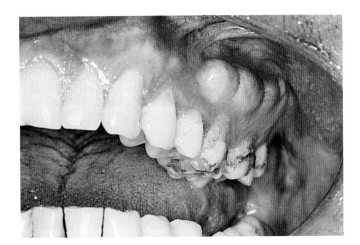

Fig. 7.13 Multiple exostoses in the maxilla.

composed entirely of dense, cortical bone or consist of cancellous bone with a shell of cortical bone. The lesions are entirely benign and need to be removed only for cosmetic reasons or before the construction of a denture.

Developmental exostoses are seen occasionally on the buccal alveolus in the molar region of the maxilla (Fig. 7.13). Irregularities of the alveolus following tooth extraction are also often described clinically as exostoses, as is enlargement of the genial tubercle in edentulous patients. Reactive exostoses may result from repeated trauma or irritation to the periosteum.

Multiple jaw exostoses (often referred to as osteomas) may be found in Gardner's syndrome (OMIM 175100). Affected patients may also have sclerotic dense bone islands, multiple odontomes, unerupted and supernumerary teeth, and hazy sclerosis of wide areas of the jaw (Fig. 7.14).

It is important to recognize this syndrome, which may come to light after lesions are identified by dental panoramic tomography (Table 7.3). Patients with Gardner's syndrome develop multiple bowel polyps that have a high risk of transforming into cancer, and require referral for medical assessment. Desmoid tumours, epidermoid cysts, and characteristic retinal pigmentation may also be present.

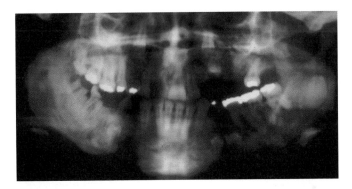

Fig. 7.14 DPT showing multiple osteomas, unerupted teeth, and hazy sclerosis in Gardner's syndrome.

Table 7.3 Genetic disorders affecting the bone of the jaws

Gardner's syndrome	Mutations of *APC*, autosomal dominant. Around 40% of cases arise as new mutations with no family history.
Osteogenesis imperfecta	Eight subtypes; majority of cases involve a mutation of type 1 collagen genes *COL1A1* and *COL1A2*. Six dominant and two recessive forms also known.
Osteopetrosis	Nine subtypes; majority arises from autosomal dominant mutations of *CLCN7*. Recessive form most often involves *TCIRG1* and the X-linked type involves *IKBKG*.
Cleidocranial dysplasia	Around 70% involve mutation of *RUNX2*; this gene is a transcription factor thought to regulate other genes responsible for bone and cartilage development. Other cases involve a mutation of *MSX-2* and there are also recessive forms.
X-linked hypophosphataemia	Over 80% of familial hypophosphataemia results from mutation of *PHEX*, which is X-linked. Various autosomal recessive forms account for the remainder of cases.
Achondroplasia	Caused by mutations of *FGFR3*, important for cartilage development. Mutations of other genes in the pathway cause similar phenotypes.
Fibrous dysplasia	*GNAS1* mutation causes McCune–Albright syndrome; post-zygotic mutation results in mosaic state with variable features.
Cherubism	Mutations of *SH3BP2* that lead to gain of function or dominant negative activity.
Noonan's syndrome	Genetically heterogeneous; 50% have mutations in *PTPN11* and some in *SOS1*. These and other mutations affect the MAP kinase pathway.
Osseous dysplasia	Variants described as periapical, focal, florid, and gigantiform cementoma may be a single familial disorder, gene unknown.

Key points Bone swellings

- Torus mandibularis and torus palatinus are common developmental abnormalities
- Tori may be composed of compact or cancellous bone
- Jaw exostoses, odontomes, and hazy sclerosis seen in Gardner's syndrome
- Intra-osseous cysts may produce bony hard swellings

- Odontogenic and primary bone tumours can cause bone expansion
- Periostitis and Garré's osteomyelitis may cause a localized swelling
- Fibrous dysplasia may present in childhood as solitary or multiple bony swellings

Fibrous dysplasia of bone

Fibrous dysplasia of bone may involve one or several bones in the body, and the terms 'monostotic' and 'polyostotic' are applied to these different forms of the disease. McCune–Albright syndrome (OMIM 174800), a severe form of polyostotic fibrous dysplasia, in which the bone lesions are accompanied by skin pigmentation, precocious puberty in females, and, occasionally, other endocrine abnormalities, is a hereditary disorder.

Monostotic fibrous dysplasia is much more common than polyostotic forms. Virtually any bone may be involved but the lesion arises most frequently in a limb bone, rib, or skull bone, particularly the jaws. Jaw lesions are more common in the maxilla than in the mandible. When the maxilla is affected, adjacent bones, such as the zygoma and sphenoid, may also be involved and the term 'craniofacial fibrous dysplasia' is then used. The majority of patients with monostotic fibrous dysplasia present in childhood or adolescence, but, occasionally, the disease is not diagnosed until adult life. Patients presenting in adult life may have been aware of a quiescent bony enlargement for some years and may give a history of recent expansion of the lesion. Reactivation of quiescent lesions may occur for unknown reasons and has been reported in pregnancy. In either jaw, the first sign of fibrous dysplasia is a gradually increasing, painless, hard swelling that is not well circumscribed and that causes a gradually increasing facial asymmetry. The enlargement is usually smooth, often fusiform in outline, and is more pronounced buccally than lingually or palatally (Fig. 7.15). Maxillary lesions commonly

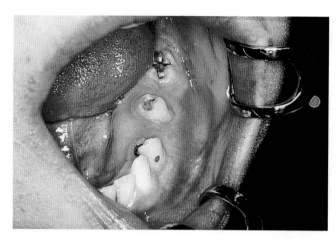

Fig. 7.16 Monostotic fibrous dysplasia of the mandible showing fusiform expansion of the buccal and lingual aspects, with displacement of the teeth.

involve the sinus, zygomatic process, and floor of orbit, and the orbital contents may be displaced. In some cases, where growth is more rapid and extensive, there may be marked swelling of the cheek with exophthalmos and proptosis. Mandibular lesions occur most frequently in the molar and premolar regions and, if the lower border is involved, there may be an obvious protuberance and increase in depth of the jaw (Fig. 7.16). In either jaw there may be some malalignment, tipping, or displacement of teeth, and in children any teeth involved by the lesion may fail to erupt.

Radiographically, the jaw lesions are variable in appearance and their borders are often difficult to define because of the gradual transition to a normal, uninvolved bone pattern. The variable appearances reflect differing amounts of bone formed within the fibrous tissue of the lesions. The lesions may be radiolucent initially but, as the degree of trabeculation increases, they become mottled and eventually opaque, the many delicate trabeculae giving a ground-glass or orange-peel-stippling effect on radiographs (Figs 7.17 and 7.18).

Polyostotic fibrous dysplasia is two to three times as common in females as males and the distribution of lesions is very variable. Bone swellings frequently occur in the bones of one limb but the skull, vertebrae, ribs, and pelvis are also often involved. Although almost any combination can occur, there is a tendency for the lesions to arise segmentally and to be localized in one limb or on one side of the body. Patients with severe polyostotic disease are usually diagnosed in childhood because of the associated bony deformities and pathological fractures. The polyostotic form may also present as McCune–Albright syndrome.

Microscopically, fibrous dysplasia shows replacement of normal bone by cellular fibrous tissue containing islands and trabeculae of woven bone. Osteoblastic rimming of trabeculae may also be seen and lamellar bone may be deposited. Typically, the newly formed trabeculae of bone are delicate and of irregular shape, resembling Chinese characters, and consist of immature, coarse-fibred woven bone (Fig. 7.19). Lesional bone merges with that of the surrounding normal bone and it is this feature, in particular, that distinguishes the lesion from ossifying fibroma. It is suggested that, with increasing age of the lesions, the amount and cellularity

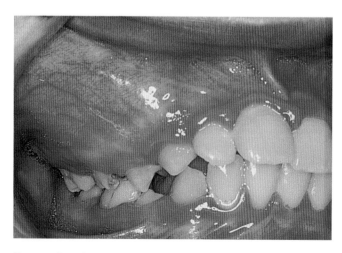

Fig. 7.15 Buccal expansion of the maxilla in monostotic fibrous dysplasia.

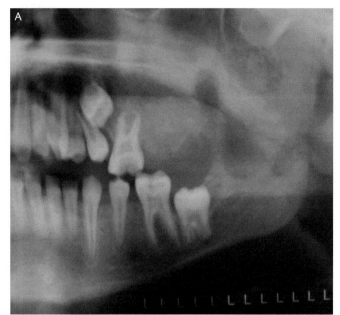

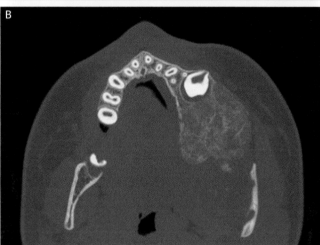

Fig. 7.17 Radiograph of the maxilla showing deformity of the maxillary tuberosity and opacification of the maxillary antrum in fibrous dysplasia. The bone has a 'ground-glass' appearance (A). Corresponding coronal CT through the lesion (B).

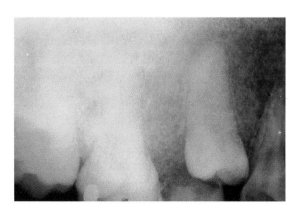

Fig. 7.18 Radiograph of fibrous dysplasia in the maxilla showing 'orange peel' stipling appearance.

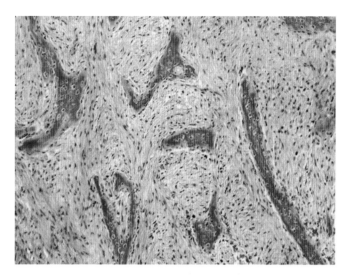

Fig. 7.19 Fibrous dysplasia showing fine curvi-linear woven bone trabeculae forming in a cellular fibrous background.

of the fibrous tissue decreases, whilst the amount of bone increases, although these are not constant features. As the lesion matures, there is progressive remodelling of the woven bone to lamellar bone.

Mutations of the *GNAS1* gene are found in the lesions of fibrous dysplasia. In McCune–Albright syndrome, germline mutations are found (i.e. all cells in the patient's body have the mutation). In the polyostotic and monostotic forms, the lesional cells have the mutations but cells from normal tissues do not, implying post-zygotic mutation and genetic mosaicism.

Fibrous dysplasia tends to expand mainly during the period of active skeletal growth and become quiescent when bone maturity is reached. Cessation of active growth can be assessed by bone scanning and the majority of cases can then be treated by conservative surgical removal of sufficient of the lesion to reduce any deformity. In cases where fibrous dysplasia causes problematic deformity or intractable bone pain, medical management using denosumab can be considered. This humanized antibody therapy targets RANKL, which is over-expressed in fibrous dysplasia cells as a result of the *GNAS1* mutation.

Key points Fibrous dysplasia of the jaws

- More common in maxilla than mandible
- May be monostotic or polyostotic; *GNAS* gene mutation
- Fusiform bony expansion; maxillary lesions also expand into sinus
- Radiographic features vary with maturation; radiolucent to ground-glass radiodensity
- Margins of lesion merge with surrounding normal bone
- Delicate trabeculae of woven bone in cellular or collagenous fibrous tissue
- Expansion usually stops with skeletal maturation (20 years old)
- Bone scanning used to show growth cessation, jaw can then be re-contoured

Osseous dysplasia

Osseous dysplasia (or cemento-osseous dysplasia) presents a range of clinical appearances. A single lesion, often associated with the apex of a tooth, is termed focal osseous dysplasia (Fig. 7.20A). Multiple, small (<1 cm) lesions associated with the apices of the mandibular incisors is called periapical osseous dysplasia. Multiple, larger lesions, involving one or more quadrants in one or both jaws, is called florid osseous dysplasia (Fig. 7.20B). Osseous dysplasia is more prevalent in women than in men, occurs predominantly in the mandible, and is seen most frequently in Black people. The condition is frequently asymptomatic and is detected by radiography, mostly in patients over 30 years of age. Osseous dysplasia shares some histological features with fibrous dysplasia, comprising fibrous tissue within which cementum-like paucicellular mineralized matrix develops (Fig. 7.21). The radiographic features of osseous dysplasias reflect the extent of mineralization and may be radiolucent, mixed, or radiopaque. Extensive multifocal osseous dysplasia of the jaws has been described in families and is called familial gigantiform cementoma (OMIM 137575; Table 7.3), such lesions may expand and distort the jaws causing facial deformity.

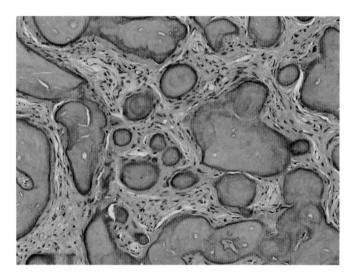

Fig. 7.21 Florid osseous dysplasia showing dense paucicellular mineralized matrix in a background of bland fibrous tissue.

Cherubism

Cherubism (OMIM 118400) is a rare disorder of bone inherited as an autosomal dominant character with variable expressivity that may be caused by mutations in the *SH3BP2* gene. The gene encodes a cell-signalling molecule involved in the regulation of inflammation and bone remodelling. Males are affected about twice as frequently as females. The descriptive term 'cherubism' relates to the unusual clinical appearance and facial deformity of patients with this disease. The condition is an important differential diagnosis for fibrous dysplasia.

Children with cherubism appear normal at birth, but painless swellings of the jaws appear between the ages of 2 and 4 years old. The swellings are usually symmetrical and always involve the mandible, either alone or in combination with the maxilla. Typically, the swellings enlarge up to the age of about 7 years old, but then become static and begin to regress, with progressive reduction in the facial deformity as the patient passes from puberty into adult life. The characteristic facial deformity is a fullness of the cheeks and jaws producing a typical chubby face. A rim of sclera may be visible beneath the iris due to stretching of the skin over the swellings or to upward displacement of the orbit by maxillary lesions, so that the eyes appear upturned to heaven. The chubby face and upturned eyes produce a cherubic appearance, often enhanced by fullness of the submandibular space due to hyperplasia of the submandibular lymph nodes. Abnormalities of the dentition include premature loss of deciduous teeth and displacement, lack of eruption, and failure of development of many permanent teeth.

Radiological examination shows multilocular radiolucencies (Fig. 7.22) with expansion and thinning of the cortical plates. Mandibular lesions often originate near the angle and then spread to involve the body and ramus of the mandible, sparing the condyle. Maxillary lesions are often confined to the tuberosities but the sinus may be obliterated.

Microscopically, the lesions consist mainly of cellular and vascular fibrous tissue containing varying numbers of multinucleate osteoclast-like giant cells. The giant cells are distributed as focal collections, often around thin-walled vascular channels. Vessels surrounded by a cuff of

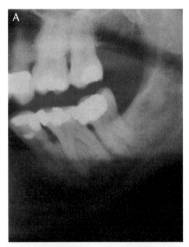

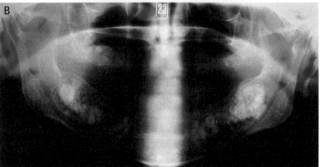

Fig. 7.20 Focal osseous dysplasia associated with the apex of a mandibular first molar (A). Multi-focal radiodense masses in a case of florid osseous dysplasia (B).

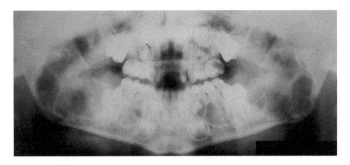

Fig. 7.22 Bilateral multilocular radiolucent lesions at the angles of the mandible in cherubism.

hyaline, eosinophilic collagen are found. As the activity of the lesions decreases they become progressively more fibrous, the number of giant cells diminishes, and varying amounts of metaplastic bone are laid down.

Cherubism is a self-limiting condition and there is progressive improvement in facial appearance from about puberty onwards, but conservative cosmetic surgery is often required. Radiographically, the improvement in appearance may be accompanied by some bony infilling of the lesions, but residual radiolucent areas can remain into old age.

> **Key points** Cherubism
> - Family history, *SH3BP2* gene mutation
> - Distinct clinical facial features
> - Bilateral, symmetrical, multilocular radiolucencies of posterior mandible
> - Histology shows a giant cell-rich lesion
> - Enlarged submandibular lymph nodes present

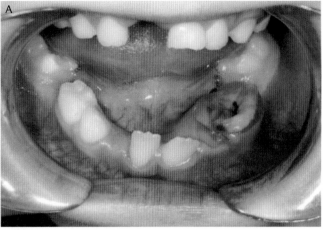

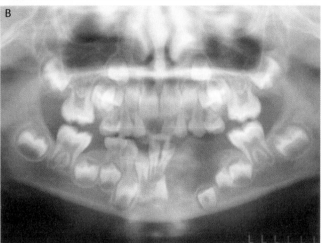

Fig. 7.23 Central giant cell granuloma in the left mandible showing expansion and perforation of the alveolus. DPT showing radiolucency with displacement of the successor teeth.

Central giant cell granuloma

Central giant cell granuloma may occur at any age but presents most frequently in the second and third decades. There is a female predominance. It involves the mandible more frequently than the maxilla and most lesions arise in the anterior part of the jaws. Central giant cell granuloma usually presents clinically as a swelling of the bone, and growth may sometimes be rapid. Some cases present as a brown or red swelling that perforates the bone cortex, often in the alveolus (Fig. 7.23A). Others are symptomless and are first detected on routine radiological examination.

Radiographically, the lesion appears as a well-defined radiolucent area with thinning, expansion, and, occasionally, perforation of the cortex. Involved teeth may be displaced and their roots may show resorption (Fig. 7.23B). Many lesions are multilocular but the radiographic appearances are not specific and diagnosis is made by biopsy.

Histological examination shows large numbers of multinucleate, osteoclast-like giant cells lying in a vascular stroma that is rich in small, spindle-shaped cells (Fig. 7.24). The giant cells may be arranged in

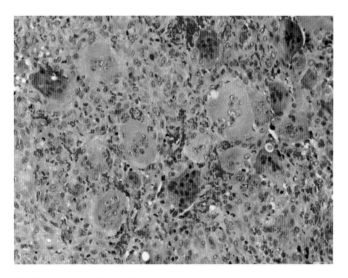

Fig. 7.24 Central giant cell granuloma showing numerous multinucleated osteoclast-like giant cells in a loose vascular stroma. There are numerous extravasated erythrocytes (red cells).

focal aggregates or be scattered throughout the lesion, although they are often related to vascular channels. The spindle-cell component probably consists predominantly of mononuclear precursors of the giant cells, but includes fibroblasts and endothelial cells. Foci of extravasated erythrocytes and deposits of haemosiderin are common in the stroma. The lesion may also contain a few trabeculae of osteoid or bone.

Key points Giant cell granuloma

- Peripheral giant cell granuloma presents as a gingival lump and is also called giant cell epulis (Chapter 2)
- Central giant cell granuloma may present as a peripheral lesion, but is usually detected by radiology
- Most lesions arise in the inter-premolar region
- Multi-nodular foci of osteoclast-like giant cells in rich vascular stroma
- Red cell extravasation and haemosiderin often present
- Hyperparathyroidism must be excluded by serology
- Central lesions treated by curettage and depot steroid injection

---

Bone tumours

Primary tumours of bone are uncommon lesions in the jaws. They may arise from any of the different cell types present in bone, including cartilage, haematopoietic marrow, and vascular and fibrous tissues. Their classification is complex, and some types are site-specific and have not been recorded in the jaws. For convenience, Langerhans cell histiocytosis has been included in the classification, since destructive lesions in the jaws are a frequent feature of this disease.

Key points Bone tumours

Primary bone tumours are rare in the jaws

Benign bone tumours
- May be radiolucent or radiodense
- Typically expand the jaws and are well circumscribed
- Are usually excised with a narrow margin

Malignant bone tumours
- Destructive lesions that may cause tooth exfoliation
- Most common malignant tumour in bone is metastatic carcinoma
- Sarcomas may be solitary but often have metastasized at presentation
- Multi-modal therapy is used for bone sarcoma
- Osteosarcoma of the jaw has better prognosis than at other skeletal sites

---

Central giant cell granuloma is a condition of unknown aetiology. It has been suggested that it could be a reaction to some form of haemodynamic disturbance in bone marrow, perhaps associated with trauma and haemorrhage. Intra-osseous giant cell granulomas respond well to injection of depot steroids, sometimes after curettage. Central giant cell granuloma is impossible to distinguish histologically from a focal lesion of hyperparathyroidism, which must be excluded by biochemical investigations (serum calcium and alkaline phosphatase) when a giant cell lesion is diagnosed on biopsy. Giant cell granuloma of the jaws can occur in Noonan's syndrome (Table 7.3). Giant cell tumour of bone does not usually affect the jaws and is defined by a specific histone gene (*H3F3A*) mutation.

Key points Differential diagnoses of giant cell lesions

- Giant cell epulis (peripheral giant cell granuloma)
- Central giant cell granuloma
- Hyperparathyroidism
- Cherubism
- Aneurysmal bone cyst
- Noonan's syndrome
- Giant cell tumour of bone (very rare in the jaws)

Benign bone tumours

Osteoma

Osteoma is a benign, slow-growing neoplasm consisting of well-differentiated mature bone (Figs 7.25 and 7.26). It may arise as a central or sub-periosteal lesion and is most frequently found in the paranasal sinuses. The majority of osteomas are diagnosed in adult life. Histologically, osteomas can be divided into compact (ivory) and cancellous types. The compact osteoma consists of a mass of dense lamellar bone with few marrow spaces; the cancellous type is made up of interconnecting trabeculae enclosing fatty or fibrous marrow. Multiple jaw osteomas are a manifestation of Gardner's syndrome (Fig. 7.14).

Chondroma

Chondromas are very rare lesions in the jaws. They tend to occur in the anterior maxilla and posterior mandible. Mature hyaline cartilage is present and bland individual chondrocytes are found. Osteocartilaginous exostosis (osteochondroma) is regarded as a benign cartilage capped tumour and occurs in the mandibular condyle. Bizarre parosteal osteochondromatous proliferation (BPOP) is a rare benign tumour that has been described in the anterior maxilla. These lesions are treated by conservative surgical excision.

Chondromyxoid fibroma

This is a very rare benign tumour in the jaws. It shows a multi-nodular appearance histologically and typically possesses loose myxoid

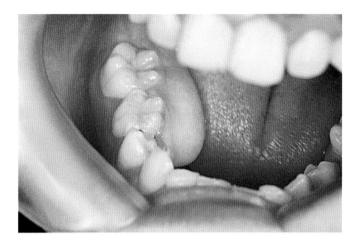

Fig. 7.25 Osteoma presenting as a swelling of the lingual plate of the mandible.

cartilaginous matrix without cytological atypia. Treatment is by surgical excision with a conservative margin.

Chondroblastoma

These uncommon benign neoplasms are characterized by eosinophilic chondrocytes in a hyaline or myxoid cartilage matrix. Chicken-wire calcification is a characteristic feature. The tumour is normally excised surgically, aiming to achieve complete removal.

Ossifying fibroma

The ossifying fibroma is a well-demarcated, occasionally encapsulated, benign neoplasm (Fig. 7.27). It occurs in the jaws and other craniofacial bones, particularly those of the sino-nasal complex and orbit. It consists of fibrous tissue containing varying amounts of bony trabeculae and rounded calcified bodies (psammona bodies). Its demarcated nature is an important feature distinguishing it from fibrous dysplasia. Clinically, ossifying fibroma presents as a slowly enlarging and progressive swelling

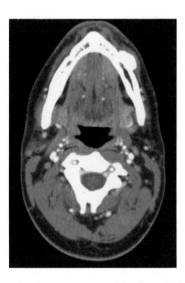

Fig. 7.26 CT scan showing an osteoma arising from the buccal cortex of the mandible.

and, when it involves the jaws, it most often affects the premolar–molar region of the mandible. Radiologically, the appearances vary with the stage of development of the lesion. Initially there is a well-demarcated radiolucent area within which, as the lesion matures, varying amounts of calcified tissue are deposited (Fig. 7.27). Juvenile and adult types are recognized. Adult-type ossifying fibromas are slow-growing but the juvenile types may show rapid growth. Histologically, the juvenile types are characterized by richly cellular, mitotically active fibrous tissue. They are separated into trabecular and psammomatous subtypes, though both patterns of mineralization may occur together. Treatment of ossifying fibroma should aim to surgically remove the entire tumour with a small margin of normal surrounding tissue. Historically, a recurrence rate of about 30–60% has been noted in juvenile cases, whereas adult types seldom recur.

In rare cases, ossifying fibroma of the jaws is associated with hereditary hyperparathyroidism as part of the hyperparathyroidism–jaw tumour syndrome (OMIM 145001).

Osteoblastoma

Osteoblastoma (osteoid osteoma) is a rare tumour in the jaws. Nocturnal bone pain is a characteristic clinical feature. Broad trabeculae

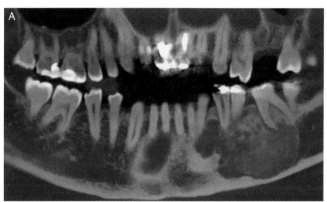

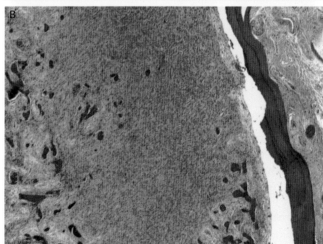

Fig. 7.27 Cone beam CT showing an ossifying fibroma in the left body of the mandible. Histology shows cellular fibrous tissue that contains islands of woven bone. The well-demarcated interface of the neoplasm with normal bone is seen on the right.

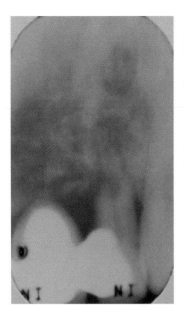
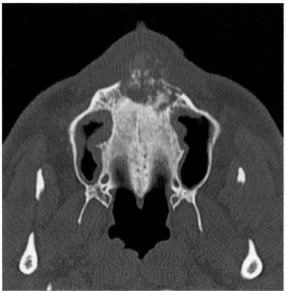

Fig. 7.28 Osteosarcoma of the anterior maxilla. The periapical radiograph shows 'moth-eaten' bone and irregular root resorption of the maxillary lateral incisor. The CT scan shows the extent of the lesion.

of unmineralized osteoid rimmed by plump osteoblasts are present. Osteoid osteoma must be distinguished from cementoblastoma, which forms in relation to the roots of teeth, most often lower first permanent molars (Chapter 6).

Vascular malformation in bone

Vascular malformation in bone ('haemangioma of bone') is a rare lesion of the jaws that is more common in the mandible than in the maxilla. Radiographically, it shows a multilocular honeycomb appearance. Aspiration will reveal fresh blood. Microscopically, most vascular malformations of bone are of the cavernous type, showing dilated, thin-walled, vascular chambers expanding the marrow cavity. Copious bleeding may follow tooth extraction, if the tooth root involves the vascular malformation. Patients should be referred to hospital for tooth extraction if an underlying vascular malformation is suspected. Intra-osseous vascular malformations may be part of the Sturge–Weber syndrome, due to mutation of the *GNAQ* gene (OMIM 185300).

Malignant bone tumours

Osteosarcoma

Osteosarcoma is the commonest primary malignant tumour of bone, but is relatively rare in the jaws. These neoplasms occur in children and adolescents, but many are seen in patients around 30 years of age, which is about a decade later than the average for juvenile osteosarcoma elsewhere in the skeleton. Occasionally, osteosarcoma presents in older patients, sometimes in association with Paget's disease of bone.

In the jaws, osteosarcoma usually presents with swelling, which may be accompanied by pain or paraesthesia, and, radiographically, it may appear as a radiolucent, radiopaque, or mixed lesion (Fig. 7.28). Widening of the periodontal ligament is a classic radiographic feature. Histologically, several subtypes are recognized but they are all characterized by direct formation of abnormal osteoid or bone by malignant osteoblasts (Figs 7.29 and 7.30). Highly atypical cartilage may be

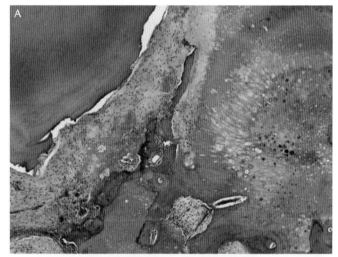
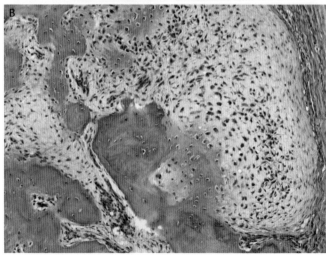

Fig. 7.29 Osteosarcoma showing malignant osteoid formation in the periodontal ligament and atypical cartilage (A). Pleomorphic malignant osteoblasts are seen on higher magnification (B).

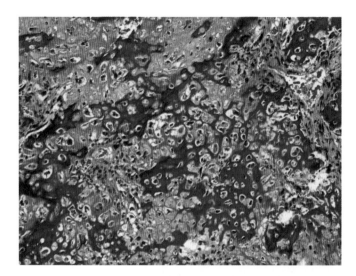

Fig. 7.30 Osteosarcoma showing malignant osteoid in a filigree pattern. Note the pleomorphic osteoblasts with hyperchromatic nuclei.

present in the chondroblastic variant. Osteosarcoma may arise centrally within the jaws or peripherally, in relation to the periosteum. Central and periosteal osteosarcomas are high-grade neoplasms. Some central neoplasms, known as telangiectatic osteosarcomas, present as rapidly expanding, high-grade tumours containing blood-filled spaces. A distinctive variant known as parosteal osteosarcoma is less aggressive.

High-grade osteosarcomas have a high rate of metastasis and patients are staged using imaging prior to treatment. Chemotherapy is normally used first and then the primary tumour is excised. Response to the drug can then be assessed; sometimes the resected tumour is completely necrotic.

Ewing's sarcoma

These distinctive bone tumours form part of the 'small, dark, round cell' neoplasms occurring in children and adolescents (Fig. 7.31A). They are rare in the jaws and when diagnosed at that site, they are often part of disseminated disease. Ewing's sarcoma typically shows a cytogenetic fusion of the *EWS-FLi1* genes, though other fusions may be present (Fig 7.31B). Like osteosarcomas, Ewing's sarcomas are treated

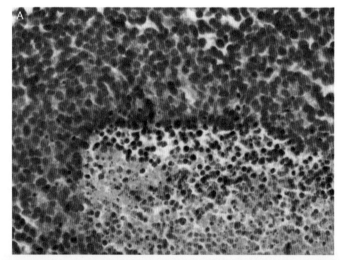

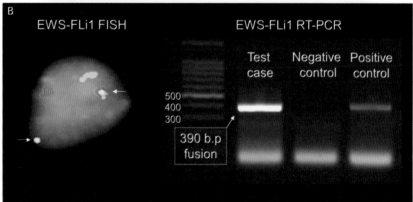

Fig. 7.31 Ewing's tumour composed of sheets of 'small round blue cells'. The tumour has the characteristic *EWS-FLi1* fusion gene. The FISH preparation shows a malignant cell with a EWS-FLi1 dual fusion. The green signal is the EWS probe hybridizing to chromosome 22q12. Red signal is the FLi1 probe hybridizing to chromosome 11q24. Yellow fusion signals (arrows) identify products of t(11;22)(q24;q12) translocation. Reverse transcriptase polymerase chain reaction (RT-PCR) shows a 390 base pair (b.p) fusion transcript. *Courtesy of Dr Nick Bown.*

by chemotherapy followed by resection. Over 50% show complete response to the chemotherapeutic agent.

Chondrosarcoma

Chondrosarcomas are rare tumours in the jaws. The anterior part of the maxilla and posterior part of the mandible are the most common sites of occurrence, but mandibular tumours may also originate in the condylar processes. Chondrosarcomas show a high degree of cellularity and possess plump, often binucleated, chondrocytes in a hyaline or myxoid cartilage matrix. Calcification and endochondral ossification may occur and this is reflected in their variable radiographic appearances. Treatment is by surgical removal, aiming to achieve complete excision with marginal clearance. The prognosis depends on histological grading, which is determined by thorough sampling of the excised specimen.

Myeloma

Myeloma is a malignant neoplasm composed of plasma cells and, generally, occurs as a disseminated disease involving many bones (multiple myeloma). Less commonly, the condition occurs as a solitary lesion within bone or, more rarely, soft tissue (solitary myeloma or plasmacytoma). Some, but not all, patients with solitary lesions eventually develop multiple myeloma.

Jaw lesions may occur as part of multiple myeloma or as a solitary lesion, and extra-medullary plasmacytoma may also occur in the oral soft-tissues, presenting as diffuse or polypoid swellings. Myeloma is the result of neoplastic proliferation of a single clone of immunoglobulin-producing cells. Abnormally high levels of a homogeneous immunoglobulin and/or its constituent polypeptide chains may appear in serum and are termed paraproteins.

Clinically, multiple myeloma occurs most frequently in patients between 50 and 70 years of age. Although any bone may be involved, the skull, vertebrae, sternum, ribs, and pelvic bones are most commonly affected. These are sites where haematopoietic marrow is normally present. Jaw lesions may be the initial manifestation of disease but, more commonly, they are purely incidental to the overall clinical presentation. The classical radiographic feature is of sharply demarcated, round, or oval osteolytic lesions with a characteristic punched-out appearance (Fig. 7.32).

Microscopically, the lesions are densely cellular and consist of sheets of pleomorphic cells that bear a striking resemblance to mature plasma cells or their immediate precursors. The neoplastic cells typically show restricted kappa or lambda light chain expression, and this clonal pattern can be demonstrated by the use of *in situ* hybridization.

Myeloma is usually treated by chemotherapy and bone marrow transplant. In addition, patients may be taking long-term bisphosphonates and are at risk of developing osteonecrosis of the jaw.

Langerhans cell histiocytosis

Langerhans cell histiocytosis (LCH) comprises a spectrum of disease with a wide range of clinical manifestations. However, it presents in one of three main ways:

(1) Disseminated multi-organ disease (Letterer–Siwe disease)

(2) Multifocal, involving bone and other organs (multifocal eosinophilic granuloma)

(3) Solitary lesion in bone (unifocal eosinophilic granuloma)

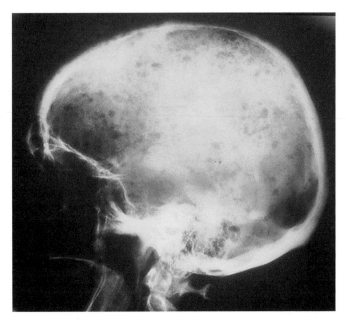

Fig. 7.32 Radiograph of the skull showing punched-out radiolucencies in multiple myeloma.

Letterer–Siwe disease occurs mainly in infants and children under 2 years of age and has a high mortality. Skin and pulmonary lesions may be present, as well as infiltration of the gingiva by neoplastic Langerhans cells.

Multifocal eosinophilic granuloma occurs in children and adolescents. Patients with multifocal eosinophilic granulomas involving the craniofacial bones, orbit, and posterior pituitary gland, present with the classic triad of Hand–Schuller–Christian syndrome: skull defects, exophthalmus, and diabetes insipidus.

Unifocal and multifocal eosinophilic granulomas occur in older children and, less commonly, in adults. The majority of patients are under 20 years of age, and males are affected about twice as commonly as females. Any bone may be involved but the cranium and jaws are common sites. Jaw lesions are more common in the mandible. Radiographs show either solitary or multiple osteolytic lesions. Multiple eosinophilic granuloma involving the jaws can result in extensive destruction and loss or loosening of teeth, which on radiographs may appear to be 'floating in air' (Fig. 7.33A).

Histologically, the lesions of LCH are characterized by sheets and aggregates of Langerhans cells, which strongly express CD1a and Langerin by immunohistochemistry (Fig. 7.33). Typically, there are large numbers of eosinophils, hence the term 'eosinophilic granuloma'.

Single lesions may respond to curettage and/or localized radiotherapy. Multifocal disease is managed by haematologists. *BRAF* mutations are present in over half of LCH cases and there are clinical trials evaluating BRAF-targeted therapies.

Metastatic tumours

It has been estimated that metastatic tumours in the oral soft-tissues and jaws account for about 1% of malignant tumours occurring in the oral cavity. Metastasis to bone is more common than to the soft tissues, the mandible being much more frequently affected than the maxilla. The most common primary tumours reported as

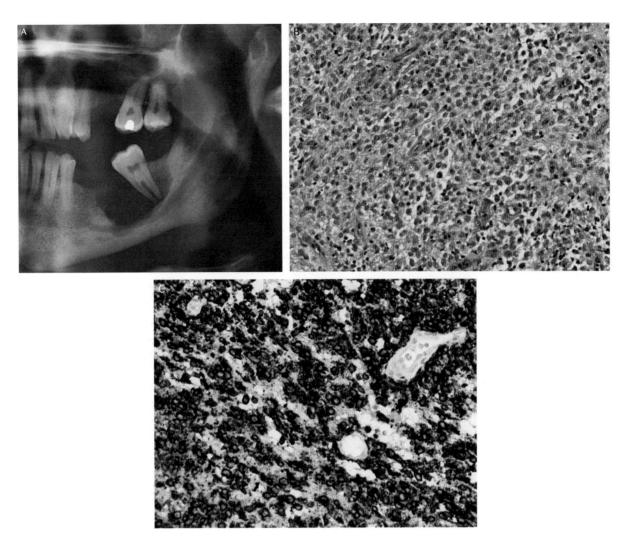

Fig. 7.33 LCH showing a radiolucent lesion associated with tooth exfoliation in the left mandible. Histology shows sheets of Langerhans cells that show strong expression of CD1a by immunohistochemistry.

metastasizing to the jaws are carcinomas of the lung, bowel, breast, prostate, and kidney. Presenting features of metastatic tumours may be pain, loose teeth, swelling, and paraethesia or anaesthesia of the lip due to involvement of the inferior alveolar nerve, but many lesions are asymptomatic. Metastatic deposits in the gingiva can resemble an epulis clinically.

Most metastatic tumours are osteolytic but some, such as carcinomas of breast and prostate, may be osteoblastic and appear radiographically as an area of radiodensity rather than radiolucency.

Genetic disorders of bone

Patients with inherited disorders of bone are seen in dental practice, although not frequently. Some of the more common inherited bone disorders that may involve the jaws are listed in Table 7.3. It should be noted that certain disorders described in previous sections of this chapter are also genetic in origin.

Osteogenesis imperfecta

Osteogenesis imperfecta (brittle bone disease; OMIM 120150) is an hereditary disease and consists of a heterogeneous group of related disorders caused principally by mutations in the genes that code for type-1 collagen. It is characterized by generalized osteoporosis, with slender bones and a tendency for the bones to fracture after minor trauma. The long bones have narrow, poorly formed cortices composed of woven bone. Fractures normally heal but exuberant callus may be formed. The sclerae may appear blue because they are so thin that the pigmented choroid shines through and there is sometimes a family history of deafness caused by distortion of the ossicles in the ears. Other abnormalities that may be present are joint hypermobility with lax ligaments, thin translucent skin, and heart valve defects. Some forms of osteogenesis imperfecta are associated with dentinogenesis imperfecta (Chapter 5). Eight main types of osteogenesis imperfecta have been described.

Osteopetrosis (Albers–Schonberg disease, marble bone disease)

This is a rare disease (OMIM 607634 and others) characterized by excessive density of all bones with obliteration of marrow cavities and the development of a secondary anaemia. There appears to be a defect in osteoclastic activity and, as normal bone formation relies on the interdependence of deposition and resorption, there is a failure in the remodelling of the developing bone. There is, therefore, an excessive formation of bone that is mechanically weak, and so fractures are common. The jaws are composed of dense bone with greatly reduced medullary spaces. Delayed eruption of teeth may occur and osteomyelitis is a common complication of tooth extraction. Radiographic examination shows an increased density of the whole skeleton with no distinction between cortical and medullary bone. The base of the skull shows marked radiodensity, whereas the vault is generally less dense. Jaw involvement is variable, the mandible being more frequently affected than the maxilla, and the density of the bone may render the roots of the teeth almost invisible on radiographs. Obliteration of the maxillary antrum may be a feature.

Cleidocranial dysplasia

Cleidocranial dysplasia (OMIM 119600) is transmitted as an autosomal dominant trait. It is characterized by abnormalities of many bones, but particularly of the skull, jaws, and clavicle. Dental anomalies are also common. A variety of abnormalities of the skull may be present, the fontanelles and sutures tend to remain open and the skull appears flat with prominent frontal, parietal, and occipital bones, producing a 'helmet-shaped' head. The nasal bridge is also depressed. Partial or complete absence of the clavicles allows the shoulders to be brought forwards until they meet in the mid-line. The maxilla may be underdeveloped with a high, narrow-arched palate. The deciduous dentition tends to be retained with delayed or non-eruption of the permanent dentition because of multiple impactions (Fig. 5.23). Supernumerary teeth and dentigerous cysts are also common. The roots of the teeth tend to be thinner than normal and secondary, cellular cementum is either absent or sparsely present on both deciduous and permanent teeth.

X-linked hypophosphataemia (vitamin D resistant rickets)

This is a type of rickets characterized by low serum phosphate levels and a lack of response to treatment with vitamin D, in contrast to nutritional

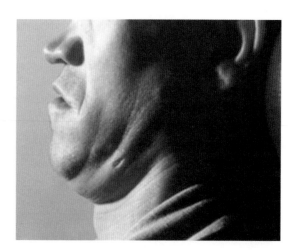

Fig. 7.34 Achondroplasia showing retrusive middle-third of the face.

rickets. The disease is caused by mutations in the *PHEX* gene (OMIM 307800). Affected individuals have short stature, and radiographs show short and squat long bones. There may be delayed eruption of teeth. The dentine fails to mineralize properly and the pulp may become infected through pulp horn defects, leading to abscess formation in the absence of dental caries. Predentine is widened, whilst the circumpulpal dentine is thinned and resembles interglobular dentine throughout its entire thickness.

Achondroplasia

Achondroplasia (OMIM 100800) may be inherited as an autosomal dominant trait, but many cases have no family history and appear to be due to spontaneous mutations. It is the most common form of dwarfism and is associated with an abnormality in endochondral ossification. There is an absence or a defect in the zone of provisional calcification of the cartilage in the epiphyses and in the base of the skull. The trunk and head are of normal size but the limbs are excessively short. The middle-third of the face is retrusive due to defective growth of the base of the skull (Fig. 7.34) and severe malocclusion is common.

Noonan's syndrome

Noonan's syndrome (OMIM 163950) is a complex genetic disorder affecting 1:2,500 live births. The features are variable and include congenital heart disease, feeding problems, speech and hearing difficulties, and disorders of behaviour and intelligence. Children affected by Noonan's syndrome have a distinctive facial appearance, including heavy eyelids, tight neck skin, and low-set ears. Giant cell lesions can develop in bones and joints, but are most frequent in the jaws where they can resemble giant cell granuloma or cherubism clinically.

Metabolic and endocrine disorders of bone

The normal process of osteogenesis may be affected by a variety of metabolic diseases or various factors as in osteoporosis. An inadequate supply of bone salts, such as in vitamin D deficiency (rickets), may affect the normal process of calcification. Homeostasis of calcium and phosphate metabolism is affected by the activity of the parathyroid glands, disturbances of which are associated with changes in bone.

Humoral hypercalcaemia of malignancy

Hypercalcaemia is relatively common in patients with cancer, occurring in approximately 20–30% of cases. It occurs in patients with both solid tumours and haematological malignancies, particularly breast and lung cancer, and multiple myeloma. Malignancy is often evident, clinically, by the time hypercalcaemia occurs, and the onset is associated with poor prognosis. Bisphosphonates or denosumab are often prescribed for patients with certain cancers to reduce the effects of hypercalcaemia and to preserve bone mass.

Osteoporosis

Bone is in a state of constant turnover and, in adult life, bone loss gradually predominates over bone apposition. Osteoporosis results either when the bone loss is excessive or when the apposition of bone is reduced. A variety of risk factors have been identified, such as alcohol abuse and steroid therapy, but the disease presents most commonly in postmenopausal women, where it is related to hormonal disturbance. The rate of loss of bone mineral is variable but in most postmenopausal women it is about 1–2% per year. In about a quarter of cases, more rapid loss, up to 5–8% per year, may occur. The rate of loss is about twice as fast in women as in men. Osteoporosis is also accentuated in several other diseases, particularly Cushing's syndrome, thyrotoxicosis, and primary hyperparathyroidism.

The jaws may be involved and osteoporosis may be detected on dental panoramic tomograms. Osteoporosis occurring in edentulous patients may result in the mandible being reduced to a thin, fragile strip of bone. Osteoporotic bone is of normal composition but it is reduced in quantity. There is an increased radiolucency of bone, the cortex is thinned, and there are more marrow spaces in the cancellous bone associated with thin trabeculae.

Primary hyperparathyroidism

This relatively common disease is seen predominantly in middle-aged women and results from excessive parathormone secretion, usually from idiopathic hyperplasia of a parathyroid gland or an adenoma, but occasionally from a parathyroid carcinoma. The effects of parathormone include stimulation of intestinal absorption of calcium, reabsorption of calcium by the renal tubules, and bone resorption by osteoclasts. Thus, excess secretion of the hormone results in hypercalcaemia and hypercalciuria. There is a generalized osteoporosis, pathological calcification of the lungs and blood vessels, and urinary calculi that cause severe renal colic (pain).

Histologically, osteoclastic activity is increased throughout the skeleton. On occasions, focal areas of bone resorption result in the formation of lesions called brown tumours, which consist of large numbers of multinucleate, osteoclast-like giant cells scattered in a highly cellular, vascular fibroblastic connective tissue stroma. There is much haemosiderin pigment present, hence the brown colour of these lesions seen macroscopically. Histologically, it is impossible to distinguish a brown tumour of hyperparathyroidism from other giant cell lesions of bone. Very rarely, a focal collection of osteoclasts (brown tumour) may occur in relation to the periosteum and be indistinguishable from a peripheral giant cell granuloma (Fig. 2.14; Chapter 2).

Radiographic examination may show no detectable changes or a generalized osteoporosis. Partial loss of the lamina dura around the teeth may occur but it is not a constant feature. If focal lesions (brown tumours) develop, they present as sharply defined, round, or oval radiolucent areas, which may appear multilocular.

Secondary hyperparathyroidism

Secondary hyperparathyroidism occurs in response to chronic hypocalcaemia, most frequently as a result of chronic renal failure, but also in association with rickets and osteomalacia. The bone changes are complex and are a mixture of those associated with osteomalacia and hyperparathyroidism. Involvement of the jaws has been reported and changes may be detected on radiographs.

Rickets and osteomalacia

Acquired rickets and its adult counterpart osteomalacia are due to deficiency of vitamin D. Deficiency may be due to lack of exposure to sunlight or dietary causes. In the UK, dietary deficiency is seen mainly among the Asian immigrant population. In addition, the high cereal content of their diet and the use of wholemeal grains containing phytates impairs calcium absorption. Other causes of hypocalcaemia, such as renal failure or malabsorption, may also be associated with osteomalacia. The radiographic changes are similar to those seen in osteoporosis but, in contrast to the latter, where the bone present is normally mineralized, in rickets and osteomalacia there is a failure of mineralization of osteoid and of cartilage. Dental abnormalities in acquired rickets include enamel hypoplasia and defective dentine mineralization.

Acromegaly

This disease is caused by prolonged and excessive secretion of growth hormone, usually due to a secreting adenoma of the anterior lobe of the pituitary developing after the epiphyses have closed. There is renewed growth of the bones of the jaws, hands, and feet with overgrowth of some soft tissues. Activation of the condylar growth centre of the mandible causes the jaw to become enlarged and protrusive, and if teeth are present, they become spaced. The soft tissues of the face, particularly the lips and nose, become thickened and enlarged (Fig. 7.35).

Paget's disease of bone

Paget's disease of bone is characterized by disorganized formation and remodelling of bone, unrelated to functional requirements. The aetiology of the disease remains unclear, but it is thought to be due to a primary dysfunction of osteoclasts. The natural history of the disease can be divided into three progressive and overlapping phases (Table 7.4).

In the first two phases, the bones become softened and distorted, and their overall size may be markedly increased. In the sclerotic phase, the distorted bones become fixed in their deformed state. Paget's disease occurs predominantly in patients over 40 years of age. Sub-clinical disease is not uncommon, and radiological surveys and autopsy studies have demonstrated an incidence of about 3% in all persons over 40 years of age. However, there are differences in geographical incidence: it is rare in Russia, Asia, and parts of Europe compared to the

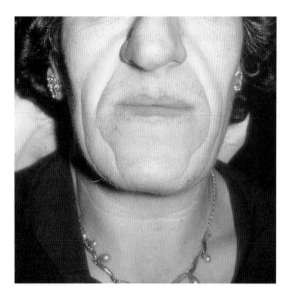

Fig. 7.35 Acromegaly showing coarsening of facial features and mandibular prognathism.

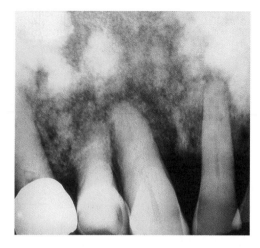

Fig. 7.36 Cotton-wool appearance of the bone in Paget's disease. Hypercementosis is often present.

United Kingdom, Australasia, and North America, although the incidence is decreasing. The lesions may involve a single or small number of bones or, less commonly, may be disseminated widely throughout the skeleton. Lesions are commonest in the weight-bearing bones of the axial skeleton, particularly the sacrum, followed by lumbar, thoracic, and cervical vertebrae. The skull and femur are the next most frequent sites. Jaw lesions are more common in the maxilla than in the mandible, and although monostotic lesions have been reported, when the jaws are involved, the calvaria is almost invariably affected.

Clinically, patients with Paget's disease show varying degrees of bony deformity and distortion of the weight-bearing portions of the skeleton, and of the skull and facial bones. However, most cases are mild, and the disease may be discovered incidentally on radiographs, or the patient may complain of bone pain. When the skull is involved, patients may also present with signs and symptoms of sensory or motor disturbances related to cranial nerve compression. With progressive enlargement of the maxilla, the alveolar ridge becomes thickened and widened, the palate flattened, and there is increasing facial deformity. The bony enlargement may lead to incompetence of the lips. Edentulous patients may complain of difficulties in wearing dentures due to progressive increase in jaw size. In dentate patients, derangement of the occlusion, spacing of the teeth, and retroclination of incisors and palatoversion of posterior teeth may be striking. The teeth often show hypercementosis and may become ankylosed, leading to difficulty in extraction. Root resorption may also occur in the osteolytic phase. In the active stages of the disease, post-extraction haemorrhage may be a problem because of the highly vascular marrow that contains extensive arterio-venous communications. In contrast, in the later sclerotic phase, the bone is relatively dense and avascular, and extraction sockets are prone to infection.

The radiographic features are variable but reflect the different stages of the disease. Osteolysis is the earliest change, followed by patchy osteosclerosis and the appearance of ill-defined and irregular radiopaque areas, producing a characteristic cotton-wool appearance (Fig. 7.36). In the skull, thickening of the outer table of the vault and loss of distinction between the tables and diploe are also typical features (Fig. 7.37). In

Table 7.4 Phases of Paget's disease of bone

Early lytic or 'hot' phase	Rarely diagnosed during this phase. Osteoclasts become active and sharply defined radiolucent areas are seen. May be detected incidentally as intense areas of uptake on bone scans.
Intermediate or 'mixed' phase	Osteolytic areas increase and disorganized osteoblastic activity lays down coarse trabeculae of woven bone. Mixed radiolucent and radiodense areas are seen and cortical thickening occurs.
Final or 'cold' phase	Previously formed woven bone remodels to form lamellar bone. Mosaic pattern appears histologically and the bone shows radiodense sclerosis.

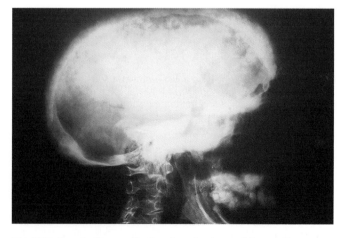

Fig. 7.37 Paget's disease affecting the calvarium and the maxilla.

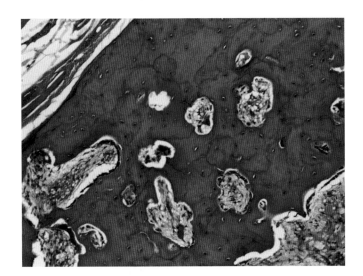

Fig. 7.38 Paget's disease of bone showing active osteoclasts and osteoblasts, and the mosaic pattern of reversal lines.

osteoblastic activity involving most of the trabeculae. As a result of the increased remodelling activity, the bone trabeculae show numerous resting and scalloped reversal lines, which stain deeply with haematoxylin, giving the bone matrix a characteristic mosaic appearance (Fig. 7.38). Investigation of the blood chemistry is important in the diagnosis of Paget's disease. The serum calcium and serum phosphorus levels are usually within normal limits but the serum bone alkaline phosphatase level is often raised, sometimes markedly so in patients with widespread active disease. Once diagnosed, Paget's disease of bone can be controlled medically; therapy often involves the use of bisphosphonate drugs. Medication-related osteonecrosis of the jaw (MRONJ) may follow invasive dental procedures in patients with Paget's disease.

the jaws, loss of the lamina dura, hypercementosis, and ankylosis may be noted.

The microscopic features of Paget's disease reflect the disorganized bone remodelling that is a feature of the disease. During the early osteolytic phase, osteoclastic resorption predominates. The resorbed areas are filled by cellular and vascular fibrous marrow, within which new bone forms, and this in turn is remodelled and replaced by further new bone. This disorganized remodelling activity is repeated, and in fully developed, active lesions, there is simultaneous osteoclastic and

> **Key points Paget's disease of bone**
> - Presents in patients over 40 years of age
> - May be symptomless and an incidental radiographic finding
> - Tooth spacing may develop as jaw expands
> - Bone pain and varying degrees of bone deformity
> - Tooth extraction complicated by hypercementosis, ankylosis, and bone sclerosis
> - Osteolytic, mixed, and osteosclerotic phases seen on radiographs
> - Disorganized remodelling of bone, and mosaic pattern seen in bone biopsies

Temporomandibular joints

The temporomandibular joints (TMJs) function as a pair of synovial joints between the mandible and the temporal bone. Due to their complex evolution, the TMJs are one of the few joints in the human body that contain upper and lower joint spaces separated by a fibrocartilaginous articular disc. The mandibular condyle is a bony ellipsoid structure with an articular surface that is covered by fibrocartilage, which is the major growth centre for the condyle, up to the age of skeletal maturity (around 20 years old). The condyle is attached to the ramus of the mandible by a thin neck. The opposing articular fibrocartilage of the TMJ lines the glenoid fossa, which is a hollow within the squamous temporal bone bounded on the anterior aspect by a ridge of bone known as the articular eminence.

Temporomandibular disorders

Temporomandibular disorders (TMDs) are the next most common cause of oro-facial pain after odontogenic pain. The term TMD encompasses a number of conditions affecting the muscles of mastication and/or the joint complex, and has recently been reclassified. There are many different types of TMD but the 12 most common are listed in Table 7.5. Signs and symptoms of TMD as a group include: joint noises (clicking, grating (crepitus)); pain affecting the joint complex and muscles of mastication, which can radiate; ear pain (otalgia) or ringing in the ear (tinnitus) without aural disease; headache located in the temporal region and exacerbated by jaw movement or (para)function; and alteration in jaw movements (subluxation, dislocation (open lock) and decreased range of movement (closed lock)).

The international consensus for initial management of the 12 most common types of TMDs, presenting for the first time with no red flag signs and symptoms of malignancy (Box 7.1), is to embark upon conservative therapy. Conservative therapy should begin with patient reassurance and explanation about TMDs, and may include: simple time-limited topical or systemic analgesics, e.g. NSAIDs; self-administered physiotherapy; thermal treatment, such as moist heat and covered ice; a short period of alteration in the individual's preparation and selection of food to help reduce pain; and full-coverage occlusal splints.

Accurate diagnosis and follow-up is important, especially if trismus is an accompanying feature of the initial presentation. If symptoms persist or are atypical, then further investigations are required to exclude malignancy, including appropriate imaging (CT and MRI scans). Malignancy

Table 7.5 Twelve most common TMDs

Category	Subcategory		
Myalgia (1)	Local myalgia **(2)**		
	Myofascial pain **(3)**		
	Myofascial pain with referral **(4)**		
Arthralgia (5)			
Intra-articular disorders	Disc displacements	With reduction **(6)**	With reduction with intermittent locking **(7)** Occasionally reducing discs cause locking (intermittent limited opening)
		Without reduction with limited opening **(8)** (acute phase)	Without reduction without limited opening **(9)** (generally over time pseudo disc formation allows acute phase to progress to this)
	Degenerative joint disease **(10)**		
	Subluxation **(11)**		
Headache attributable to TMDs (12)			

Source data from *Journal of Oral & Facial Pain and Headache*, 28, Schiffman E, Ohrbach R, Truelove E. et al., Diagnostic Criteria for Temporomandibular Disorders (DC/TMD) for Clinical and Research Applications: Recommendations of the International RDC/TMD Consortium Network and Oro-facial Pain Special Interest Group, pp. 6–27.

invading the infratemporal fossa, e.g. squamous cell carcinoma and adenoid cystic carcinoma, may cause TMD-like signs and symptoms.

Disc displacements

Displacement of the articular disc, most often in an anterior direction, may or may not reduce back to its original position. If the disc reduces, it produces an audible click with or without intermittent locking, as well as possible deviation of jaw movement to the unaffected side. If the disc does not reduce, then it can interfere with jaw movements, most notably decreasing translation of the condylar head on the

Box 7.1 Red flag signs and symptoms that are suggestive of a malignancy mimicking a TMD

- Recurrent epistaxis
- Anosmia
- Persistent nasal obstruction or purulent discharge
- Objective hearing loss
- Near complete trismus precluding oral examination
- Signs of oral malignancy
- Previous head and neck cancer
- Cervical lymphadenopathy
- Cranial nerve dysfunction (especially trigeminal and facial nerves)
- Pre-auricular mass
- Failure to respond to management or progression despite intervention

affected side, restricting opening. In some circumstances, the condylar head on the affected side will function on the retrodiscal lamina. The latter is a neurovascular area of the articular disc and, consequently, causes pain and limited mouth opening (to around 10–15 mm interincisal distance).

There are, therefore, two main clinical diagnoses that can be made in respect of disc displacements: disc displacement with reduction and disc displacement without reduction. The latter can cause limited opening in the acute phase, but over time, remodelling of the disc occurs with formation of a 'pseudo-disc', and nearly a full range of movement is restored to the affected TMJ.

A painless click is common in the general population (around 30%) and is not necessarily an indication for therapy, because progression to disc displacement without reduction is rare.

Surgery for disc displacements does not produce predictable results nor are the results necessarily stable over the longer term. If surgery is considered, the most minimally invasive option (arthrocentesis or arthroscopy) should be used, only if conservative management has failed and there are still significant functional deficits.

Arthritic disorders affecting the TMJ

For clinical purposes, osteoarthritis and osteoarthrosis are no longer separated and the term 'degenerative joint disease' is used to group the two conditions together. Degenerative joint disease is diagnosed clinically when crepitus is present on TMJ movement with or without pain.

Osteoarthritis and osteoarthrosis

Osteoarthritis most commonly affects the weight-bearing joints of the hips, knees, and spine, but also involves the fingers, thumb, and great toe. Osteoarthritis is rare in the TMJ and is most likely a result of previous

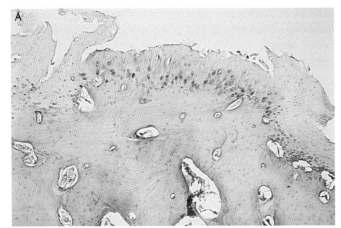

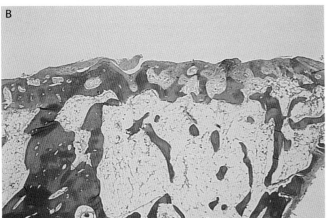

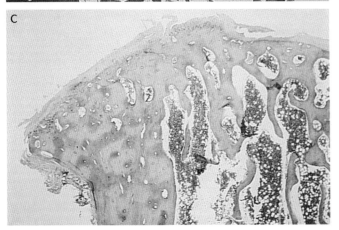

Fig. 7.39 Osteoarthritic changes in the temporomandibular joint showing fibrillation and fragmentation of articular cartilage (A), denudation and exposure of underlying bony end-plate (B), and osteophytic lipping of the condyle (C).

and if crepitus remains, the diagnosis becomes osteoarthosis. Both conditions may respond to anti-inflammatory drugs or physiotherapy. Surgical intervention would follow the same rationale as that described in the section Disc displacements.

Rheumatoid arthritis

In rheumatoid arthritis, there is inflammation of the synovial lining of several joints and the TMJs are involved in around half of those affected. The condition is an autoimmune disorder with a wide range of manifestations. Whilst this type of arthritis has some genetic basis, at least half of the risk is attributed to environmental factors, particularly smoking and viral infection. The initial phase of the disease is due to non-specific inflammation affecting the synovial membrane. There is then an amplification phase due to T-cell activation. This is followed by a chronic inflammatory phase with tissue injury due to release of the cytokines IL-1, IL-6, and TNF-alpha. Microscopically, proliferation of the synovial lining, often in a villous pattern, leads to the formation of granulation tissue termed pannus. Destruction of bone and cartilage results from the release of cytokines from the pannus. The TMJs become swollen, tender, and painful, with stiffness and limitation of opening. Destruction of the mandibular condyle may result in anterior open bite. Systemic disease is present and primary treatment is by 'disease modifying anti-rheumatic drugs' (DMARDs), which are wide-ranging in activity. Non-steroidal anti-inflammatory drugs may also be used.

Juvenile chronic (rheumatoid) arthritis shows early onset (typically around 5 years old) and there is usually severe systemic involvement. Mandibular growth may be severely reduced leading to anterior open bite and a 'bird face' appearance, due to marked mandibular retrusion. Periods of remission typically occur and there may be some regeneration of the joint tissue in the quiescent phase.

Septic arthritis

Infection of the TMJ by bacteria such as *Staphylococcus aureus* usually arises by haematogenous spread from a distant focus of infection. The affected joint is red, swollen, and painful. On aspiration, the joint fluid may be thick and yellow due to the high neutrophil content. Crystal arthropathy should be excluded. Management is usually by antibiotic therapy and elimination of the distant focus of infection.

Ankylosis

Fusion across the TMJ (ankylosis) can severely limit jaw opening and may result from longstanding severe arthritic diseases, trauma, or even mastoid infection. Ankylosis can be treated by prosthetic joint replacement. In children a costo-chondral rib graft may be used to increase growth potential.

trauma. Loss of articular cartilage is characteristic, leading to bone erosion. New osteocartilaginous proliferations (osteophytes) form at the periphery of the condyle (Fig. 7.39). Pain, crepitus, tenderness, and limitation of opening may be present. Imaging shows articular erosion, most commonly affecting the mandibular condyle, but imaging is not necessary to make the diagnosis. Marginal bony proliferations are present and these can break away to form loose bodies in the joint space. If pain is absent, the inflammatory component of the osteoarthritis is quiescent,

---

Key points Temporomandibular joint

- TMJs are unusual in having an interarticular disc
- TMDs are the most common cause of oro-facial pain after odontogenic pain
- Maxillary cancers in the pterygoid space can mimic TMDs
- Uncommon TMJ diseases may be overlooked clinically

Uncommon disorders of the TMJ

Ganglion cyst

Weakness of the TMJ capsule can lead to distension of the joint wall leading to a pre-auricular cystic swelling. The cyst content resembles synovial fluid. Microscopically, ganglion cyst is composed of bland fibrous tissue, and multiple cystic chambers containing mucoid material are present. Synovial fluid is thought to be able to pass from the joint space into the cyst, but reverse flow is not possible. Ganglion cyst is very common in the wrist but is rare in the TMJ. Surgical removal is normally required.

Crystal arthopathy

Gout is a common metabolic disorder that leads to elevated serum uric acid levels with deposition of urate crystals in joints and other tissues. Needle-like crystals may be present in fluid aspirated from the joint and there is usually an acute inflammatory infiltrate. The condition is rare in the TMJ and usually widespread urate crystal deposits are present elsewhere. Deposition of calcium pyrophosphate dihydrate crystals in a joint is known as pseudogout. Inflammatory cells are also present in affected joint, which becomes red, swollen, and painful. Pseudogout can affect the TMJ, but the condition is very rare in that location.

Synovial chondromatosis

This disorder affects mainly large joints but can rarely occur in the TMJ. The affected TMJ shows restriction of movement and stiffness, but radiological imaging may appear normal. Cartilaginous or osteocartilaginous nodules form around the synovial lining and can be shown by MRI. Numerous nodules containing chondrocytes that may appear atypical, even though synovial chondromatosis is benign, may be present. No cure is known but surgical resection of part of the synovial lining may improve function and symptoms.

Pigmented villo-nodular synovitis

Pigmented villo-nodular synovitis (PVNS) is also known as giant cell tumour of tendon sheath and, although it more commonly affects large, weight-bearing joints, it has been described in the TMJ. There is destruction of the condyle and articular tissue, often with involvement of adjacent soft-tissue. Surgical excision is indicated. The diseased tissue shows a characteristic orange-brown colour and, microscopically, there are multinucleated osteoclast-like giant cells, foamy macrophages, fibrotic areas, and haemosiderin deposits.

Condylar hyperplasia

Condylar hyperplasia is an uncommon benign process that begins between the first and third decades. It is also a feature of acromegaly. The mandibular condyle enlarges unilaterally or bilaterally, and the overgrowth results in facial asymmetry and occlusal derangement (Fig. 7.40). The condyle may be grossly enlarged and continues to grow when skeletal maturity has been reached. Various patterns of condylar hyperplasia are recognized, the most common type is also known as hemi-mandibuar hypertrophy. Imaging with scintiscanning

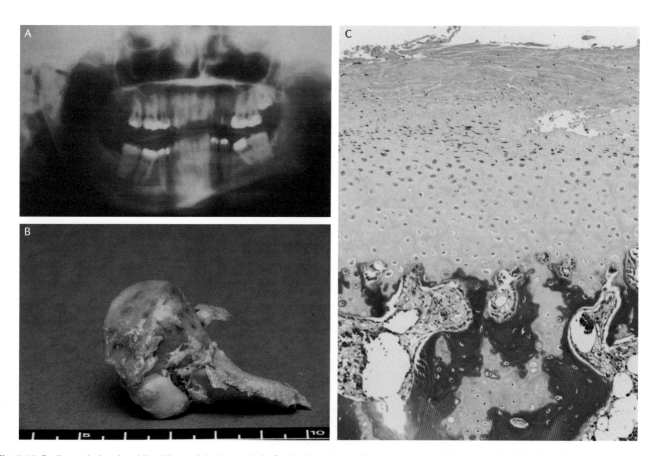

Fig. 7.40 Radiograph showing right-side condylar hyperplasia. Surgical specimen of an enlarged mandibular condyle. Histology shows increased thickness of the articular hyaline cartilage and endochondral ossification.

can be used to confirm ongoing growth activity, and the involved condyle may be excised, with reconstructive surgery used to correct the mandibular deformity.

Neoplasms

True neoplasms are very rare in the TMJ and around two-thirds of reported cases are malignant, comprising sarcomas and metastatic carcinomas. This may reflect publication bias and the true prevalence of neoplasia in the TMJ being unknown. All of the benign or malignant neoplasms described earlier in the chapter have been reported to occur in the TMJ. In addition, osteochondromas (osteocartilaginous exostosis) are benign tumours with a cartilage cap that may interfere with function and have been described in the TMJ as solitary lesions or as part of multiple osteochondromas (OMIM 133700). Treatment is by excision of the bony exostosis.

8

Skin diseases affecting the oro-facial region

Chapter contents

Introduction

Examination of the face and hands can identify significant skin diseases and also provide clues to the presence of underlying systemic disease. Many patients ignore even malignant skin tumours because they are often painless, subtle in appearance, and may be slow-growing. Dental healthcare professionals should be aware of how to recognize malignant skin tumours. If suspicious, but unsure of the nature of the lesion, the patient should be referred to their general medical practitioner for further evaluation. If malignancy is obvious, then an urgent referral to an appropriate specialist (dermatologist, plastic surgeon, or oral and maxillofacial surgeon) should be made using the '2-week wait' (2WW) pathway (Chapter 1). Benign lesions and inflammatory diseases are more common and are important considerations in the differential diagnosis of head and neck skin abnormalities.

Skin infections

It is important that the dental healthcare professional should be able to recognize common skin infections involving the oro-facial region. Some infections, such as erysipelas, can mimic cellulitis associated with a dental infection. When infection is diagnosed, it is vital to consider the underlying or predisposing factors, as these may be not only important diagnoses, but also may require treatment to achieve an effective clinical outcome. The adage 'infection is the disease of the diseased' is a useful reminder when dealing with patients presenting with infection.

Bacterial infections

Erysipelas

Direct inoculation of *Streptococcus* into skin through minor trauma is the most common initiating factor for erysipelas, which occurs in isolated cases. Infection involves the upper dermis and, characteristically, spreads to involve the dermal lymphatic vessels. Clinically, the disease starts as a red patch that extends to become a fiery red, tense, and indurated plaque. Erysipelas can be distinguished from cellulitis by its advancing, sharply defined borders and skin streaking due to lymphatic involvement. The infection is most common in children and the elderly, and whilst classically a disease affecting the face, in recent years it has more frequently involved the leg skin of elderly patients. Although a clinical diagnosis can be made without laboratory testing, and treatment is antibiotic therapy, when the diagnosis is suspected in dental practice, referral to a medical practitioner is recommended.

Impetigo

Impetigo is a bacterial infection most often seen in children but also encountered in adults, particularly if predisposing factors, such as immunosuppression, are present. Classically, the disorder is associated with *Staphylococcus aureus*, but infection often commences with group A beta haemolytic *Streptococci* (*Streptococcus pyogenes*) that become replaced by *S. aureus* as the infection progresses. Impetigo occurs in bullous and non-bullous forms and is highly contagious. Clinically, impetigo commences as a single erythematous patch that rapidly evolves into a vesicle that ruptures and dries to produce a characteristic golden crust (Fig. 8.1). Lesions commonly occur on the vermillion lip borders, and nasal and circumoral skin. Reactive cervical lymphadenitis is common. Diagnosis is based on the clinical features and treatment normally involves application of topical agents combined with systemic antibiotics. The antibiotic must cover both *S. aureus* and *S. pyogenes*; impetigo is, fortunately, very rarely associated with methicillin resistant *S. aureus* (MRSA).

Angular cheilitis

Patients commonly present complaining of soreness and cracking of the skin at the angle of the mouth. Erythema is often present. This condition is referred to as angular cheilitis. Often a mixed infection is present: *S. aureus* and *Candida albicans* are often recovered from the lesion, though other organisms may be found.

A number of underlying systemic conditions are known to predispose to angular cheilitis. Nutritional deficiencies include iron, riboflavin (B_2), folate, and B_{12} deficiencies, giving rise to anaemia. Diseases that may be associated include diabetes mellitus, Crohn's disease and oro-facial granulomatosis, Sjögren's syndrome, HIV, and Down's syndrome. Dermatological conditions such as eczema and perioral dermatitis can also predispose to angular cheilitis.

Local factors may also predispose to angular cheilitis and the overgrowth of the infecting organisms can be related to the creation of a moist local environment in a skin crease. Loss of vertical dimension due to extreme attrition or worn dentures leads to overclosure and is a common predisposing factor that can be corrected by dental treatment. Habitual licking of the angle of the mouth and conditions where drooling of saliva occurs, such as hypersalivation or neurological disorders, also may cause a moist local environment. Poor denture hygiene is a

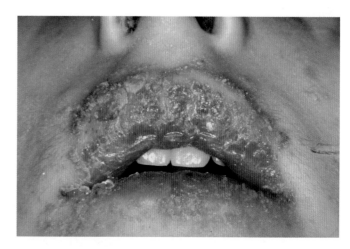

Fig. 8.1 Impetigo showing 'golden crusts' and lip swelling.

common cause where *Candida* infection under the upper denture acts as a reservoir for continuous re-infection.

Treatment usually involves topical application of anti-fungal and anti-bacterial cream, often with hydrocortisone to reduce inflammation. Elimination of any local or systemic predisposing factors is essential. To maintain health, good denture hygiene is vital, including leaving the dentures out at night; application of petroleum jelly to the angle of the mouth may be useful if saliva tracks on to the skin.

Actinomycosis

Cervicofacial actinomycosis is a chronic condition characterized by abscess formation, draining sinus tracts, fistulae, and tissue fibrosis (Fig. 8.2). The condition is caused by branching Gram-positive bacteria belonging to the genus *Actinomyces* ('ray fungus'), though mixed infection is usually present. Chronic actinomycosis can occur in other

locations but over half of cases occur in the cervicofacial region. The condition may follow dental abscess, periodontal suppuration, or osteonecrosis (Chapter 7), and initially presents as swelling in the submandibular triangle. Multiple sinus tracts may then form and these typically discharge pus containing small yellowish granules, known as sulphur granules. The overlying skin is typically erythematous and has a 'lumpy' texture. Biopsy or microbiological testing can be used to confirm the diagnosis of actinomycosis. Treatment is by elimination of any underlying cause of sepsis and prolonged antibiotic therapy.

> **Key points** **Bacterial infections on the face**
> - Present as red and often excoriated patches
> - Cervical lymphadenitis often present
> - Impetigo common in children and young adults
> - Angular cheilitis may be caused by *Staphylococcus* or *Candida*
> - Underlying systemic disease should be considered

Viral infections

Squamous cell papilloma (common wart)

Warts mainly occur in children on the oro-facial skin, possibly related to finger sucking, which can spread the virus from lesions on the digits to the lips, particularly the angle of the mouth. Intra-oral tissues may be affected in the same way (Chapter 2). Warts are caused by human papillomavirus and are spread by direct contact with infected persons or contaminated surfaces. The lesions vary in size between 1 and 10 mm and show a verrucous, papillary, or cauliflower-like architecture. Often, multiple lesions are present. Spontaneous resolution may occur but treatments, including cryotherapy, chemical and mechanical removal, and cautery, are available.

Molluscum contagiosum

Molluscum contagiosum presents with multiple, small, firm, raised papules that often develop on the facial skin. The lesions are not painful but are typically pruritic. Molluscum contagiosum most commonly affects children and young adults, although it can occur at any age. It is highly contagious and easily spread. The molluscum contagiosum virus can be spread through skin-to-skin contact with an infected person, or it can be transmitted by contact with contaminated objects, such as a flannel or towel. Lesions usually resolve within 12–18 months, though may persist in immunocompromised patients. Patients should be advised to avoid spreading the disease to others and also not to squeeze the lesions, as this may lead to scarring and infection at other sites touched.

Slapped cheek syndrome

Slapped cheek syndrome is common in children, usually affecting them between the ages of 3 and 15 years old. Most cases develop during the late winter months or early spring. A distinctive erythematous rash appears on the cheeks, though lesions may also develop at other skin sites. Slapped cheek syndrome is caused by parvovirus B19, which is

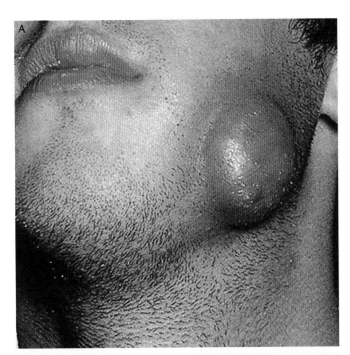
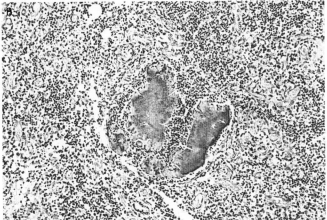

Fig. 8.2 Actinomycosis and a sample of pus containing a colony of actinomyces (sulphur granule).

an airborne virus that spreads by droplets. The condition is usually self-limiting and resolves in a few days, though it may rarely persist for 3–4 weeks. Management is by reassurance, maintaining fluid intake and possibly analgesics and antihistamines. More serious infection may develop in immunocompromised patients and in anaemia (such as sickle cell anaemia). Pregnant women without immunity are at increased risk of miscarriage and should avoid contact with infected individuals.

Measles

Prior to immunization with the MMR (measles, mumps, and rubella) vaccine, measles was a relatively common childhood infection. Although rarely presenting to the dentist nowadays, it is important to be able to recognize measles, as it is a highly unpleasant viral illness that can lead to significant morbidity. The measles virus spreads very easily by droplets or contact with a contaminated surface. The initial symptoms of measles include flu-like symptoms, red eyes and sensitivity to light, fever, and greyish white vesicles (Koplik spots) in the mouth and throat (Chapter 2). After a few days, a red-brown vesicular rash will appear on the facial skin, usually starting behind the ears, then spreading around the head and neck. If the diagnosis is suspected, affected children should be kept away from school and parents should seek advice about management. Measles can be a serious disorder in adults and immunocompromised patients, and medical advice should be sought.

Chickenpox

Infection with varicella zoster virus is very common and most of the population acquire the infection in childhood, though many cases are not recognized clinically. A rash of red itchy spots that quickly turn into blisters appears. The blisters rupture and crust over. Lesions are most likely to appear on the face, ears, and scalp, but often also involve the axilla, chest, abdomen, arms, and legs. Chickenpox is self-limiting and contact with others should be avoided to limit spread. Pregnant women, new-born babies and immunocompromised people are at a particular risk. Varicella zoster virus can lie dormant in the ganglia and may be reactivated, resulting in shingles in later life.

Shingles

Activation of varicella zoster virus in a ganglion can lead to infection of a nerve. The virus becomes reactivated following childhood chickenpox in older, stressed, or immunocompromised patients. Most often, shingles affects a spinal nerve and lesions encircle one-half of the trunk. However, shingles can be reactivated in the trigeminal ganglion. There are three distinct phases. In the pre-eruptive phase, the patient will complain of pain, burning, or itching in the affected dermatome. This can lead to an erroneous diagnosis of dental pain if the maxillary or mandibular dermatomes are affected, as no skin lesions are present. After a few days the eruptive phase begins and a vesicular crusted rash appears over the

dermatome. This does not cross the mid-line and neuritic pain is typically present. The lesions crust over and resolve over a few weeks. The disease may then enter a third phase known as post-herpetic neuralgia, where pain persists long after the cutaneous lesions have resolved. If the ophthalmic division of the trigeminal nerve is affected, then the eye may be affected and referral to a specialist is advised.

Ramsay Hunt syndrome is caused by activation of varicella zoster virus in the geniculate ganglion of the facial nerve. Vesicular eruptions may appear on the pinna, in the auditory canal, on the tympanic membrane, or, occasionally, on the hard palate. There may be unilateral loss of taste of the anterior two-thirds of the tongue. Facial palsy and pain may occur and there may, rarely, be central nervous system involvement.

Anti-viral therapy may be prescribed for both shingles and Ramsay Hunt syndrome. Referral to a medical practitioner is advised when these conditions are suspected.

Herpes simplex infection

Infection by Herpes simplex virus, most often type 1, can lead to herpetic gingivo-stomatitis. The lips and circumoral skin are frequently involved by the vesicular rash (Chapter 2).

Key points Viral infections on the face

- Most are self-limiting childhood infections, but may occur in adults
- Likely to present to doctor rather than dentist
- Measles less common due to MMR vaccine
- Underlying systemic disease should be considered

Fungal infections

Angular cheilitis

Angular cheilitis is a common disorder that presents in dental practice and is usually a mixed infection of *Candida albicans* and bacteria, most often *Streptococcus* and *Staphylococcus*. The condition is described in the section on bacterial infections.

Dermatophyte infections

Fungal infections caused by *Tinea* (ringworm) are very common on the scalp and may also be spread to the face as circular erythematous patches. The infection may be acquired from infected persons or animals, such as pets and cattle. The condition is self-limiting and is readily treated by topical agents and appropriate hygiene measures.

Common benign skin lesions

Acne

Acne vulgaris is characterized by areas of scaly red skin, comedones, papules, pustules, and nodules, sometimes with scarring. Acne affects

the face in areas where the follicles are dense. The condition occurs most commonly during adolescence and may continue into adult life. In adolescence, an increased level of testosterone in both sexes is thought to be an important predisposing factor. It is important to know that the main concern is psychological, as there may be reduced self-esteem, or even depression and suicidal thoughts. In such cases, referral to a medical practitioner is advised.

Rosacea

Rosacea is a very common chronic facial skin condition seen in patients over 30 years old, which is associated with facial flushing. As rosacea progresses, patients may experience burning and stinging sensations, permanent redness, telangiectasia, papules, and pustules. In severe cases, the facial skin can thicken and enlarge, usually on and around the nose. The cause is unknown and, although no cure is known, patients can benefit from medical advice to prevent progression and control symptoms.

Seborrhoeic keratosis

Seborrhoeic keratosis or seborrhoeic wart is a common lesion that presents mainly on the head, neck, and trunk. Lesions may be multiple or solitary, and occasionally patients have numerous lesions. Most lesions are symptomless or mildly itchy and patients may experience parts of the lesions tearing away. Seborrhoeic keratosis often has a verrucous surface. Characteristically, it has a 'stuck on' appearance over normal skin and is often described as 'greasy'. Pigmentation is common and can vary from dark brown to pale yellow. On close inspection, comedo-like openings (blackheads) may be present. Lesions typically range between 10 and 30 mm and some may be larger. Seborrhoeic keratosis presents most frequently in patients aged over 40 years old and is common in elderly patients. Lesions can be treated effectively by curettage, followed by pathological examination to confirm the diagnosis.

Actinic keratosis

Actinic keratosis is a very common disorder and it has been estimated that around one-quarter of the population over 60 years old in the UK have lesions. Actinic keratosis is characteristically scaly due to hyperkeratosis. The disorder is induced by sun exposure and artificial UV radiation. Individuals with fair skin, blue eyes, and blond hair are at higher risk than others. Men are affected more frequently than women. Lesion distribution is related to sun exposure and the scaly patches are most often seen on the face, head, neck, forearms, and hands (Fig. 8.3). The background skin often shows spidery vessels (telangiectasia), yellow-grey areas (elastosis and collagenosis), and redness. Lesions of actinic keratosis are usually less than 10 mm and are covered by a rough, white scale. Other variants include erythematous, pigmented, lichenoid (smooth), hypertrophic lesions, or keratin horns. Actinic keratosis shows cytological atypia in the epidermis. Severe dysplasia is seen in the Bowenoid-type. Actinic keratosis may transform to squamous cell carcinoma. Where there is clinical suspicion of carcinoma, urgent referral must be made. Actinic keratosis is often treated in primary medical care by cyrotherapy or with a cytotoxic topical agent. Actinic keratosis affecting the vermillion border of the lip is referred to as actinic cheilitis (Fig. 8.3). Squamous cell carcinoma can be subtle at that location and referral to a specialist is indicated for suspicious lesions.

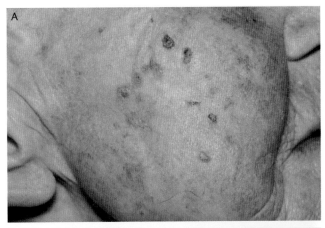

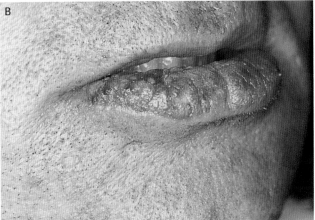

Fig. 8.3 Actinic keratosis on the skin of the cheek and actinic cheilitis on the lower lip.

Ephelis

The ephelis or freckle is a common lesion in childhood and is most prominent in red-haired or fair-skinned individuals. Clinically, freckles are macular (flat) pale brown areas, often in crops, and usually pose no diagnostic problem. Melanin pigment production is stimulated by UV light. Freckles, therefore, become most prominent during summer and tend to fade in the winter months. This helps to distinguish them from lentigos, which remain pigmented. Freckles arising on the vermillion border of the lips are often termed oral melanotic macules.

In contrast to freckles, simple lentigines tend to be more heavily pigmented, may occur in very large numbers, and do not fade during the winter months. Typically, they are sharply demarcated melanotic macules ranging between 3 and 5 mm, with a uniform pigment distribution. They tend to arise in childhood and may increase in number in young adults, sometimes 'erupting' dramatically. They are not restricted to sun-exposed areas. Solar lentigo is common on the face and may be difficult to distinguish from melanocytic naevus or lentigo maligna, clinically. Specialist referral is then indicated. Multiple circumoral melanotic macules are seen in Peutz–Jeghers syndrome (OMIM 175200) (Fig. 8.4), where macules may also be present in oral mucosa, toes, and fingers, along with intestinal polyposis. Pigmented labial and intra-oral macules with streaky nail pigmentation is seen in Laugier–Hunziker syndrome.

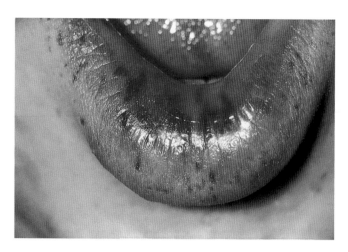

Fig. 8.4 Melanin pigmentation of the lip in Peutz–Jegher syndrome.

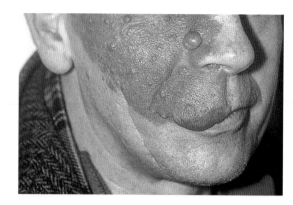

Fig. 8.5 Sturge–Weber syndrome.

No systemic manifestations are associated, and many authors now refer to this disorder simply as Laugier–Hunziker pigmentation. Most simple lentigines remain static or regress in adult life.

Benign melanocytic naevus

Unlike freckles and simple lentigines, where pigmentation is largely due to accumulation of melanin in dermal macrophages ('melanin drop out'), the benign melanocytic naevus is formed by aggregations of melanocytes. Benign melanocytic naevi are also known as moles. Histologically, there are many variants, and the most common microscopically recognized types are junctional, intra-dermal, and compound. Clinically, two variants are recognized. The acquired melanocytic naevus arises in patients generally up to the age of 30 years old and is typically flat or slightly raised, symmetrical, and most often brown, although the colour can vary from pink to black. The intra-dermal naevus is typically firmer in texture and tends to protrude from the surface, resulting in a dome-shaped or papillomatous lesion. Intra-dermal naevi are typically pigmented and lighten with age. Removal of benign melanocytic naevi causing a clinical or cosmetic problem can be undertaken by shave biopsy, but, as with all pigmented lesions, the tissue should be submitted for pathological examination. If there is any clinical suspicion of malignant melanoma, then an urgent referral should be made using the 2WW pathway (Chapter 1).

Superficial vascular malformations

Superficial arterio-venous malformations are caused by the abnormal development of blood vessels. On facial skin, they may be confused, clinically, with other pigmented lesions, but typically blanch under pressure as blood is displaced. In Sturge–Weber syndrome, one or more trigeminal dermatomes are involved, producing an extensive vascular lesion (Fig. 8.5). There may be intra-osseous extension in the underlying jaw bone, which is important, as tooth extraction may be followed by torrential bleeding (Chapter 2).

Inflammatory disorders of the facial skin

A large number of inflammatory disorders may occur on the facial skin. Many are self-limiting or transitory, whilst others, such as lupus

erythematosis, are clinically important lesions with possible systemic associations. Some of the more common inflammatory lesions are listed in Box 8.1. Inflammation causing lip swelling is common and the differential diagnosis is listed in Table 8.1.

Box 8.1 Inflammatory skin diseases presenting on the face

Infections

Bacterial

- Erysipelas
- Impetigo
- Actinomycosis

Viral

- Verruca vulgaris (common wart)
- Molluscum contagiosum
- Slapped cheek syndrome
- Measles
- Chickenpox/shingles
- Herpes labialis (cold sore)

Fungal

- Angular cheilitis

Inflammatory diseases

- Acne
- Rosacea
- Psoriasis
- Lichen planus
- Discoid/systemic lupus erythematosus
- Bullous pemphigoid
- Pemphigus vulgaris
- Sarcoidosis

Table 8.1 Differential diagnosis of lip swelling

Hereditary/developmental	Hereditary angioedema
	Superficial vascular malformations
	Lymphangiomatous malformations
Infection	Acute alveolar abscess
	Impetigo
	Erysipelas
	Herpes labialis
Inflammatory	Allergic angioedema
	Insect sting/bite
	Erythema multiforme
	Oro-facial granulomatosis
	Crohn's disease
	Sarcoidosis
Trauma	Haematoma
	Mucocoele
Neoplastic	Minor salivary gland tumour
	Other benign and malignant neoplasms
Iatrogenic	Cosmetic fillers
	Surgical emphysema

Common skin cancers

Epidermal tumours

Basal cell carcinoma

This is the most common cancer in humans and frequently occurs in the mid-face and adjacent sun-exposed skin, including the ears and scalp. Risk factors include a fair complexion, blue eyes, and fair hair. However, basal cell carcinoma can develop on sites of minimal sun exposure and also in areas of previous traumatic injury. Most basal cell carcinomas arise in patients over 40 years of age, but, increasingly, basal cell carcinoma is encountered in younger patients. Clinically, basal cell carcinoma is slow-growing, typically enlarging by only 2–3 mm a year. Characteristically, patients report the lesion as 'never healing' and they may experience spontaneous bleeding or production of a scab or crust that may be shed, only to subsequently re-appear (Fig. 8.6A).

Basal cell carcinoma is locally invasive and metastatic spread is very rare, occurring in less than 0.1% of cases. Several clinical and histological subtypes are recognized (Table 8.2). Microscopically, basal cell carcinomas are composed of sheets and islands of squamous cells resembling those in the basal layer of the epidermis, referred to as 'basaloid' cells (Fig. 8.6B). The cells are dark-staining and are supported by fibrous stroma. Often, the islands of tumour cells retract from the stroma in histological sections and this can be a useful diagnostic feature. The basaloid cells often form a peripheral palisade and there may be squamous differentiation with formation of keratin whorls in the more central areas. Interestingly, basal cell carcinoma has a high mitotic rate

but this is partly counterbalanced by a high apoptotic rate, resulting in overall slow growth. Nodular basal cell carcinoma is the most common histological subtype, accounting for around 65%. The other subtypes are more prone to recurrence than the nodular-type and those with a malignant squamous component behave as squamous cell carcinoma.

Basal cell carcinomas are normally readily treated by surgical removal with a margin of surrounding tissue. Radiotherapy and local ablative methods can also be used and all methods achieve high cure rates. If left untreated, basal cell carcinomas can progress to invade and destroy deeper soft-tissues and bone, resulting in a destructive lesion clinically termed 'rodent ulcer'. When basal cell carcinoma involves orbital or other important structures, specialized surgical techniques, such as Moh's surgery, where marginal tissue is examined by frozen section during the operation, can be used to ensure clearance whilst preserving normal tissue. Recognition of basal cell carcinoma and prompt referral is a useful service to the patient, and dental healthcare professionals can expect to encounter several cases during their careers. Basal cell carcinomas can be multiple and also are a feature of basal cell naevus syndrome (OMIM 109400) (Chapter 7).

Squamous cell carcinoma

Cutaneous squamous cell carcinoma of the head and neck most frequently involves the lower lip, external ear, periauricular region, scalp, and forehead (Figs 8.7 and 8.8A). Microscopically, squamous cell carcinoma is made up of sheets of squamous cells (keratinocytes) that show

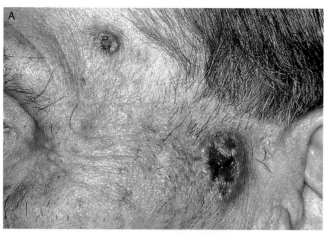

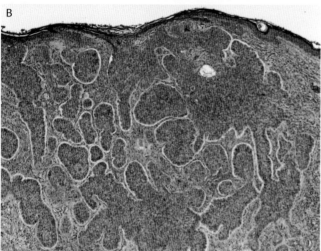

Fig. 8.6 'Rodent ulcers' on the temple and pre-auricular skin. Histology shows islands of malignant basaloid cells invading the dermis, consistent with basal cell carcinoma.

Table 8.2 Basal cell carcinoma variants

BCC variant	Clinical features
Solid (nodular)	Non-healing and slowly enlarging, bleeds or scabs; shiny or translucent nodule, rolled edge, becomes more irregular with time
Superficial	Slowly expanding pink/red patch, fine raised 'whipcord' edge, surface becomes crusted with time; more common on the abdomen
Mixed types	Poorly defined apparently multifocal lesions with mixed superficial and nodular features
Morphoeic (infiltrative)	Occur mostly on the face, especially central area; slowly enlarging yellow-white waxy patches; ill-defined edges, firm texture, fine surface vessels
Basi-squamous (metatypical)	Features of both basal cell carcinoma and squamous cell carcinoma
Other types	Rarely origin in sebaceous naevus and linked to BCNS syndrome

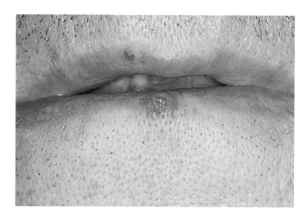

Fig. 8.7 Squamous cell carcinoma on the lower lip at the muco-cutaneous border, mimicking a cold sore.

nuclear and cellular pleomorphism, hyperchromatism, and frequent mitosis. Well-differentiated squamous carcinomas (Fig. 8.8B) form abundant keratin and often have a cohesive invasive front. Poor outcome due to local recurrence and/or metastatic spread to lymph nodes

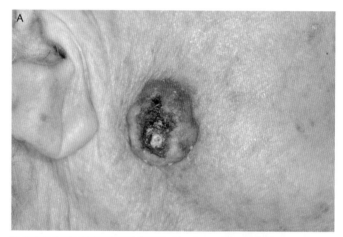

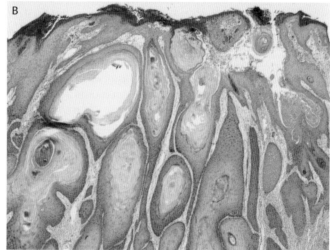

Fig. 8.8 A large, nodular, and ulcerated lesion on the cheek. Histology shows a well-differentiated squamous cell carcinoma expanding and invading the dermis.

is associated with squamous cell carcinomas that are poorly differentiated, have a non-cohesive invasive front, are large in size and thickness, have perineural invasion, or show lympho-vascular spread. Frequently, the development of squamous carcinoma is preceded by actinic keratosis, which is a precancerous lesion that appears as a small, scaly plaque or papule, sometimes with an erythematous base. Actinic keratosis is very common and is often multiple (Fig. 8.3A).

Squamous cell carcinoma of the vermillion border of the lip is easily overlooked in the early stages and is often asymptomatic (Fig. 8.7). It frequently arises in actinic keratosis, which is referred to as actinic cheilitis on the lip. The prognosis of squamous carcinoma of the lip is generally better than that of its intra-oral counterpart. Surgical treatment is normally performed but radiotherapy can also be used. Prompt recognition and rapid referral of suspicious lip lesions can reduce morbidity.

Melanocytic tumours

Lentigo maligna

Lentigo maligna is an important lesion to recognize. It occurs most frequently in sun-exposed skin, is most commonly found on the face, and can be difficult to distinguish from other pigmented lentigines. Seen most often in late middle-aged and elderly patients, lentigo maligna is typically flat, dark brown or black, and suspicion is raised by its irregular shape and steady progressive enlargement. A special technique known as dermatoscopy can be useful to aid identification in the dermatology clinic. Histological examination shows short runs and nests of atypical melanocytes at the epidermal–dermal interface. Lentigo maligna is regarded as a precancerous lesion. If left untreated, lentigo maligna will grow steadily over years and may transform into malignant melanoma. Clinically, a raised nodule develops and the lesion is then referred to as 'lentigo maligna melanoma'.

Malignant melanoma

Malignant melanoma is less common than carcinoma and only around one-fifth of all cutaneous melanomas occur in the head and neck. A number of clinically distinct variants are well recognized (Table 8.3). Superficial spreading melanoma accounts for up to half of all head and neck melanomas. The lesions have a slow-growing initial phase (radial growth phase) for the first few months. Such lesions are regarded as melanoma *in situ*, but with continued growth, an invasive component develops. Superficial spreading malignant melanoma is typically flat, dark brown or variegated, and some lesions develop a red halo. The outline may become irregular with time, and dermal invasion (vertical growth phase) is often signified by a raised nodular appearance (Fig. 8.9A). Invasive malignant melanoma has a high metastatic potential and a number of histological factors, including thickness (Breslow thickness), depth, mitotic rate, and ulceration, are predictive of prognosis. Nodular melanoma is an aggressive disease that accounts for around one-quarter of melanomas and is most common in males in the fifth and sixth decades. They may occur at any site but are most common in sun-exposed skin. As the name suggests, nodular malignant melanoma presents as a firm, deeply pigmented, raised lesion showing invasive (vertical) growth from the outset. Lentigo maligna melanoma is typically a flat form of melanoma and makes up around one-fifth of head and neck melanomas. The precursor lesion is known as lentigo maligna. Some malignant melanomas are non-pigmented and are referred to as amelanotic melanomas. Desmoplastic melanoma is a rare subtype

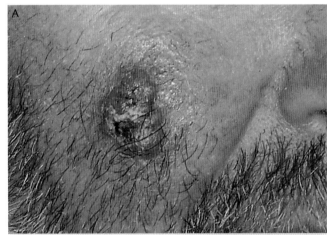
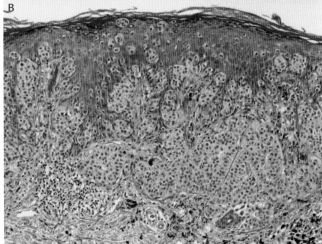

Fig. 8.9 An ulcerated nodular malignant melanoma on the cheek. Histology shows nests of malignant melanocytes in the dermis along with melanin deposits.

Table 8.3 Malignant melanoma types in head and neck

Type of melanoma	Features
Superficial spreading melanoma	Flat, dark brown, red halo, irregular outline
Nodular melanoma	Firm, intensely pigmented, raised, often multinodular, irregular margin
Lentigo maligna melanoma	Flat, variably pigmented, irregular margin
Amelanotic melanoma	Non-pigmented, flat or raised, irregular margin
Desmoplastic melanoma	Innocuous indurated discoid papule, plaque or nodule, non-pigmented

Table 8.4 ABCDE scheme for recognition of malignant melanoma

Asymmetry	Non-matching halves across the diameter
Border	Edges are ragged, indented, or indistinct
Colour	Non-uniform pigmentation: tan, brown, black, white, red, blue
Diameter	Greater than 6 mm is typical (may be smaller)
Evolving	Changes in the lesion over time

Reproduced from *CA: Cancer Journal for Clinicians*, 35, 3 Friedman RJ, Rigel DS, Kopf AW, Early detection of malignant melanoma: The role of physician examination and self-examination of the skin, pp. 130–151. Copyright © 1985 American Cancer Society, published by John Wiley and Sons

of melanoma with a poor prognosis that is found mostly on the sun-exposed skin of the head and neck.

Clinically, a new or changing 'mole' is the most common presentation of malignant melanoma, but bleeding, itching, and ulceration may also be presenting features. The 'ABCDE scheme' is a useful guide to diagnosis (Table 8.4); however, examination of any pigmented lesion that simply 'looks different' from other moles is also advocated. Any change in a pre-existing melanocytic naevus (mole) warrants investigation. Surgery is the treatment of choice for malignant melanoma and lesion thickness is one of the critical factors that determines outcome. Prompt recognition and referral can be lifesaving, as thicker tumours have very poor outcomes. In the UK, vemurafenib, an oral tyrosine kinase inhibitor, has been approved by NICE (National Institute for Health and Care Excellence) as a possible treatment for unresectable or metastatic melanoma harbouring a BRAF V600E mutation.

Other malignant tumours

A variety of other malignant tumours may arise in the skin of the hands, head, and neck, including carcinomas of sweat glands, Merkel cell carcinoma, cutaneous lymphoma, angiosarcoma, dermatofibrosarcoma, and other less common lesions. Referral is usually made on the basis of a 'clinically malignant tumour' and diagnosis relies on histopathological examination of a representative biopsy. Critical clinical features are steady progressive or rapid growth of a new lesion, change in a pre-existing lesion, ulceration, bleeding, or change in pigmentation.

Referring for a suspected skin cancer

National Institute for Health and Care Excellence (NICE) recently published guidelines on the recognition and referral of suspected cancer, including skin cancers (Box 8.2). It is essential to adopt a reassuring and professional manner when referring a patient with a suspected skin cancer, most likely noticed as an incidental finding in the dental clinic. Severe psychological trauma may result from unguarded comments. A sympathetic approach is important. In the first instance, where the diagnosis is unclear, a referral to the patient's general medical practitioner is appropriate. If the lesion is obviously malignant, then offering to arrange a referral to a medical expert (dermatologist, plastic surgeon, or oral and

Box 8.2 Suspected cancer: recognition and referral. Skin cancers

Malignant melanoma of the skin

Refer people using a suspected cancer pathway referral (for an appointment within 2 weeks) for melanoma if they have a suspicious pigmented lesion with a weighted 7-point checklist score of 3 or more.

Weighted 7-point checklist

Major features of the lesion (scoring 2 points each):

- Change in size
- Irregular shape
- Irregular colour

Minor features of the lesion (scoring 1 point each):

- Largest diameter 7 mm or more
- Inflammation
- Oozing
- Change in sensation

Squamous cell carcinoma

Consider a suspected cancer pathway referral (for an appointment within 2 weeks) for people with a skin lesion that raises the suspicion of squamous cell carcinoma.

Basal cell carcinoma

Consider a routine referral for people if they have a skin lesion that raises the suspicion of a basal cell carcinoma.

Only consider a suspected cancer pathway referral (for an appointment within 2 weeks) for people with a skin lesion that raises the suspicion of a basal cell carcinoma if there is a particular concern that a delay may have a significant impact, because of such factors as lesion site or size.

Reproduced from *Suspected cancer: recognition and referral*, page 22/23 © NICE 2015. All rights reserved. Last updated July 2017

maxillofacial surgeon) to have a lesion checked, but without being alarmist, may be appropriate. It is a matter of individual professional judgement to choose the right form of words in any particular clinical circumstance.

Key points Skin cancer

- Skin cancer commonly affects the head and neck region
- Basal cell carcinomas are very common, but treatment is usually effective
- Squamous cell carcinoma may develop from actinic keratosis
- Squamous cell carcinoma may metastasize to cervical lymph nodes and intra-parotid lymph nodes
- Malignant melanoma is less common but life-threatening—early diagnosis and treatment is essential

9
Neck lumps

Chapter contents

Introduction

Whilst dental healthcare professionals naturally focus on assessment of the teeth and the supporting tissues, they also have an important role in assessing the whole oro-facial complex and the neck. Assessment of the neck is particularly important, not least, because it contains the regional lymph nodes that are involved in immune surveillance of the head and neck region. The neck also contains the major salivary glands: the submandibular gland and the tail of the parotid gland. Mid-line structures include the hyoid bone, larynx, and trachea, along with the thyroid gland and parathyroid glands. The assessment of these anatomical structures should form part of the routine clinical examination. The discovery of an abnormality in the neck, which may not have been noticed by the patient, may expedite the diagnosis of significant disease and facilitate a timely intervention.

Systematic examination of the neck

A through understanding of the anatomy of the neck is essential and informs the clinical examination. It is also important to understand the concept of the anatomical levels that map out the lymph node groups of the neck (Chapter 1; Fig. 1.2). Accurate assessment of the neck is usually best achieved by a combination of visual inspection and palpation, with the patient in a slightly reclined position, the clinician standing behind the patient. Any lumps, e.g. enlarged lymph nodes, are described by anatomical site, size, consistency (cystic, soft, rubbery, hard), whether the lump is mobile or fixed to the underlying tissue, and if palpation elicits pain or discomfort. The combination of these parameters will help to formulate the differential diagnosis; for example, an isolated hard lump that is fixed to underlying structures is likely to represent metastatic cancer, whereas, bilateral soft lumps that are mobile and painful to palpation are likely to represent lymphadenitis as a consequence of systemic infection.

> **Key points Lymphadenopathy**
> - Always examine the neck by visual inspection and palpation
> - The differential diagnosis includes infective and malignant diseases
> - Infective causes are the most common
> - Transient lymphadenopathy is common in children
> - Detailed history may reveal likely cause
> - Persistent cervical lymphadenopathy (>2 weeks) requires further investigation
> - Red flag signs and symptoms should prompt an urgent referral (Box 9.1)

Ancillary tests for neck lumps

Ultrasound examination can be used to ascertain important information about a neck lump such as the site (precise anatomical location, superficial or deep), size, consistency (solid or cystic), and multi-focality (Fig. 9.1). Doppler settings can help to establish the vascularity of a lesion and its proximity to major vessels. Ultrasound can be used during fine-needle aspiration biopsy (FNAB) to ensure accurate sampling of a lesion; for example, aspiration of cyst content is usually inadequate for cytological diagnosis, whereas sampling of the cyst wall may be more informative. FNAB material can be used to prepare direct smears on glass slides or can be placed in a proprietary liquid-based fixative for cytological examination (Fig. 9.2A). If an infective cause is suspected, and pus or serous fluid is obtained, then the sample should be sent to the microbiology laboratory for culture and sensitivity testing. Tissue diagnosis can be approached using either a core biopsy or open biopsy of the neck lump. Core biopsy is usually sufficient for histopathological diagnosis and has the advantage of being less invasive than an open biopsy (Fig. 9.2B). Second-line imaging techniques like CT, MRI, and PET–CT are reserved for cases where there is diagnostic uncertainty

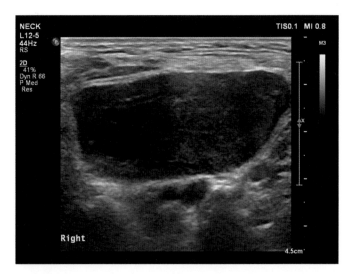

Fig. 9.1 Ultrasound scan showing an enlarged lymph node in a patient with metastatic oro-pharyngeal squamous cell carcinoma.

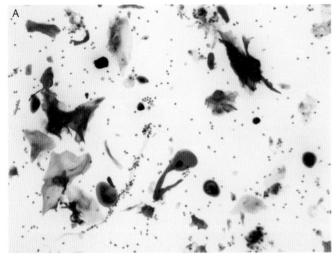

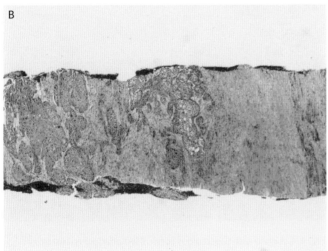

Fig. 9.2 Cytology of squamous cell carcinoma showing large, abnormal, pink and blue keratinocytes, and tiny neutrophils in the background (PAP stain) (A). A core biopsy of a lymph node showing islands of metastatic squamous cell carcinoma (B).

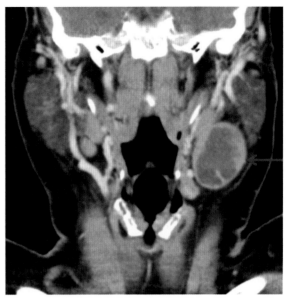

Fig. 9.3 CT scan showing an enlarged, cystic lymph node in a patient with metastatic oro-pharyngeal squamous cell carcinoma.

or a high index of suspicion for malignancy (Fig. 9.3). In the latter case, upper aerodigestive tract endoscopic examination under general anaesthetic with surveying biopsies may be required. Haematological tests (e.g. FBC) may be useful to establish general health, likelihood of infection (leucocytosis), immunocompromised state (leucopenia), and leukaemia.

Lymphadenopathy

Lymphadenopathy is the term used for enlarged lymph nodes as a consequence of disease. The most common cause of lymphadenopathy is loco-regional infection or systemic infection; in these cases, the term lymphadenitis is also used. The other major cause of lymphadenopathy is metastatic cancer or haematological malignancy: leukaemia and lymphoma (Table 9.1). Therefore, it is important that persistent neck lumps are thoroughly investigated to establish the cause. It is worth emphasizing that lymphadenopathy is common in children and is usually a consequence of a self-limiting infection. It is not always possible to identify the infective agent and, therefore, in the absence of other signs and symptoms, treatment is usually supportive: fluids and analgesics, with a 'watch and wait' policy in the first instance.

Bacterial infections causing lymphadenitis

The most common cause of bacterial lymphadenitis is dental infection: acute apical abscess, pericoronitis, necrotizing ulcerative gingivitis, lateral periodontal abscess, and osteomyelitis. Other causes include sinusitis, streptococcal pharyngitis, bacterial sialadenitis, and staphylococcal skin infections. These infections are usually transient and are either self-limiting or respond to local measures: removal of the cause (e.g. exodontia of a carious tooth) and drainage of pus. Antimicrobial agents are required if there is spreading infection and/or systemic signs of infection, such as malaise, pyrexia, and lymphadenitis.

Table 9.1 Differential diagnosis of cervical lymphadenopathy

Infections	Neoplastic	Miscellaneous
Bacterial	*Primary*	*Granulomatous disease*
Dental infection	Hodgkin lymphoma	Sarcoidosis
Streptococcal pharyngitis	Non-Hodgkin lymphoma	Crohn's disease
Bacterial sialadenitis	Leukaemia	*Connective tissue disease*
Staphylococcal skin infection	Langerhans cell histiocytosis	Rheumatoid arthritis
Tuberculosis		Scleroderma
Atypical tuberculosis		Systemic lupus erythematosus
Cat scratch disease		Sjögren's syndrome
Brucellosis		
Syphilis		
Leprosy		
Lyme disease		*Drug reactions*
		e.g. Phenytoin
Viral	*Secondary (metastases)*	
Pharyngitis/ common cold	Head and neck squamous cell carcinoma	*Rare causes*
Primary herpetic stomatitis		Castleman disease
Chickenpox	Head and neck adenocarcinoma	Kawasaki disease
Shingles		Kikuchi–Fujimoto syndrome
Herpangina	Head and neck melanoma	Cherubism
Hand, foot, and mouth disease	Thyroid cancer	
Measles	Distant malignant neoplasms, e.g. lung, colorectal, breast, prostate	
Glandular fever		
HIV infection		
Parasitic	Unknown (occult) primary malignancy	
Toxoplasmosis		

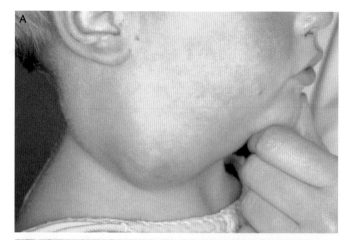
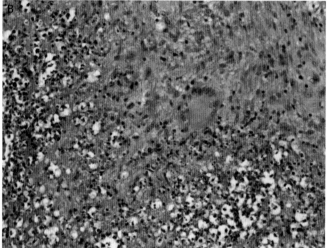

Fig. 9.4 A child with tuberculous cervical lymphadenitis. Histology shows necrotizing granulomatous inflammation and a Langhans giant cell (centre of field).

Some bacteria cause chronic granulomatous lymphadenitis. Granulomatous inflammation is characterized by the formation of focal collections of epithelioid macrophages called granulomas. The granulomas usually have a rim of lymphocytes and plasma cells. The macrophages often fuse to form multinucleate giant cells. Foreign-body giant cells have randomly distributed nuclei, Langhans giant cells have nuclei arranged in a horse-shoe configuration, and Touton giant cells have a ring of nuclei and voluminous lipid-laden cytoplasm. Tuberculosis, caused by *Mycobacterium tuberculosis*, is the prototypic granulomatous infection and usually infects the lungs. However, occasionally it causes cervical lymphadenitis, which historically was called scrofula (Fig. 9.4A). Pulmonary tuberculosis and tuberculous cervical lymphadenitis are most prevalent in the developing countries of Asia and Africa. Typically, the infected lymph nodes become enlarged, firm, and matted. Tuberculosis is characterized by necrotizing granulomatous inflammation, and the lymph node architecture is replaced with caseous (cheese-like) necrotic debris (Fig. 9.4B). Sinus tracts may develop from the necrotic lymph node to the skin surface, producing a so-called 'collar stud' abscess. Suspected tuberculosis is investigated with chest radiography to identify any pulmonary involvement. A tuberculin skin test (Mantoux test) is used to assess the immunological response to *Mycobacterium tuberculosis*. Sputum samples and a fresh tissue sample from the affected lymph node can be collected for microbiological testing; however, the bacterium is very slow-growing and it may take several weeks to identify any colonies. Successful growth facilitates antibiotic-sensitivity testing. The organisms can be identified in tissue samples using the Ziehl–Neelsen stain for acid-fast bacilli—a staining technique that stains the tiny bacilli red. Molecular biological tests (e.g. polymerase chain reaction) can also be used to identify bacterial DNA. Prolonged antibiotic therapy is required to clear the infection, and combinations of antibiotics, such as isoniazid and rifampicin, are usually required.

In the UK, infectious granulomatous lymphadenitis in children is usually caused by an 'atypical' non-tuberculous mycobacterium, e.g. *Mycobacterium avium-intracellulare*. Children with atypical tuberculosis often respond to surgical excision of the infected lymph node or group of lymph nodes. Other bacterial infections causing granulomatous lymphadenitis are rather uncommon, but include cat scratch fever (*Bartonella henselae*), brucellosis (*Brucella melitensis*), syphilis (*Treponema pallidum*), leprosy (*Mycobacterium leprae*), and Lyme disease (*Borrelia burgdorferi*).

Viral infections causing lymphadenitis

Viral-induced lymphadenitis is very common and typically occurs following adenovirus infection of the upper respiratory tract: viral pharyngitis and the common cold. Mucocutaneous infection with herpes simplex virus, varicella zoster virus, the coxsackie viruses (herpangina; hand, foot, and mouth disease), and paramyxovirus causing measles are also associated with generalized cervical lymphadenitis (Chapter 2). Glandular fever is caused by the Epstein–Barr virus (EBV) and typically presents with fever, malaise, and weight loss, accompanied by pharyngitis, cutaneous rashes, and cervical lymphadenopathy. This disease is common in children and young adults, and is transmitted in saliva. It is sometimes referred to as 'kissing disease' or infectious mononucleosis. Patients are tested using a panel of laboratory assays that include the Paul Bunnel test, the Monospot test, and specific tests for EBV viral capsid antigen. If these tests are equivocal, another aetiological agent, such as cytomegalovirus and HIV, should be considered.

Rarely, toxoplasmosis (*Toxoplasma gondii*), a protozoal infection, can cause similar signs and symptoms. *Toxoplasma gondii* may be acquired from the faeces of domestic animals, particularly cats, and contaminated soil and foods, e.g. inadequately cooked meat. The infection is usually self-liming, but it also responds to a prolonged course of tetracycline. Toxoplasmosis can be a life-threatening illness in immunocompromised patients and infection during pregnancy is associated with congenital abnormalities.

Other inflammatory causes of cervical lymphadenitis

Sarcoidosis is a granulomatous inflammatory disease of unknown cause. The disease produces non-specific symptoms, such as low-grade fever, malaise, and weight loss, but typically causes pulmonary signs and symptoms: cough, dysponea, and bilateral hilar lymphadenopathy. Other clinical features include cervical lymphadenitis (Fig. 9.5A), skin rashes and subcutaneous nodules, eye lesions (uveitis), oral mucosal disease (lip swelling and ulceration), and salivary gland disease (sialosis and xerostomia; Chapter 4). The combination of uveitis, parotitis, and facial palsy caused by sarcoidosis is called Heerfordt's syndrome (uveoparotid fever). Diagnosing sarcoidosis is challenging and thorough systemic investigation is usually only prompted following the diagnosis of granulomatous inflammation from a tissue biopsy. The granulomas tend to be small, well defined, and often confluent (Fig. 9.5B). The term 'naked' granuloma is sometimes used to describe the paucity of lymphocytes, as other granulomatous diseases tend to have a dense lymphocytic component. Sarcoid granulomas also lack the necrosis typically seen in tuberculosis. Investigations include chest radiography to screen for pulmonary disease. Haematological tests may reveal anaemia, increased plasma viscosity, and erythrocyte sedimentation rate, along with elevated serum angiotensin-converting enzyme, and calcium levels. Trans-bronchial biopsy is required to sample any enlarged

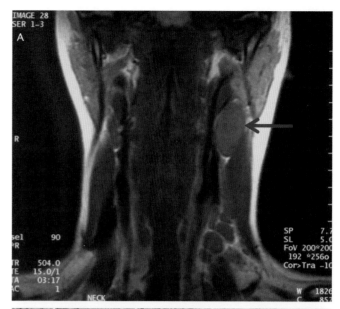

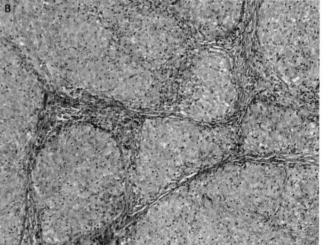

Fig. 9.5 MRI scan showing an enlarged left jugulo-digastric lymph node in sarcoidosis. Histology shows non-necrotizing granulomatous inflammation in a lymph node.

hilar lymph nodes. The disease is managed using immune-modulating drugs, such as systemic steroids.

Malignant causes of lymphadenopathy

The main malignant neoplasms causing lymphadenopathy are listed in Table 9.1. Red flag signs and symptoms of malignant lymphadenopathy are listed in Box 9.1.

Lymphomas tend to cause generalized lymphadenopathy or enlargement of groups of lymph nodes, and are usually accompanied by constitutional symptoms such as fatigue, malaise, weight loss, pyrexia, and night sweats. Enlarged lymph nodes feel rubbery and may be matted together. Lymphomas are a diverse group of malignant neoplasms characterized by the proliferation and accumulation of malignant lymphoid cells within lymph nodes. Lymphomas are traditionally classified into Hodgkin and non-Hodgkin lymphomas.

Hodgkin lymphoma accounts for about 10% of all lymphomas. It is predominantly a disease of young adults and typically presents with cervical lymphadenopathy, which may be the first sign of the disease. Early diagnosis is associated with excellent prognosis. Histological diagnosis depends on the identification of Reed–Sternberg cells, which are large cells that have a double or bi-lobed nucleus producing a 'mirror image' or 'owl eye' appearance (Fig. 9.6). The aetiology of the disease is unknown but genetic factors, immune competency, and EBV infection are considered to be important factors. Prognosis depends on the histological subtype and clinical staging; however, in early stage disease, chemoradiotherapy provides cure rates of around 80%.

Non-Hodgkin lymphomas are most commonly derived from the B lymphocyte lineage and are either high-grade B cell lymphomas (e.g. diffuse large B cell lymphoma, Burkitt lymphoma) or low-grade B cell lymphomas (e.g. small lymphocytic lymphoma, follicular lymphoma,

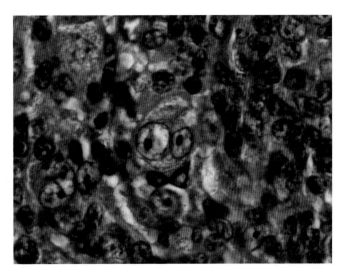

Fig. 9.6 Hodgkin lymphoma showing a Reed–Sternberg cell with 'owl eye' nuclei (centre of field).

marginal zone lymphoma, mantle cell lymphoma). T cell lymphomas are uncommon, but nasal-type NK/T cell lymphoma has a predilection for head and neck sites, and usually presents with mucosal lesions called extra-nodal lymphoma. Whilst leukaemias may cause lymphadenopathy, other stigmata are usually already well established; for example, constitutional symptoms (fatigue, malaise, weight loss, pyrexia, and night sweats), pallor (due to anaemia), abnormal bleeding (petichae, bruising, purpura; due to thrombocytopenia), intercurrent infection (due to leukopenia), and skin and oral mucosal lesions. The exception is chronic lymphocytic leukaemia, which evolves from small lymphocytic lymphoma and may primarily present as cervical lymphadenopathy. Examination of the peripheral blood demonstrates a leukaemic component of abnormal circulating B cells. The diagnosis and classification of lymphoma and leukaemia is a specialist area and precise diagnosis relies on the accurate assessment of the morphological features (type of malignant cells and ancillary cells) in combination with the identification of specific molecular markers and staging information (e.g. involvement of other lymph node groups, spleen, bone marrow, and blood).

Squamous cell carcinoma (SCC) is the most common malignant neoplasm to metastasize to the lymph nodes of the neck. Metastatic disease is usually ipsilateral: on the same anatomical side as the primary tumour. Metastasis to the contralateral side is a poor prognostic factor and this is reflected in tumour staging systems. Another major indicator of poor prognosis is when the metastatic carcinoma breaches the lymph node capsule and spreads into the adjacent parenchymal tissues of the neck, which is referred to as extra-nodal extension. The sites of metastasis are often predictable and reflect the lymphatic drainage of the head and neck region. SCCs derived from head and neck skin are usually located on sun-exposed areas of the scalp, ears, face, and lips. The majority of scalp and ear SCCs metastasize to para-parotid and intra-parotid lymph nodes and then to level II lymph nodes. SCC of the lip tends to metastasize to level I lymph nodes: submental and submandibular lymph nodes. Oral cavity SCC initially spreads to level I lymph nodes. Oro-pharyngeal SCC metastasizes to level II lymph nodes. Nasopharyngeal carcinoma classically presents with bilateral lymphadenopathy. Laryngeal SCC tends to metastasize to lymph nodes at levels III, IV, and VI. An isolated metastasis of SCC in level V is very uncommon and raises the possibility of a distant primary tumour, most commonly from the lung.

Adenocarcinomas of the major and minor salivary glands and thyroid cancers (e.g. follicular thyroid carcinoma, papillary thyroid carcinoma, medullary carcinoma, and anaplastic thyroid carcinoma) may metastasize to cervical lymph nodes. It is not unusual for papillary thyroid carcinoma to present as an isolated lateralized neck lump in the absence of obvious thyroid disease. In young adults, the lump may be dismissed as reactive lymphadenitis in the first instance, delaying diagnosis. Metastasis to the head and neck region from distant sites is uncommon and usually represents the progression of already advanced malignant disease. Virtually any 'distant' malignant tumour can metastasize to the cervical lymph nodes; however, the most prevalent cancers are the ones most likely to be encountered: lung, colorectal, breast, and prostate cancer. Occasionally, following a diagnosis of cervical lymph node metastasis (usually SCC), no primary tumour can be identified. These patients are labelled as having 'unknown' or 'occult' primary tumours. Despite rigorous investigation, including modern imaging techniques (CT, MRI, and PET–CT), and close follow-up, the location of the primary tumour site may remain an enigma.

Other causes of lumps in the neck

Developmental cysts

The embryological development of the head and neck is complex and involves the folding of the branchial arches, which results in trapped, enclaved epithelial remnants that can form developmental cysts later in life.

Epidermoid cyst

The epidermoid cyst can occur anywhere on head and neck skin. Typically, there is a modest, pea-sized cyst just below the skin surface, which, on close inspection, has a punctum (black dot) on the skin surface that represents the ostium of a blocked pilosebaceous follicle. The cyst contains keratin debris and is lined by an attenuated orthokeratinized squamous epithelium. The wall of the cyst is composed of compressed fibrous tissue. Occasionally, the cyst becomes infected and produces an acute skin abscess. If the cyst ruptures, extravasated keratin causes an intense foreign-body giant cell response. The lesion is treated by conservative surgical excision.

Dermoid cyst

The dermoid cyst usually presents with a swelling in the mid-line in the floor of the mouth and, classically, produces a 'double-chin' appearance (Fig. 9.7A). The cyst probably arises from the enclaved epithelium in the mid-line as a result of fusion of the mandibular and hyoid branchial arches. It is similar to the epidermoid cyst, in that it mainly contains keratin debris and is lined by an attenuated orthokeratinized squamous epithelium; however, it is the presence of skin adnexal structures (pilosebaceous follicles, erector pilli muscles, and eccrine sweat glands) in the wall of a dermoid cyst that separates the two entities. The treatment is conservative surgical excision.

Branchial cyst

The branchial cyst is a lympho-epithelial cyst; it is lined by squamous epithelium and the wall contains organized lymphoid tissue (Fig. 9.8). It arises between the anterior border of the sternocleidomastoid muscle and the angle of the mandible (Fig. 9.9). Although the branchial cyst is thought to be derived from remnants of the branchial arches or pharyngeal pouches, it is possible that it arises from salivary gland or tonsil

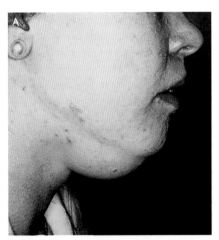
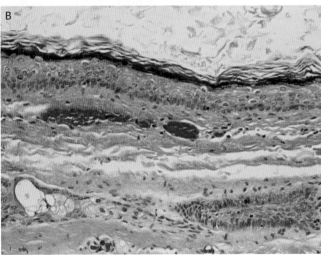

Fig. 9.7 Dermoid cyst presenting as a submental swelling. The lining of the cyst is composed of orthokeratinized squamous epithelium and there are pilosebaceous follicles in the cyst wall.

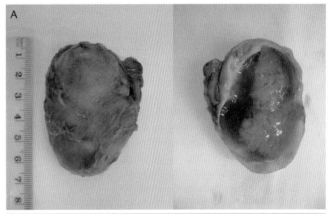
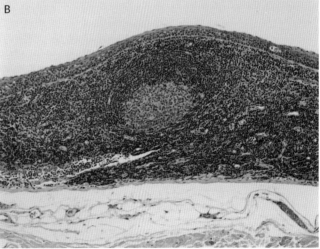

Fig. 9.8 The cut surface of a branchial cyst. Histology shows a squamous epithelial lining with lymphoid tissue in the wall (lympho-epithelial cyst).

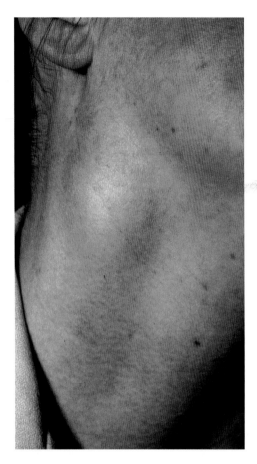

Fig. 9.9 Branchial cyst.

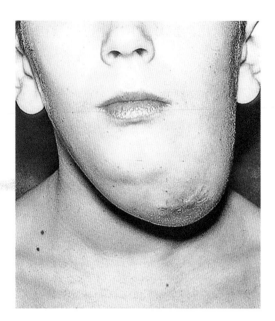

Fig. 9.10 Cystic hygroma.

tissue enclaved during development. The branchial sinus originates in the same position and, rather than developing into a cyst, produces a blind ending tract from the skin surface into the deep tissues of the neck.

Thyroglossal cyst

The thyroglossal cyst is derived from residues of the embryonic thyroglossal duct. The latter is formed during development by the migration of cells destined to form the follicular exocrine structures of the thyroid gland. The cells migrate caudally in the mid-line from the tuberculum impar of the tongue into the lower part of the neck. Consequently, thyroglossal cysts arise in the mid-line of the neck, typically in the region of the hyoid bone, and have a distinctive clinical sign; the lump moves upwards with swallowing. The cyst is effectively treated by surgical removal, along with dissection of the tract. The mid-portion of the hyoid bone is often removed as part of the operation (Sistrunk procedure), which reduces the chance of recurrence. Histopathological examination of the specimen reveals a cyst/tract lined by respiratory-type epithelium. A careful search of the cyst wall by the pathologist is undertaken to look for scattered thyroid follicles.

Cystic hygroma

The cystic hygroma (Fig. 9.10) is a lymphangiomatous malformation that occurs early in the development of the lymphatic system and most frequently affects the neck. Most are present at birth and present as large, fluctuant swellings, often up to 10 cm in diameter. They may extend to involve the base of tongue, floor of mouth, and, less commonly, buccal mucosa.

Thyroid and parathyroid lesions

The thyroid and parathyroid glands are located in the mid-line of the neck just below the laryngeal eminence. Swelling of the thyroid gland is called a goitre, the principal causes are listed in Box 9.2. A thyroid lesion may present as an isolated nodule or a multi-nodular swelling.

> **Box 9.2 Thyroid disease**
> **Non-neoplastic lesions**
> - Hyperplastic/colloid nodule
> - Thyroid cyst
> - Multi-nodular goitre (e.g. iodine deficiency)
> - Hashimoto thyroiditis (autoimmune hypothyroidism)
> - Graves' disease (autoimmune hyperthyroidism)
>
> **Neoplastic lesions**
> *Benign*
> - Follicular adenoma
>
> *Malignant*
> - Papillary carcinoma
> - Follicular carcinoma
> - Medullary carcinoma
> - Anaplastic carcinoma

They are variably associated with normal systemic levels of thyroid hormone (euthyroid), hyperthyroidism, and hypothyroidism. Parathyroid lesions are usually either hyperplasias or adenomas and are associated with signs and symptoms of hyperparathyroidism. Parathyroid carcinomas are uncommon.

Diffuse swelling of the neck

Diffuse swelling of the neck is usually associated with spreading infection, trauma, or surgical intervention (Table 9.2). Angioedema is characterized by a rapidly developing, diffuse neck swelling that can compromise the airway and result in asphyxiation. There are two distinct variants: allergic angioedema, caused by a type I hypersensitivity reaction, and non-allergic types. Non-allergic angioedema includes hereditary angioedema caused by a deficiency of C1-esterase inhibitor (an inhibitor of the complement pathway that is part of the inflammatory cascade) and acquired causes, which may be idiopathic but are commonly associated with medications, including angiotensin-converting enzyme (ACE) inhibitors and NSAIDSs. Distinction between the diseases is important because the management of the conditions can be different. Hereditary angioedema is treated with androgenic steroids to boost endogeneous levels of C1 esterase inhibitor, whereas acute allergic angioedema is managed with antihistamines and responds to intramuscular adrenaline in an emergency.

Carotid paraganglioma

Paragangliomas are rare neuroendocrine neoplasms. The carotid paraganglioma (carotid body tumour) arises from the carotid bodies located at the bifurcation of the common carotid artery. It typically presents as a slow-growing mass in the lateral part of the neck.

Table 9.2 Causes of diffuse neck swelling

Infection	Cellulitis
	Ludwig's angina
	Necrotizing fasciitis
Trauma	Oedema
	Haematoma
Iatrogenic	Surgical emphysema
Allergic	Allergic angioedema
Non-allergic	Hereditary angioedema
	Acquired angioedema

10

Oral manifestations of systemic disease

Chapter contents

Introduction

This chapter emphasizes the importance of oral disease in the context of systemic disease. Oral disease may be the first sign of an underlying systemic disorder, which should trigger further investigations or referral to a medical or specialist practitioner, expediting early diagnosis and appropriate clinical care. In those patients with known illnesses, dental healthcare professionals should have an appreciation of the effects of these diseases on the oro-facial complex; patients can then benefit from the supportive care of the dental team.

Gastrointestinal disease

Coeliac disease

Coeliac disease (gluten-induced enteropathy) is a genetically determined inflammatory small bowel disease that is induced by gluten in the diet. Gluten is present in wheat, rye, and barley. The inflammatory reaction results in malabsorption due to morphological abnormalities in the small intestinal mucosa. It was once thought of as a rare disease of childhood, but now it is understood to be a common disease that can be diagnosed at any age. Studies undertaken since the advent of serological screening indicate a prevalence of 0.5–1% in the population, with adult presentations now more frequent than childhood ones. This new appreciation has led to the concept of the 'coeliac iceberg' (Fig. 10.1). At the tip of the iceberg are those with overt disease, with the lower groups classified in order as: silent coeliac disease, latent coeliac disease, and healthy individuals with genetic susceptibility. Severe presentations in childhood classically were of diarrhoea, failure to thrive, and weakness. However, it is now understood that patients with coeliac disease may have minimal gastrointestinal symptoms of malabsorption at presentation and experience other rather non-specific symptoms of the disease. The increasing recognition of the disease is attributed to several factors, including new serological assays, advances in flexible endoscopy allowing clinicians to take duodenal biopsies more easily, and an increased index of suspicion in looking for the disease. The disease is associated with an increased rate of osteoporosis, infertility, autoimmune diseases, and malignancy, especially lymphoma. Treatment should involve a gluten-free diet, which is a major undertaking and for which dietetic advice is essential. The mortality rate in untreated disease exceeds that in the general population, but with a gluten-free diet, the mortality rate returns to normal.

Immunological markers in blood (anti-endomysial antibody and tissue tranglutaminase antibody) are now widely used to identify patients with coeliac disease with a high degree of sensitivity and specificity. Definite diagnosis still requires the demonstration of characteristic mucosal abnormalities on small bowel tissue, usually obtained by endoscopy.

Oral manifestations of coeliac disease include enamel hypoplasia, recurrent aphthous-type ulceration, and, on occasions, other oral manifestations of malabsorption. Enamel hypoplasia in coeliac disease is typically generalized, and symmetrically and chronologically distributed. Horizontal grooves and roughening of the enamel surface occur together with opacities and discoloration. The enamel lesions can be mild and not easily identified on cursory inspection.

Recurrent aphthous-type ulceration is thought to occur more frequently in patients suffering with coeliac disease. Malabsorption may result in anaemia or haematinic deficiency (iron, vitamin B_{12}, folic acid), which, clinically, may manifest as recurrent aphthous-type ulceration, recurrent candidosis, angular cheilitis, or glossitis. In patients with sufficiently severe aphthous-type ulceration to be referred for secondary care management, approximately 4% have coeliac disease as the underlying cause. It is thus common practice to undertake a full blood count and haematinic assay on patients presenting with these conditions and some oral medicine specialists also routinely check for a coeliac-associated antibody for patients presenting with recurrent aphthous-type ulceration. Treatment with a gluten-free diet is curative for many patients, although some continue to suffer with aphthous ulceration, even when on the diet. In these circumstances, the ulceration is managed as described previously for patients with recurrent aphthous stomatitis in Chapter 2.

Crohn's disease

Crohn's disease was first described as regional ileitis affecting the terminal ileum, usually in young adults, and characterized by chronic granulomatous inflammation. Since then our understanding of the disease has increased and it is now recognized as a disease that can affect every part of the gastrointestinal tract. In addition, the disease can affect extra-gastrointestinal sites, including the skin, joints, liver, and bone marrow. The disease is more common in the Western world compared to underdeveloped countries. Symptoms can start at any age, with a peak in early adulthood. Many environmental triggers have been postulated, including food constituents and specific infections; however, none has been conclusively established as the cause. The natural history of Crohn's disease is of relapsing and remitting episodes of bowel inflammation, with accompanying episodes of abdominal pain and nutritional deficiency due to malabsorption. Histological examination of affected

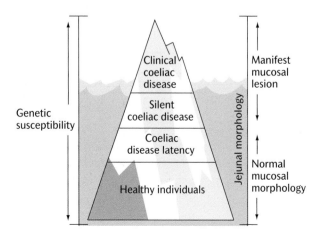

Fig. 10.1 The coeliac iceberg and spectrum of gluten sensitivity.

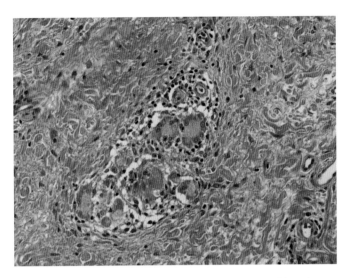

Fig. 10.2 Granulomatous inflammation in Crohn's disease. There is a granuloma containing multinucleate giant cells in the centre of the field.

shows fibrosis and a dense infiltration of the mucosa and submucosa with lymphocytes and plasma cells. (Fig. 10.2). Non-caseating granulomas (aggregates of macrophages, frequently including multinucleated and mononuclear types and without necrosis), are typically present.

Lymphoedema and dilated lymphatics may be a prominent feature and, when present, account for the tissue oedema seen in some of the oral manifestations, such as swollen lips and bucco-labial mucosa.

Oral manifestations of Crohn's disease are observed in less than 10% of patients diagnosed with the disease; however, oral symptoms may precede intestinal symptoms in some cases by many years. The oral manifestations of Crohn's are shown in (Fig. 10.3) and include:

Non specific
- Aphthous or linear fissure-like ulcers affecting non-keratinizing mucosa surfaces
- Glossitis secondary to deficiency or malabsorption of iron, vitamin B_{12}, or folic acid
- Angular cheilitis

Characteristic
- Persistent, diffuse swelling of the lips and cheeks
- Oedematous and hyperplastic thickening of the bucco-labial mucosa together with fissuring producing a 'cobble-stone' appearance'
- Oedematous and hyperplastic enlargement of the bucco-labial mucosa presenting as polypoid tag-like lesions or deep folds of mucosa that can mimic denture irritation hyperplasia
- Redness and swelling of attached gingiva

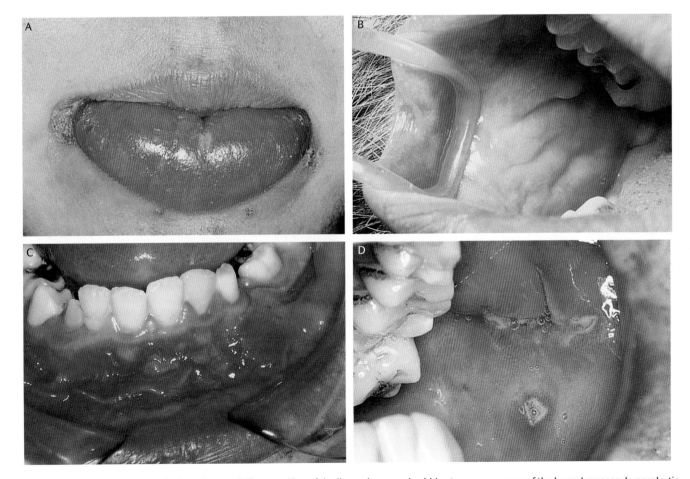

Fig. 10.3 Oral manifestations of Crohn's disease. Diffuse swelling of the lip, oedema, and cobble-stone appearance of the buccal mucosa; hyperplastic tags in the labial sulcus, aphthous-like ulcers, and linear fissured ulcers.

Systemic management of Crohn's is based around 5-aminosalicylic acid products, corticosteroids, and immunosuppressive agents, including azathioprine and methotrexate. More recently, biological agents such as infliximab and adalimumab, which are forms of anti-tumour necrosis factor alpha (anti-TNF-alpha) antibodies, have been increasingly used for severe cases. Where lesions are limited to the mouth, topical and intra-lesional steroids are usually tried first, before systemic agents are used.

Oro-facial granulomatosis

Oro-facial granulomatosis is a term used to describe a clinico-pathological picture of oral changes similar to that found in oral Crohn's disease, namely swelling of the face, lips, and oral tissue in association with histological evidence of non-caseating granulomatous inflammation within these tissues. Such changes can be found secondary to several systemic disorders: Crohn's disease, sarcoidosis, granulomatous infections, and foreign-body reactions, but can also occur where the aetiology and any systemic associations remain unclear at presentation (Box 10.1). Oro-facial granulomatosis encompasses the disorders described as Melkerson–Rosenthal syndrome and its incomplete form, cheilitis granulomatosa, where only the lips are affected. Melkerson–Rosenthal syndrome consists of the triad of facial swelling, fissured tongue, and unilateral lower motor neuron facial palsy. It is rarely seen in its complete form. There is some evidence emerging that oro-facial granulomatosis is more likely to present with lip and buccal swelling compared to other oro-facial lesions.

Assessment of patients presenting with these manifestations is necessary to exclude a systemic association, although it needs to be borne in mind that subsequent development of a systemic disease may become apparent, especially when the disease onset is in childhood. Diagnosis is made on the basis of the characteristic clinical presentation and biopsy to demonstrate the non-caseating granulomas. Granulomas may only be present at the level of the underlying muscle,

so it is advisable to extend the biopsy beyond the superficial mucosa. To minimize morbidity at the biopsy site, the buccal mucosa is preferred over the lip. Occasionally, granulomas are not found, but this does not exclude a clinical diagnosis of oro-facial granulomatosis. To confirm a diagnosis of oro-facial granulomatosis, the biopsy should show peri-lymphatic chronic inflammation, lymphoedema, and small granulomas. Stains for acid-fast bacilli are negative and there is no evidence of foreign material in the granulomas. Haematological and biochemical investigations (full blood count and haematinics) will usually be normal with only infrequent evidence of raised levels of inflammatory markers, such as erythrocyte sedimentation rate (ESR) or C reactive protein. By contrast these results are frequently abnormal in Crohn's disease. Serum levels of angiotensin-converting enzyme (ACE) and, if indicated, chest radiography will usually be normal, effectively excluding sarcoidosis.

The aetiology of oro-facial granulomatosis remains unclear. Sensitivity to food has been observed in some patients and dietary manipulation is an approach that is increasing being used as part of treatment. Where facilities allow, patch testing for contact urticaria and contact dermatitis to possible food allergens can be undertaken. The most commonly implicated food substances are cinnamon and benzoate, a commonly used preservative, especially in carbonated drinks. A cinnamon- and benzoate-free diet is frequently tried empirically for a 3-month trial period. If successful in reducing signs and symptoms, then excluded foods can be re-introduced in a controlled manner. Should dietary manipulation be unsuccessful, then the management is similar to that used for oral manifestations of Crohn's disease. Topical and intra-lesional steroids can lead to a reduction in the soft-tissue swelling, but the effect is frequently short-lived and repeated injections are usually needed. Many systemic drugs have been tried with a variety of success, although azathioprine has emerged as the one most frequently used. Others include clofazamine and thalidomide. Topical steroids, and antiseptic and analgesic mouthwashes can be helpful for managing the oral ulceration in oro-facial granulomatosis, while angular cheilitis and lip fissures can be improved by the use of an antimicrobial cream.

Ulcerative colitis

Ulcerative colitis is a relapsing and remitting disease characterized by acute non-infectious inflammation of the colorectal mucosa. The rectal mucosa is invariably involved with confluent inflammation and shallow ulceration, extending proximally from the anal margin. Patients often present with bloody diarrhoea. The disease may also affect extra-gastrointestinal sites, including the skin, eye, liver, and joints. In some cases it can be difficult to distinguish ulcerative colitis from Crohn's disease.

Oral manifestations of ulcerative colitis are far less common than found in Crohn's disease. Recurrent aphthous-type ulceration has been associated with the disease. The most characteristic oral manifestation is pyostomatitis vegetans (Fig. 10.4). This is a rare disorder, where the lips and cheeks are diffusely inflamed with erosions, fissured ulcers, and pustules, separating papillary projections and

---

Box 10.1 Granulomatous inflammation of the oral mucosa

- Oro-facial granulomatosis
  - Melkerson–Rosenthal syndrome
  - Cheilitis granulomatosa
- Crohn's disease
- Sarcoidosis
- Infection
  - Tuberculosis
  - Syphilis
  - Leprosy
  - Deep mycosis
- Extrinsic foreign material

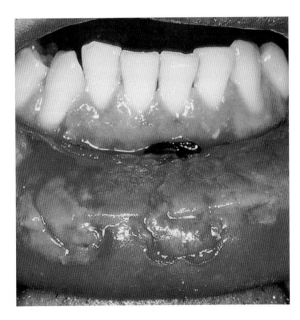

Fig. 10.4 Pyostomatits vegetans.

irregular outgrowths (vegetations) from the mucosal surface. Skin lesions (pyodermatitis vegetans) may occur at the same time as the oral lesions. Histological examination shows acanthosis and multiple micro-abscesses containing numerous neutrophils and eosinophils at the tips of the connective tissue papillae and within the epithelium. Very rarely, pyostomatitis gangrenosum has been reported as an oral manifestation of ulcerative colitis. The patient typically presents with irregular, deep, foul-smelling ulcers, on the lips.

Systemic management of ulcerative colitis is similar to Crohn's disease and based around 5-aminosalicylic acid products, corticosteroids, and immunosuppressive agents, including azathioprine. Oral lesions of aphthous-type ulceration and pyostomatitis vegetans will frequently respond to topical steroids, although management of the ulcerative colitis will often improve the oral lesions.

Nutritional deficiency

Scurvy is due to deficiency of vitamin C (ascorbic acid) found in fresh fruit and vegetables. It is rarely seen today, but cases still occur in elderly and neglected patients, and younger patients who have a markedly restricted diet. Skin manifestations include capillary fragility, leading to spontaneous bruising. Oral manifestations include friable and swollen gingiva with marked false pocketing and mobility of the teeth. Management is with ascorbic acid tablets.

Liver disease

Jaundice

Jaundice is a condition characterized by excess bilirubin in the bloodstream. The bilirubin accumulates in the skin, which results in a yellowish discoloration to the skin and mucosa, including the oral cavity (Fig. 10.5). Jaundice can occur due to many causes, including prehepatic and post-hepatic diseases. Management depends on finding the cause of the jaundice.

Liver dysfunction

Abnormal liver function may result from a wide variety of causes, including hepatitis virus infection, alcohol abuse, and drug reactions. Hepatitis C infection has been linked to oral lichen planus and hyposalivation. Abnormal liver function is important in dentistry in relation to prescribing, because drug metabolism may be impaired. Further, synthesis of blood coagulation factors may be reduced, resulting in prolonged bleeding after dental extraction. In addition, the ability of the hepatitis B virus to be contracted through the practise of dentistry has led to hepatitis B vaccination for dental healthcare workers and universal cross-infection control precautions.

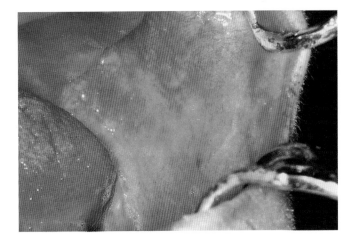

Fig. 10.5 Yellow pigmentation of the buccal mucosa in a patient with jaundice.

Genitourinary disease

Many muco-cutaneous diseases with oral involvement may have associated genital lesions. These include lichen planus, vesiculobullous disorders, and aphthous-type ulceration, which are discussed in Chapter 2.

Reiter's syndrome

Reiter's syndrome is a triad of polyarthritis, urethritis, and eye manifestations, including conjunctivitis. It usually occurs in young men as a reaction to non-specific urethritis, frequently due to chlamydia infection in a genetically susceptible individual. Skin lesions resemble psoriasis on the palms and soles. Various oral lesions have been described in a proportion of cases, including painless erythematous papules on the palate and, most commonly, lesions that resemble migratory stomatitis (erythema migrans). Some patients with Reiter's syndrome experience spontaneous resolution, whilst others have chronic symptoms that wax and wane. For patients with urethritis, a course of a tetracycline may help.

Genitourinary infections

Sexually transmitted diseases, including syphilis, herpes simplex, and condyloma acuminatum, may occur in the oral cavity and are discussed in Chapter 2. High-risk human papillomavirus in relation to oro-pharyngeal malignancy is discussed in Chapter 3.

Cardiorespiratory disease

Sarcoidosis

This is a systemic disease of unknown aetiology that usually presents with shortness of breath and skin or eye lesions. Chest radiography reveals bilateral hilar lymphadenopathy and pulmonary lesions. It most commonly affects young adults. Histological examination of affected tissue shows small, well-defined, non-caseous granulomas composed of groups of epitheliod macrophages, often with Langhans giant cells. The level of serum angiotensin converting enzyme is frequently raised in the active phase of the disease. Hypercalciuria is also common. Treatment is with corticosteroids and immunosuppressive agents.

Oral manifestations of sarcoidosis are uncommon, but it may present as oro-facial granulomatosis. Other manifestations include submucosal, painless, red nodules covered by normal epithelium or as erythematous granular hyperplastic gingiva (Fig. 10.6). Major salivary gland involvement may occur, presenting as a painless persistent enlargement of the gland with a reduction in salivary flow. Heerfordt's syndrome (uveoparotid fever) is a rare disease and comprises uveitis, parotitis, and low-grade fever in sarcoidosis. Cervical lymphadenopathy caused by sarcoidosis is discussed in Chapter 9.

Infections

Chronic pulmonary infections, such as tuberculosis and histoplasmosis in endemic areas, may produce secondary infections in the oral cavity.

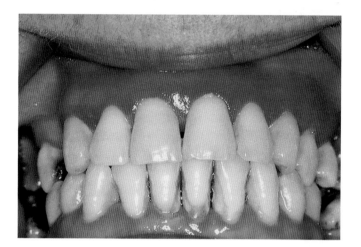

Fig. 10.6 Sarcoidosis of the gingiva.

Organisms are coughed up and produce masses or ulcers, most often in the palate or dorsal tongue. Histochemical stains for acid-fast bacilli may be positive on biopsy material.

Renal disease

Renal failure

Renal failure can have several manifestations in the mouth. Patients with renal failure have elevated levels of urea and other nitrogenous products in the blood, which is associated with ureamic stomatitis. This can appear as white patches distributed predominantly on the buccal mucosa, tongue, and floor of the mouth, which may be associated with an unpleasant taste. Sometimes widespread painful ulcerations can occur (ulcerative ureamic stomatitis). Treatment with renal dialysis will clear the oral lesions. Dryness of the mouth, and an increased susceptibility to ascending parotid gland infections, are associated with severe fluid restriction, where this is required. Renal disease can impair drug excretion. Renal disease-associated anaemia may result in pallor of the mucosa, and platelet deficiency may cause mucosal purpura and haemorrhage.

Renal failure can lead to secondary hyperparathyroidism (see the section Endocrine disease). The kidney processes vitamin D, which is necessary for calcium absorption from the gut. Reduced vitamin D levels results in lowered serum calcium and excess production of parathyroid hormone. Renal patients are now usually treated with vitamin D supplements to prevent this happening.

Renal transplantation

Patients who receive a transplanted kidney require immunosuppression to prevent rejection of the transplant. Ciclosporin has been traditionally used, but can cause significant gingival overgrowth as a complication.

Tacrolimus and mycophenolate mofetil are now increasingly being used as alternative immunosuppressants. Calcium channel blockers, given to prevent concomitant hypertension in renal disease, can also cause gingival overgrowth (Chapter 5). Immunosuppressive drugs can cause a variety of oral complications, including the development of viral, bacterial, and fungal infections. These infections may manifest themselves with an atypical appearance due to the deficient host immunological response. Immunosuppression also predisposes the patient to skin cancers, particularly squamous cell carcinoma of the lip, and patients are usually regularly monitored for these effects.

Haematological disease

Anaemia

Anaemia is a general term for either a decrease in the volume of red blood cells (erythrocytes) or in the concentration of haemoglobin. It can result from a decrease in production of erythrocytes or an increased destruction or loss of erythrocytes. The general symptoms of anaemia are typically related to reduced oxygen-carrying capacity of the blood, causing tiredness and shortness of breath. It can also exacerbate intercurrent cardiovascular disease causing palpitations and angina pectoris. Pallor of the mucous membranes is an important clinical sign. Treatment depends on identifying the cause of the anaemia and its correction.

Anaemia is often a sign of an underlying disease and the causes of anaemia are diverse (Box 10.2). Erythrocytes are formed in the bone marrow and require a number of nutritional factors, including iron, vitamin B_{12}, and folic acid, collectively called the haematinics. These nutritional factors are all absorbed from the gastrointestinal tract. Hence red cell production (erythropoiesis) depends on an adequate amount of the haematinics in the diet and absorption via a normal mucosa in the small intestine. In addition, vitamin B_{12} absorption depends on the production of intrinsic factor from the gastric parietal cells in the stomach. Lack of any of the haematinics will thus lead to anaemia.

Iron-deficiency anaemia is the most common cause of anaemia worldwide and develops when the amount of iron available to the body cannot keep pace with the need for iron in haemopoesis. This results in a hypochromic (reduction in haemoglobin within the erythrocyte) and microcytic (reduction in size of the erythrocyte) anaemia. It can occur due to:

- Decreased dietary intake of iron
- Decreased absorption of iron (e.g. Coeliac disease)
- Excessive blood loss (e.g. menstrual or gastrointestinal bleeding)
- Increased demand for red blood cells (e.g. pregnancy)

A small portion of iron is present in the plasma, bound to the protein, transferrin. Prior to iron-deficiency anaemia becoming manifest, the body will use up this plasma store of iron. Reduction in the iron plasma store, prior to the development of frank anaemia, is known as latent iron-deficiency and is enough to produce oral manifestations and other symptoms.

Folic acid and vitamin B_{12} deficiency cause a macrocytic (increase in the size of the erythrocyte) anaemia. Pernicious anaemia is an uncommon autoimmune condition caused by failure of production of intrinsic factor by the gastric parietal cells. Vitamin B_{12} binds to the intrinsic factor and the combined complex is necessary for absorption across the small intestine mucosa. Causes of vitamin B_{12} and folate deficiency include dietary deficiency, malabsorption, or increased physiological demand, e.g. during pregnancy.

A range of oral signs and symptoms can occur in patients with anaemia, the great majority occurring in those due to an underlying haematinic deficiency (Box 10.3).

Leucopenia

Leucopenia is a reduction in the white cell population of the blood. This may be due to general reduction in haemopoetic precursor cells in the

---

Box 10.2 Causes of anaemia

Disorders of haemoglobin

- Sickle cell anaemia
- Thalassaemia

Iron-related anaemia

- Iron-deficiency anaemia
- Sideroblastic anaemia

Megaloblastic anaemia

- Pernicious anaemia
- Folic acid deficiency

Anaemia associated with chronic disease

- Anaemia of chronic inflammation (connective tissue disorders and chronic infection)
- Anaemia associated with malignancy

Failure of production

- Aplastic anaemia

Haemolytic anaemia

- Spherocytosis
- Splenomegaly
- Red cell autoantibodies
- Red cell abnormalities

bone marrow, such as in aplastic anaemia, or secondary to autoimmune disorders, viral infection (e.g. HIV; see the section Immunodeficiency) or as a side-effect of drug therapy (e.g. carbamazepine). The most common selective reduction in white cells concerns neutrophils. Neutropenia can be secondary to a genetic disorder or, more commonly, caused by viruses, metabolic disorders, and as a side-effect of drug therapy. The latter sometimes causes agranulocytosis, a condition where the cells of the granulocytic series, particularly neutrophils, are absent. In neutropenia, the effect is to increase the susceptibility of the patient to infection, especially bacterial. Alongside sore throat and fever, the oral mucosa may display widespread atypical ulceration and inflammation. Gingival infection resembling necrotizing ulcerative gingivitis may occur. Treatment depends on identifying the cause of the leucopenia and its correction.

Cyclic neutropenia is a rare condition, which is characterized by regular periodic reductions in the patient's neurophil population. Gingivitis and aphthous-type ulceration may occur during the neutropenic episodes.

Bleeding diathesis

Haemophilia, von Willebrand's disease, and liver dysfunction do not usually initially manifest in the oral cavity, unless they cause excessive bleeding following tooth extraction. Platelet disorders, where the number of the platelets in the circulating blood are reduced (thrombocytopenia) or their function affected, can, however, cause spontaneous haemorrhage to occur within tissues. Causes include leukaemia, liver and renal disease, idiopathic thrombocytopenic purpura, and an adverse reaction to a medication. Thrombocytopenia causes bleeding under the skin or mucous membranes producing petechiae (small red dots), ecchymoses (bruising), and purpura (purple patches), and spontaneous gingival bleeding. Treatment depends on the cause.

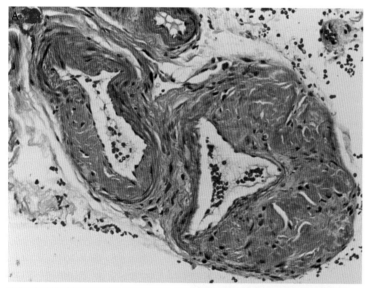

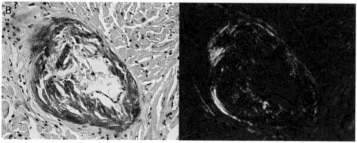

Fig. 10.7 Perivascular amyloid deposits (A). The amyloid stains pink with Congo red (B) and has a characteristic apple-green colour when viewed with cross polarized light (C).

Amyloidosis

Amyloidosis represents a heterogenous group of conditions characterized by the deposition of an extracellular proteinaceous substance called amyloid. It can be associated with multiple myeloma or chronic inflammatory diseases. All body organs may be affected by amyloid deposits. In the oral cavity, amyloidosis may cause thickening, swelling, and decreased mobility of the tongue. The lips may also be affected. Diagnosis is by biopsy and the identification of amyloid by various staining techniques. Classically, amyloid is positively stained by Congo red, and when viewed by polarized light produces a characteristic apple-green birefringence (Fig. 10.7). Management is by treatment of the underlying cause.

Immunodeficiency

Human immunodeficiency virus (HIV) infection and AIDS

HIV is a global epidemic with around 37 million people affected in 2014. Many patients are living longer due to anti-retroviral therapy and, although the global prevalence of HIV builds year on year, the new infection rate may actually be decreasing. The disease is relevant to dentistry because it may present with oral manifestations and there are also cross-infection considerations. HIV is a highly variable virus that mutates very readily and, although two main types are recognized, with most affected by HIV type 1, there can be several strains, even in an individual patient. The infection is transmitted by the exchange of blood or body fluids, principally through sexual contact, the injection of blood (e.g. intravenous drug-abusers sharing needles), or from mother to child (perinatal infection). Transmission of the virus may be followed by infection that is detected by the appearance of HIV antibodies in the blood (seroconversion). This generally occurs within 3 months of exposure. A few patients have an acute HIV infection at this time, the clinical features of which include pyrexia, skin rash, headache, diarrhoea, sore throat, and erythema of the buccal and palatal mucosa.

Following seroconversion, most patients remain symptom-free for many years (average 10 years). In this group of chronic HIV infection patients, the balance between viral replication and host immune response reaches an equilibrium, though millions of CD4 cells and billions of virions are produced and destroyed daily. Eventually, the CD4 count falls and viral load increases; patients then develop clinical acquired immune deficiency syndrome (AIDS), defined by either diagnosis of one of the AIDS-defining conditions, or by measurement of CD4 levels <200 cells/μl. Patients with AIDS often have lymphadenopathy, persistent pyrexia, diarrhoea, weight loss, fatigue, and malaise. Opportunistic infections, Kaposi sarcoma, non-Hodgkin lymphoma, thrombocytopenia, and neurological disease are also frequent features. The list of AIDS-defining diseases and diagnostic criteria is regularly updated and the websites of the US Centers for Disease Control and Prevention (CDC) and World Health Organization (WHO) are good sources of current information (see additional resources).

Oral manifestations of HIV infection

The oral manifestations of HIV infection are numerous and have been divided into three groups based on the strength of their association with HIV infection. The main lesions in each group are listed in Box 10.4.

Box 10.4 **Classification of oral lesions associated with HIV infection**

Group I: Lesions strongly associated with HIV infection

- Candidosis
  - Erythematous
  - Hyperplastic
  - Pseudomembranous
  - Linear gingival erythema
- Hairy leukoplakia (EBV)
- HIV-associated periodontal disease
  - HIV-gingivitis
  - Necrotizing ulcerative gingivitis
  - HIV-periodontitis
  - Necrotizing stomatitis
- Kaposi sarcoma
- Non-Hodgkin lymphoma

Group II: Lesions less commonly associated with HIV infection

- Atypical ulceration (oropharyngeal)

- Idiopathic thrombocytopenic purpura
- Salivary gland disorders
  - Dry mouth, decreased salivary flow rate
  - Uni- or bilateral swelling of major glands
- Viral infections (other than EBV)
  - Cytomegalovirus
  - Herpes simplex virus
  - Human papillomavirus
  - Varicella-zoster virus

Group III: Lesions possibly associated with HIV infection

- Bacterial infections other than gingivitis/periodontitis
- Fungal infection other than candidosis
- Melanotic hyperpigmentation
- Neurologic disturbances
  - Facial palsy
  - Trigeminal neuralgia

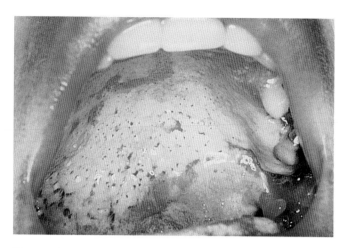

Fig. 10.8 Severe pseudomembranous candidosis associated with HIV.

However, the prevalence of some of these lesions, particularly those associated with opportunistic infection, notably oral candidosis, hairy leukoplakia, Kaposi sarcoma, and necrotizing periodontal disease, is now markedly reduced following the introduction of 'highly active anti-retroviral therapy' (HAART).

Oral candidosis

Infection of the oral cavity by *Candida* is the most frequent oral manifestation of HIV infection. *Candida albicans* is the commonest cause but other species, including azole-resistant strains, are occasionally involved. The pseudomembranous and erythematous varieties are seen most frequently but, unlike their counterparts in non-HIV infected patients, they may persist for months. Pseudomembranous candidosis (Fig. 10.8) may involve any part of the oral mucosa but the palate, cheeks, lips, and dorsum of the tongue are the most frequently affected sites. Erythematous candidosis (Fig. 10.9) presents as a red lesion, and most commonly affects the palate and dorsum of the tongue, where it is also associated with loss of the filiform papillae and can resemble median rhomboid glossitis. Chronic hyperplastic candidosis is most frequently seen on the buccal mucosa but the commissures are rarely

> **Box 10.5 HIV-associated periodontal diseases**
> - Linear gingival erythema
> - Necrotizing ulcerative gingivitis (NUG)
> - Necrotizing ulcerative periodontitis (NUP)

involved, in contrast to non-HIV cases. The prevalence of oral candidosis in HIV infection varies but is about 20% in HIV-positive patients who have not developed AIDS, compared to 70% or more in those with AIDS. However, the prevalence is decreasing due to the use of HAART.

HIV-associated periodontal diseases

HIV infection may be associated with atypical and sometimes severe periodontal diseases. The reported prevalence varies but is generally less than 10% and is decreasing since the introduction of HAART. Three main clinical types are recognized Box 10.5. Linear gingival erythema presents as a red band involving the free gingival margins that is often associated with *Candida* infection. Necrotizing ulcerative periodontitis is a severe, rapidly destructive process resulting in necrosis of gingival and periodontal tissues, sometimes with necrosis, exposure, and sequestration of alveolar bone (Fig. 10.10). It is associated with severe impairment of local defence mechanisms, probably involving significant reductions in CD4 activity and defective functioning of polymorph neutrophils. Necrotizing ulcerative gingivitis in HIV-positive patients may be persistent and extensive, and may not respond to conventional treatment.

Viral infections

Infections with herpes simplex and varicella-zoster viruses in association with HIV infection are more severe and extensive than when occurring in an HIV-seronegative patient, and frequently recur. Anti-viral drugs, such as aciciclovir, can be prescribed for prophylaxis, as these disorders can be troublesome. Viral warts are often seen in the mouths of patients infected with HIV, and unusual types of human papillomavirus have been identified in some of these lesions. Disseminated cytomegalovirus

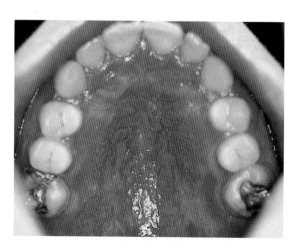

Fig. 10.9 Erythematous canidfosis associated with HIV.

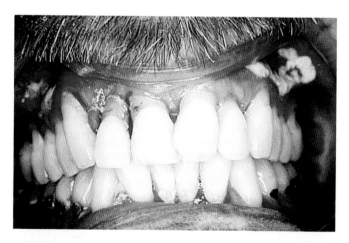

Fig. 10.10 HIV-associated necrotizing ulcerative periodontitis (NUP) and areas of pseudomembranous candidosis.

(CMV) infection may be seen in AIDS, and Epstein–Barr virus (EBV) is the cause of hairy leukoplakia and may be associated with some lymphomas. Kaposi sarcoma is associated with a herpesvirus, HHV8 (see Chapter 2). The prevalence of some of the lesions associated with viral infection, particularly hairy leukoplakia, has reduced significantly since the introduction of HAART. In contrast, the prevalence of oral warts has increased.

Hairy leukoplakia

Hairy leukoplakia (HL) presents as a white patch that cannot be removed. It occurs most frequently on the lateral borders of the tongue, bilaterally, but occasionally other areas of the oral mucosa are affected. The most characteristic lesions present as vertical white folds on the lateral border of the tongue with a raised, corrugated, or hairy surface (Fig. 10.11). However, the lesions may also have a smooth, flat surface. Histological examination of HL typically shows acanthotic, parakeratinized epithelium (Fig. 10.12A), often with long, finger-like surface projections of parakeratin, producing the hairy or corrugated appearance seen clinically. Candidal hyphae are often present in the parakeratin, but the candidosis is a secondary, rather than a causal, infection. There is an absence of associated inflammatory cells, both in the epithelium and in the lamina propria. Swollen keratinocytes with clear, glassy cytoplasm and prominent cell boundaries are present as a band in the prickle cell layer beneath the parakeratin. Some show darkly staining or expanded, pale grey staining nuclei, and perinuclear vacuoles. Chromatin clumping is a characteristic feature (Fig. 10.12C). *In situ* hybridization using the EBER (EBV-encoded RNA) test can be used to demonstrate the presence of EBV in these koilocyte-like cells (Fig. 10.12B).

HL is seen in HIV-infected patients from all risk groups, with a prevalence of about 20–25% overall, which is reduced to about 12% in patients taking HAART. However, the prevalence rate increases as the CD4-lymphocyte count falls and immunocompetence declines. HL also occurs in non-HIV-infected patients receiving immunosuppressive therapy and in response to potent topical steroids used in the oral cavity. HL has been described in other groups of patients with systemic immunosuppression, such as those receiving organ transplantation. The disease has also been reported in apparently immunocompetent

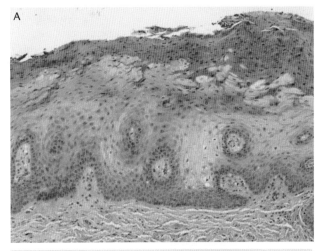

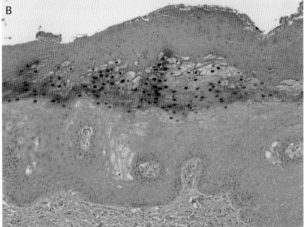

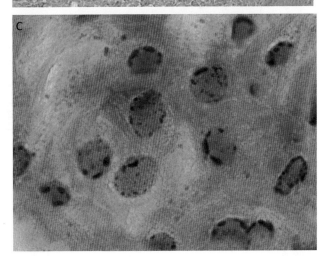

Fig. 10.12 Hairy leukoplakia showing hyperkeratosis (A). There is evidence of Epstein–Barr virus by *in situ* hybridization (blue nuclei in B). Individual keratinocytes showing viral-induced chromatin clumping in the nuclei (C).

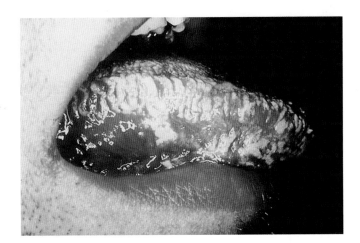

Fig. 10.11 HIV-associated hairy leukoplakia.

individuals, where there is an association with steroid inhaler usage. There is no evidence that HL is an oral potentially malignant disorder, the term 'leukoplakia' is used in this context simply to mean 'white patch'.

Kaposi sarcoma

Although Kaposi sarcoma (KS) is the commonest tumour associated with HIV infection, its prevalence is low, particularly for patients on HAART. KS is more common in males than in females and in patients whose behaviour is associated with increased risk of male-to-male transmission of HIV infection. KS is associated with infection by human herpesvirus 8 (HHV8), which appears to have a causal role.

KS is a multifocal tumour involving skin and mucosal surfaces, and presents first as reddish-purple patches, which then become nodular. Oral lesions may be the presenting feature and are seen most frequently on the palate, although other sites may be involved (Fig. 10 13). The tip of the nose is the most frequent facial site.

Early lesions of KS consist of proliferating endothelial cells and atypical, often cleft-like, vascular channels together with extravasated erythrocytes, haemosiderin, and inflammatory cells. A few atypical spindle-shaped cells may be seen in the interstitial tissues. Distinction from granulation tissue and other vascular lesions, such as haemangiomas and pyogenic granulomas, may be difficult. However, in the later stages, the vascular component decreases and the atypical spindle cells predominate, with the lesions evolving from flat lesions through plaque and nodular stages. KS can be treated by radiotherapy, surgery, or chemotherapy, and newer targeted monoclonal antibody agents are being used in clinical trials.

Non-Hodgkin lymphoma

An increased incidence of non-Hodgkin lymphoma is seen in AIDS patients (as in other groups of immunocompromised patients), and oral mucosal involvement has been described. Some of these lymphomas are associated with EBV infection.

Neurological disturbances

HIV is neurotropic and may directly involve the central nervous system leading, for example, to peripheral neuropathy or dementia. Facial nerve palsy may follow involvement of neurons in the central nervous system.

Atypical ulceration

Atypical ulceration, particularly of the oropharynx, has been described in AIDS and may resemble aphthous-type stomatitis (Fig. 10.14). Some may be associated with viral infection, such as CMV.

Idiopathic thrombocytopenic purpura

Small purpuric lesions or larger areas of bruising may be seen on the oral mucosa, associated with thrombocytopenia resulting from an auto-immune response.

HIV-associated salivary gland disease

Salivary gland disease may be a feature in a small proportion of adults with HIV infection. The prevalence may be higher in infected children. HIV-associated salivary gland disease is characterized by xerostomia and/or swelling of the major glands, almost invariably the parotid. The xerostomia may be caused by a Sjögren's syndrome-like disease associated with a salivary lympho-epithelial lesion histologically, but the patients do not show the autoantibody profile commonly seen in Sjögren's syndrome. Parotid swelling may be due

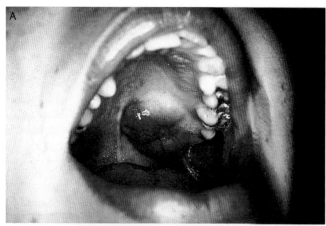

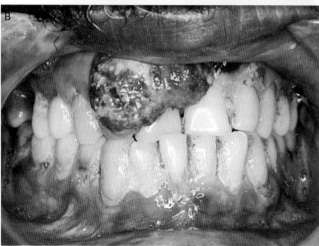

Fig. 10.13 Kaposi sarcoma associated with HIV.

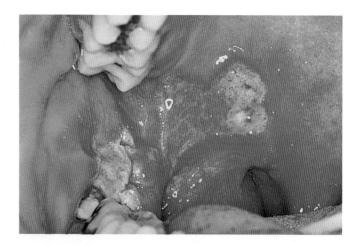

Fig. 10.14 Atypical oral ulceration associated with HIV.

to enlargement of intra-parotid lymph nodes or development of multiple lympho-epithelial cysts of varying size (HIV-associated parotid cysts).

Oral pigmentation

Melanin pigmentation of the oral mucosa has been described in patients with HIV, but whether this is directly related to the infection, or associated with drug therapy, or adrenal gland insufficiency, has not been determined.

> **Key points   HIV infection**
> - Oral signs and symptoms may be the initial manifestation
> - Wide variety of oral manifestations described
> - Opportunistic infections are a major feature
> - HAART has decreased the prevalence of opportunistic infections
> - Oral *Candida* infection is the most prevalent oral lesion
> - HL is caused by EBV infection
> - Severe periodontal breakdown occurs in some patients
> - Kaposi sarcoma is associated with HHV8 infection
> - Patients with HIV can receive dental treatment using standard infection control precautions

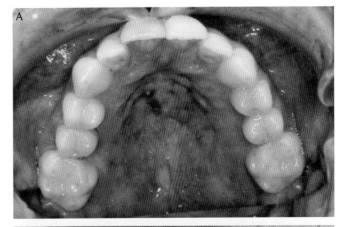

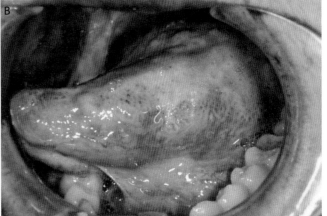

Fig. 10.15 Graft versus host disease (GVHD) after a haematopoietic stem cell transplant showing lichenoid-type lesions.

Primary immunodeficiency

Primary immunodeficiencies are disorders in which part of the immune system is absent or does not function normally. Almost all primary immunodeficiency disorders are genetic and most are diagnosed in children under the age of 1 year old, although milder forms may go unrecognized until later life. Treatment ranges from providing prophylactic antibiotics to replacement antibodies, but severe immunodeficiency has to be treated by haematopoetic stem cell transplantation. In patients with severe combined immunodeficiency (SCID), who survive because of transplantation, severe abnormalities of the developing dentition may occur, including chronological enamel hypoplasia and root growth arrest.

Stem cell and bone marrow transplantation is increasingly used for acquired disease such as leukaemia. Dental abnormalities are due partly to damage to the tooth germs from the intense chemotherapy and radiotherapy used, and partly from the disturbance due to the transplant. It is estimated that up to 80% of stem cell or bone marrow transplant patients develop graft versus host disease (GVHD). This varies from mild and transient to severe, chronic, and even life-threatening. GVHD is caused by the damage to the host cells mediated by immune cells from the donor tissue that has been grafted. The graft cells recognize the HLA antigens on the host cells as foreign. GVHD can be acute, chronic, late acute, and overlap types. Acute GVHD occurs within 100 days of the transplant and usually involves a skin rash and,

sometimes, the gastrointestinal tract, including the oral cavity, can be affected. Chronic GVHD also affects the oral cavity, skin, and gastrointestinal tract, but it can also involve other organs such as liver, eye, lungs, and joints. In the oral cavity, chronic GVHD results in lichenoid-like lesions in the oral mucosa (Fig. 10.15) and can also affect the salivary glands, causing dry mouth and parotid swelling.

Immunodeficiency associated with organ transplantation

Transplantation of organs has been made possible by the availability of immunosuppressive drugs, but the intensity of immunodeficiency can result in oral manifestations similar to those found in HIV. Most common of these are opportunistic infections due to fungal and viral microorganisms. Therapeutic immunosuppression may also lead to post-transplant lympho-proliferative disorder (PTLD) that can affect cervical lymph nodes and tonsils. There is B cell polyclonal hyperplasia that may respond to reduction in drug dose, but in a proportion of cases, the B cells acquire mutations and malignant lymphoma develops. The risk of developing skin cancers, particularly squamous cell carcinoma of the lip, is also increased (Chapter 8).

Endocrine disease

Acromegaly

Acromegaly is caused by prolonged and excessive secretion of growth hormone, after closure of the epiphyseal plates in the affected individual (excessive growth hormone in childhood before the closure of the epiphyseal plates causes gigantism). The excess growth hormone is usually due to a secreting adenoma of the anterior lobe of the pituitary. This causes renewed growth of the bones in the jaws, hands, and feet, together with soft-tissue thickening. The condylar growth centre in the mandible causes the mandible to become enlarged and protrusive, and if teeth are present, they can become spaced. The soft tissues of the face become thickened and enlarged, as does the tongue. (Fig. 7.35). Management is usually surgical removal or stereotactic ablation of the hormone-secreting adenoma, although somatostatin analogues or growth hormone receptor antagonists can be used.

Adrenocortical diseases

Addison's disease

Oral mucosal pigmentation can be due to a variety of causes (Chapter 2). An important but rare cause is the pigmentation associated with Addison's disease, most commonly due to autoimmune disease. Adrenal insufficiency results in elevated secretion of adrenocorticotrophic hormone (ACTH) by the pituitary, with the associated melanocyte-stimulating properties being responsible for the pigmentation. The pigmentation is most common in areas subjected to masticatory trauma, including the gingiva, palate, and buccal mucosa. Management is with appropriate replacement of mineralocorticoid (fludrocortisone) and glucocorticoid (hydrocortisone).

Cushing's disease

This is due to a sustained increase in glucocorticoid levels produced by the adrenal cortex, usually as a result of an ACTH-secreting pituitary adenoma. Similar effects are much more commonly seen due to corticosteroid therapy for medical purposes (Cushing's syndrome). Manifestations include weight gain and fatty tissue deposition in the facial area resulting in the characteristic rounded facial appearance of a 'moon face'. Treatment of Cushing's disease is usually by surgical removal of the hormone-secreting adenoma.

Thyroid disease

Hypothyroidism

This is a condition characterized by decreased levels of thyroid hormone. If it occurs congenitally, it results in cretinism. Oral manifestations include macroglossia. In adults, the most common causes are autoimmune disease or iatrogenic factors, such as radioactive iodine therapy or following thyroid gland surgery. Hypothyroidism occurs more frequently in patients with primary Sjögren's syndrome. General signs and symptoms mainly relate to a decreased metabolic rate in these patients, including weight gain and inability to tolerate the cold. Oral manifestations may include sensations of a burning mouth and there is sometimes impaired immune function. Treatment is with administration of thyroxine.

Hyperthyroidism

This is a condition characterized by an excess production of thyroid hormone. Causes include autoimmune disease and thyroid tumours, both benign and malignant. Treatment can be medical or surgical according to the cause. The most common cause is the autoimmune-triggered Graves' disease, which classically involves the eye and manifests as eyelid retraction, lid lag, and exophthalmos. Whilst there are no mucosal changes, dentists may be the first to recognize these eye signs. The excess thyroid hormone production causing an increased metabolic rate results in many signs and symptoms, including weight loss and heart palpitations.

Diabetes mellitus

Diabetes mellitus is a common endocrine disorder that occurs because of a deficiency of insulin, or resistance to insulin, resulting in an increase in the blood glucose level. Type I (insulin dependent) diabetes mellitus is characterized by a lack of insulin production and typically is diagnosed in childhood. Treatment is by administration of insulin. Type II (non-insulin dependent) diabetes mellitus is characterized by a resistance to the effects of insulin and tends to occur in older, obese adults, although with the increasing incidence of obesity, is now also being seen from teenage years onwards. Treatment is with dietary modification, hypoglycaemic medication, and, in some cases, insulin. The rise in the obese population in the developing and developed world accounts for the increasing incidence of type II diabetes. Diabetes is an important disease with many complications resulting in a significant economic effect on healthcare and society. Complications are multiple and include macrovascular changes (increase in atheroma formation, ischaemic heart disease, and peripheral vascular disease), microvascular changes (diabetic retinopathy, nephropathy, and neuropathy), and a general increase in susceptibility to infection. Studies suggest that strict control of the blood glucose levels results in a slowing of the late complications of diabetes and reduces the frequency of these complications, including the oral manifestations.

The oral manifestations of uncontrolled diabetes mellitus are varied, but there are no specific oral signs or symptoms (Box 10.6). The less well-controlled the diabetes is, then the more likely are the signs and symptoms of the disease. An increased susceptibility to infection, partly due to impaired neutrophil function, results in a more frequent incidence of periodontal disease and a more rapid progression, where it occurs. Interestingly, there is now evidence that periodontal treatment and a strict oral hygiene regime in diabetic patients can also help with the medical control of the disease—an example of oral disease control having a systemic effect. Healing after oral surgery can be delayed and an increased susceptibility to oral candidosis occurs (Fig 10.16). Diffuse, non-tender, bilateral enlargement of the parotid glands (sialosis) can occur. Dryness of the mouth, due to dehydration secondary to polyuria, or neuropathy of the parasympathetic nerve supply to the glands, may also be a feature. Occasionally, diabetes can be the cause of a widespread burning sensation in the mouth, which initially may be diagnosed as burning mouth syndrome. Rarely, a patient with uncontrolled diabetes may present with a generalized stomatitis resulting from a combination of dryness of the mouth, candidosis, and glossitis.

Parathyroid disease

Hypoparathyroidism

A deficiency in the production of parathyroid hormone (PTH) is rare but usually due to autoimmune disease or inadvertent surgical removal of the parathyroid glands during thyroid surgery. The hormone regulates calcium in extracellular tissues in conjunction with vitamin D. Hypocalcaemia secondary to hypoparathyroidism can cause hypoplastic enamel and hypomineralization of dentine, if it occurs during odontogenesis.

Hyperparathyroidism

An excessive production of PTH, can be primary, due to uncontrolled production from an abnormal parathyroid gland, or secondary, when PTH is continuously produced in response to chronic low levels of serum calcium. This is usually due to renal disease or lack of vitamin D production. The classical signs and symptoms produced are 'stones, bones, and abdominal groans'. Bones refers to a variety of osseous changes, including generalized osteoporosis, causing loss of lamina dura around the roots of the teeth, along with loss of distinction of the normal trabecular pattern. Persistent disease may cause 'brown tumours' of hyperparathyroidism, which is a giant cell rich lesion of the jaws (Chapter 7). These lesions appear radiographically as well-demarcated unilocular or multilocular radiolucencies.

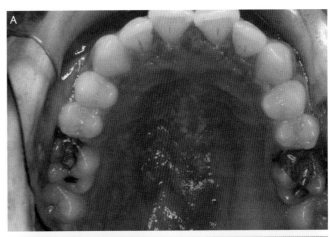

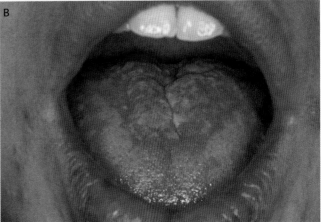

Fig. 10.16 Oral candidosis in a patient with diabetes mellitus, note the 'kissing lesion' where the dorsum of the tongue contacts the palate.

Multiple endocrine neoplasia syndrome

Multiple endocrine neoplasia syndrome type IIB is an inherited or spontaneous mutation of the *RET* proto-oncogene (MEN IIB OMIM 162300). Affected individuals have a Marfanoid appearance and develop medullary carcinoma of the thyroid gland and phaeochromocytoma of the adrenal gland in childhood. The development of multiple tumour-like malformations of peripheral nerves (mucosal neuromas) in the oral cavity is also a feature.

Connective tissue disease

This is a term used to describe a variety of conditions with an immunological basis, including primary Sjögren's syndrome (Chapter 4). Many of the conditions are more common in females, are autoimmune in origin, and involve several body systems. Secondary Sjögren's syndrome is a frequent complication of other connective tissue disorders. Many involve the skin or mucous membranes, although both primary and secondary Sjögren's syndrome, do not, other than through secondary effects due to dryness. Management is usually based around corticosteroids and immunosuppressive agents, including azathioprine, although treatment regimes vary widely according to the specific connective tissue disease involved. Oral mucosal lesions can also be helped by topical steroids.

Lupus erythematosus

This autoimmune disorder can exhibit a variety of clinical forms ranging from systemic lupus erythematosus (SLE) to discoid lupus erythematosus (DLE). SLE causes widespread changes in the connective tissues with secondary effects in most other systems, including the cardiovascular and renal systems. Characteristic skin lesions include light-sensitive erythematous lesions in the malar regions of the face (butterfly facial rash) and hands. Secondary Sjögren's syndrome can occur. Involvement of the vermillion zone of the lower lip with thickening and a white margin (lupus cheilitis) is sometimes seen. Oral signs and symptoms are diverse when they occur. Sometimes they appear as lichenoid areas and can affect the palate—a site uncommonly affected in lichen planus. The lesions, however, may look non-specific and simply appear as erythematous patches with superficial erosions. DLE is a form of the disease restricted to the skin and without the systemic associations. The skin lesions present as scaly red patches, frequently in sun-exposed skin, that heal with scar formation and hypopigmentation or hyperpigmentation. Lip and oral lesions occur, with the oral lesions frequently appearing as lichenoid areas (Fig. 2.70A). Whilst, the histopathological appearances of lichen planus and lupus erythematosus are very similar, a deeper chronic inflammatory infiltrate with a perivascular distribution would support a clinical diagnosis of lupus erythematosus (Fig. 2.70B).

Systemic sclerosis

Systemic sclerosis is a multisystem disorder in which there is widespread fibrosis of the skin and other body organs. Milder variants can be classified as limited cutaneous systemic sclerosis, including CREST syndrome (calcinosis cutis, Raynaud's phenomenon, esophageal dysfunction, sclerodactyly, and telangiectasia), and when purely limited to the skin, morphoea. In systemic sclerosis, the skin develops a diffuse hard texture with a smooth surface. This can result in a characteristic taut, 'mask-like' face, and involvement of the perioral tissues can lead to restricted mouth opening and difficulty with oral hygiene and dental treatment. Secondary Sjögren's syndrome can occur. On dental radiographs, diffuse widening of the periodontal ligament space is often present, although the extent of the widening is variable.

Mixed connective tissue disease

This is a rare condition whose clinical features represent an overlap of other connective tissue disorders. Oral lesions can appear lichenoid in nature. Secondary Sjögren's syndrome can occur.

Rheumatoid arthritis

This is a common, multisystem, autoimmune disorder. There are no mucosal lesions but oro-facial manifestations include secondary Sjögren's syndrome and temporomandibular joint involvement. This may result in pain, stiffness, and difficulty in joint movement, limiting jaw opening. Rarely, destruction of the condyles may lead to development of an anterior open bite, or ankylosis may occur. Difficulty in manipulating a toothbrush may result in poor oral hygiene.

Vascular disease

Granulomatosis with polyangitis

This rare systemic disease of unknown aetiology is characterized by necrotizing, destructive granulomatous inflammation, principally involving the respiratory tract, and a generalized necrotizing vasculitis. The disease is associated with an autoantibody directed against cytoplasmic constituents of neutrophils (c-ANCA). Many patients present with respiratory tract symptoms. Oral lesions occur and, rarely, may be the presenting feature. Oral manifestations include a florid and hyperplastic gingival lesion (strawberry gingivitis; Fig. 5.58), with heavily inflamed granular exophytic lesions and deep, necrotic oral ulceration. Classical histological features that help to secure the diagnosis are a leukoclastic vasculitis with necrosis and granulomatous inflammation. There are usually scattered small angular multinucleated macrophages. In some cases, the biopsy only shows evidence of a chronic inflammatory process. In these circumstances, close clinico-pathological correlation with the clinical features and other laboratory tests are required to make a definitive diagnosis. Management is with corticosteroids and immunosuppressive drugs, e.g. cyclophosphamide, methotrexate, and rituximab.

Giant cell arteritis and polymyalgia rheumatica

Giant cell (temporal) arteritis and polymyalgia rheumatica are systemic diseases of the elderly associated with large vessel vasculitis. Temporal arteritis may present with severe headaches, tenderness of the temple, and claudication of the jaws on eating, and can cause sudden painless visual loss. It can also cause tongue necrosis, if the lingual artery is affected. Treatment is with corticosteroids.

Polyarteritis nodosum

Vasculitic disease such as polyarteritis nodusum, affecting medium-sized arterial vessels, may result in deeply necrotizing oral lesions. The tip of the tongue can undergo necrosis if the lingual artery is affected. Treatment is with corticosteroids.

Vascular malformations

Capillary and cavernous vascular malformations are common in the oral mucosa, particularly in the tongue and lips. Some vascular malformations are part of syndromes—important examples include Sturge–Weber syndrome (Fig. 8.5) and hereditary haemorrhagic telangiectasia.

Neurological disease

Oral manifestations of neurological disease are mainly secondary. These include dry mouth secondary to abnormality of parasympathetic supply to major salivary glands, and abnormality of motor functions, such as dyskinesia, bruxism, and tongue thrusting disorders, which may result in tooth mobility or loss and ulceration. Degenerative neurological disease is increasingly important in the ageing population and is important in dentistry because patients may have problems with drooling, denture wearing, and maintenance of oral hygiene.

Drug-related and iatrogenic oral disease

Many drugs can produce adverse reactions in the mouth. Some of these are oral lesions and manifestations that mimic local or systemic disease. The majority of adverse lesions arise from prescribed medication, although recreational and over-the-counter drugs can also cause adverse effects. The diagnosis of an adverse drug reaction is not always easy, with limited utility of laboratory tests. The association of the drug and its adverse effect frequently relies on the disappearance of the oral manifestation following discontinuation of the drug, and much of our knowledge in this area is based on case reports in the literature and the reporting of suspected adverse reactions to national regulatory agencies, such as the 'yellow card' scheme run by the Medicines and Healthcare products Regulatory Agency (MHRA) in the UK.

When an adverse drug reaction is suspected, it is important for the dentist to liaise with the patient's medical practitioner. Unless the reaction is acute and severe, the patient should be advised to continue with the prescribed drug until a decision about whether to cease therapy, reduce dose, or maintain the therapy and treat the unwanted effects is reached.

Oro-facial manifestations of adverse drug reactions are numerous, and can produce many signs and symptoms. The most common manifestations include xerostomia, taste disturbances, mucosal ulceration, mucosal white patches, mucosal pigmentation, gingival enlargement, and facial angioedema and osteonecrosis.

Xerostomia

Xerostomia, or dry mouth, is the most common adverse drug-related effect seen in the mouth, and drugs are the most common cause of xerostomia. Many drugs have been implicated as causing a dry mouth or its sensation, and for some, the mechanism of action remains unclear. Many elderly patients are now taking multiple medications and these may work synergistically to cause a dry mouth. This problem is likely to increase with an ageing population taking an increasing polypharmacy of medication. The principal mechanisms of drug-induced dry mouth are through anti-cholinergic effects. Drugs implicated include tricyclic antidepressants, antipsychotics, antihistamines, and drugs used in the treatment of an overactive bladder. Other mechanisms of drug-induced dry mouth include mild dehydration induced by diuretics. The common causes of xerostomia are listed in Box 10.7.

Taste disturbance

Taste disturbance as a consequence of an adverse drug reaction is well recognized. Many drugs have been implicated but their mechanism of action to cause this adverse effect is poorly understood. Mechanisms suggested include the interfering effect of the drug or its metabolites on the composition of saliva, or by affecting taste receptor function or signal transmission. Drugs particularly implicated include amiodarone, ACE inhibitors, carbimazole, metformin, metronidazole, and penicillamine. Loss of taste (ageusia), reduction in taste (hypogeusia), and abnormal perception of taste (dysgeusia) are all possible.

Mucosal ulceration

Drug-related mucosal ulceration is well recognized (Box 10.8). Such lesions are frequently singular or persistent, rather than recurrent. They include chemically induced ulceration due to direct application of a caustic medication on the mucosa, such as aspirin or a bisphosphonate, and fixed drug eruptions, reported following the use of medication such as fluconazole. Drug-related aphthous-type ulcers are uncommon, but drugs implicated include NSAIDs and nicorandil. Cytotoxic drugs, used in chemotherapy regimes for the treatment of cancer, commonly result in oral ulceration and mucositis e.g. methotrexate and melphalan. Immunosuppressive drugs can also lead to ulceration, where opportunistic infection is frequently the cause. Vesiculo-bullous disorders such as pemphigoid, pemphigus, and erythema multiforme can be caused, or more commonly triggered, by a variety of drugs, including ACE inhibitors or penicillamine.

Mucosal white patches

Drugs have been implicated in lichenoid reactions since anti-malarials were first described as a possible cause following World War II. Since then many drugs have been implicated in cutaneous lichenoid reactions, but few have been shown to be associated with oral lesions. The drugs most commonly associated with oral lichenoid reactions include the NSAIDs, gold, and allopurinol. Lichenoid reactions to restorative dental materials may also occur, with dental amalgam being the most

Box 10.7 Common causes of xerostomia
- Medications
- Diabetes mellitus
- Sjögren's syndrome
- Radiotherapy to head and neck region

Box 10.8 Drug-related oral mucosal ulceration
- Drug-related chemical burns of the mucosa
- Fixed drug eruptions
- Drug-related mucositis
- Drug-related opportunistic infection in immunosuppression
- Drug-related vesiculobullous disease
- Drug-related aphthous-like or non-specific ulceration

commonly implicated material. Immunosuppressive drugs may also lead to white lesions, including candidiasis secondary to corticosteroids and hairy leukoplakia secondary to immunosuppressive drug regimes used in solid organ transplantation.

Mucosal pigmentation

Various drug mechanisms can induce pigmentary changes in the oral mucosa. Mechanisms include drug material becoming lodged within the mucosa, such as with phenothiazines, and stimulation of melanocytes by drugs such as oral contraceptives. The effect of the tetracycline on developing teeth is a well-recognized cause of tooth discoloration; however, similar changes to bone and the roots of teeth can sometimes give the overlying mucosa a pigmented appearance as well.

Drug-induced gingival overgrowth

Gradual and generalized overgrowth of the fibrous component of the gingiva is found as an adverse reaction to several drugs. Poor oral hygiene is a contributing factor. This adverse effect was first noticed with the use of phenytoin and, subsequently, ciclosporin and calcium channel blockers (Fig. 10.17).

Facial angioedema

Facial angioedema is a rapid oedematous swelling of the lips and adjacent structures. It is a common clinical manifestation of allergy (such as

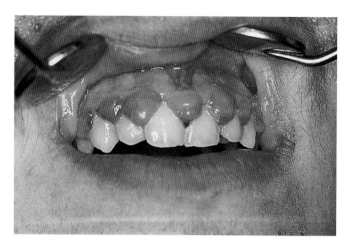

Fig. 10.17 Ciclosporin-induced gingival overgrowth in a renal transplant patient.

with penicillin allergy) or due to non-allergic mechanisms. Drugs predisposing to this reaction by non-allergic mechanisms include NSAIDs and ACE inhibitors.

Medication-related osteonecrosis of the jaw

Bisphosphonate and denosumab-related osteonecrosis of the jaw is discussed in Chapter 7.

Additional resources

Bibliography

Banerjee A, Watson TF. *Pickard's Manual of Operative Dentistry*, 10th Edition. Oxford University Press, Oxford, UK, 2015.

Barnes L, Eveson JW, Reichart P, Sidransky D. *World Health Organization Classification of Tumours. Pathology and Genetics of Head and Neck Tumours*. IARC Press, Lyon, France, 2005.

Bridge JA, Hogendoorn P, Fletcher CDM. *World Health Organization Classification of Tumours of Soft Tissue and Bone*. IARC Press, Lyon, France, 2013.

Brierley JD, Gospodarowicz MK, Wittekind C. *UICC International Union Against Cancer TNM Classification of Malignant Tumours*, 8th Edition. Wiley–Blackwell, 2017.

Cawson RA, Odell EW. *Cawson's Essentials of Oral Pathology and Oral Medicine*, 8th Edition. Churchill Livingstone, 2008.

Chiang NYZ, Verbov J. *Dermatology. A Handbook for Medical Students and Junior Doctors*. British Association of Dermatologists, 2014. http://www.bad.org.uk/shared/get-file.ashx?id=3632&itemtype=document (accessed 7 November 2017).

Coulthard P, Horner K, Sloan P, Theaker ED. *Master Dentistry. Volume 1: Oral and Maxillofacial Surgery, Radiology, Pathology and Oral Medicine*, 3rd Edition. Churchill Livingstone, 2013.

Cross S. *Underwood's Pathology: a Clinical Approach*, 6th Edition. Churchill Livingstone, 2013.

Greenwood M, Seymour RA, Meechan JG. *Textbook of Human Disease in Dentistry*. Wiley–Blackwell, 2009.

Hanahan D and Weinberg RA. The hallmarks of cancer. *Cell* 2000 **100**: 57–70.

Hanahan D and Weinberg RA. Hallmarks of cancer: the next generation. *Cell* 2011 **144**: 645–647.

Kumar V, Abbas AK, Aster JC. *Robbins & Cotran Pathologic Basis of Disease*, 9th Edition. Saunders, 2014.

LeBoit PE, Burg G, Weedon D, Sarasin A. *World Health Organization Classification of Tumours. Pathology and Genetics of Skin Tumours*. IARC Press, Lyon, France, 2005.

Leemans CR, Braakhuis BJ, Brakenhoff RH. The molecular biology of head and neck cancer. *Nature Reviews Cancer* 2011 **11**: 9–22.

Lindhe J, Lang NP. *Clinical Periodontology and Implant Dentistry*, 6th Edition. Wiley–Blackwell, 2015.

Marsh PD, Martin MV, Lewis MAO, Williams DW. *Oral Microbiology*, 5th Edition. Churchill Livingstone, 2009.

Nanci A. *Ten Cate's Oral Histology*, 6th Edition. Mosby, 2003.

Orchard G, Nation B. *Histopathology (Fundamentals of Biomedical Science)*. Oxford University Press, Oxford, UK, 2011.

Scully C. *Oral and Maxillofacial Medicine*, 3rd Edition. Churchill Livingstone, 2013.

Scully C. *Scully's Medical Problems in Dentistry*, 7th Edition. Churchill Livingstone, 2014.

Shear M, Speight P. *Cysts of the Oral and Maxillofacial Regions*, 4th Edition. Wiley–Blackwell, 2007.

Thompson LDR, Wenig B. *Diagnostic Pathology: Head and Neck*, 2nd Edition. Elsevier, 2016.

Waites E, Drage N. *Essentials of Dental Radiography and Radiology*, 5th Edition. Churchill Livingstone, 2013.

Welbury R, Duggal MS, Hosey MT. *Paediatric Dentistry*, 4th Edition. Oxford University Press, Oxford, UK, 2012.

Guidelines

Cancer of the upper aerodigestive tract: assessment and management in people aged 16 and over. NICE guideline 2016.

Helliwell T, Woolgar J. Standards and datasets for reporting cancers. Datasets for histopathology reporting of mucosal malignancies of the oral cavity. The Royal College of Pathologists 2013.

Odell EW, Farthing PM, High A, Potts J, Soames J, Thakker N, Toner M, Williams HK. British Society for Oral and Maxillofacial Pathology, UK: minimum curriculum in oral pathology. *European Journal of Dental Education* 2004; **8**: 177–184.

Schiffman E, Ohrbach R, Truelove E *et al*. Diagnostic Criteria for Temporomandibular Disorders (DC/TMD) for Clinical and Research Applications: recommendations of the International RDC/TMD Consortium Network and Orofacial Pain Special Interest Group. *Journal of Oral & Facial Pain and Headache* 2014; **28**(1): 6–27.

Suspected cancer: recognition and referral. NICE guideline 2015.

Web resources

British National Formulary	https://www.bnf.org/products/bnf-online/
Cancerstats. Cancer Research UK	http://www.cancerresearchuk.org/cancer-info/cancerstats/
Cochrane Library	http://www.cochranelibrary.com/
Online Mendelian Inheritance in Man	http://www.omim.org/
Pubmed	http://www.ncbi.nlm.nih.gov/pubmed
US Centers for Disease Control and Prevention (CDC)	http://www.cdc.gov/
World Health Organization (WHO)	http://www.who.int/en/

Professional associations

British Society for Oral and Maxillofacial Pathology	http://www.bsomp.org.uk/
British Society for Oral Medicine	http://www.bsom.org.uk/
General Dental Council	http://www.gdc-uk.org
Royal College of Pathologists	https://www.rcpath.org/
Royal College of Physicians and Surgeons of Glasgow	https://rcpsg.ac.uk/
Royal College of Surgeons of Edinburgh	https://www.rcsed.ac.uk/
Royal College of Surgeons of England	https://www.rcseng.ac.uk/

Index

Boxes, figures and tables are noted with italic letters *b*, *f* and *t*, respectively after the page number.